VITAMINS AND HORMONES

VOLUME 45

VITAMINS AND HORMONES
ADVANCES IN RESEARCH AND APPLICATIONS

Editor-in-Chief

G. D. AURBACH

Metabolic Diseases Branch
National Institute of Arthritis,
Diabetes, and Digestive and Kidney Diseases
National Institutes of Health
Bethesda, Maryland

Editor

DONALD B. MCCORMICK

Department of Biochemistry
Emory University School of Medicine
Atlanta, Georgia

Volume 45

ACADEMIC PRESS, INC. Harcourt Brace Jovanovich, Publishers

San Diego   New York   Berkeley   Boston
London   Sydney   Tokyo   Toronto

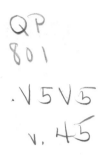
ACADEMIC PRESS, INC.
San Diego, California 92101

United Kingdom Edition published by
ACADEMIC PRESS LIMITED
24-28 Oval Road, London NW1 7DX

LIBRARY OF CONGRESS CATALOG CARD NUMBER: 43-10535

ISBN   0-12-709845-3   (alk. paper)

PRINTED IN THE UNITED STATES OF AMERICA
89 90 91 92   9 8 7 6 5 4 3 2 1

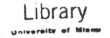

Contents

Experimental Obesity: A Homeostatic Failure due to Defective Nutrient Stimulation of the Sympathetic Nervous System

G. A. BRAY, D. A. YORK, AND J. S. FISLER

Estrogen Regulation of Protein Synthesis and Cell Growth in Human Breast Cancer

KEVIN J. CULLEN AND MARC E. LIPPMAN

Calcium Homeostasis in Birds

SHMUEL HURWITZ

Pyrroloquinoline Quinone: A Novel Cofactor

JOHANNIS A. DUINE AND JACOB A. JONGEJAN

Folylpolyglutamate Synthesis and Role in the Regulation of One-Carbon Metabolism

BARRY SHANE

Biotin

KRISHNAMURTI DAKSHINAMURTI AND JASBIR CHAUHAN

Preface

This volume of *Vitamins and Hormones* provides excellent reviews on an array of interesting and currently important subjects. G. A. Bray, D. A. York, and J. S. Fisler review the topic of experimental obesity. They provide an exhaustive review of neuroanatomic and physiological responses to the intake of foods and the control systems regulating body nutrient stores.

K. J. Cullen and M. E. Lippman present an important review of estrogen control of protein synthesis and cell growth in breast cancer. Tumors responsive to estrogen produce an array of protein growth factors that are implicated in the growth of breast cancer cells.

S. Hurwitz has prepared an authoritative review of calcium homeostasis in birds. This subject is of particular interest in calcium metabolism given the remarkable observation that the shell of each egg contains mineral equivalent to ten percent of the bird's entire body stores of calcium. B. Shane presents a detailed analysis of folylpolyglutamates. Synthesis and metabolism of polyglutamate derivatives of folate are important aspects of one carbon metabolism.

It has been some time since biotin has been reviewed in this series. K. Dakshinamurti has summarized this topic for us, translating from the biochemical cofactor functions of biotin in CO_2-fixing carboxylases to the mammalian manifestations of biotin deficiency. The study of pyrroloquinoline quinones, a class of compounds only recently discovered, is a rapidly moving field. J. A. Duine and J. A. Jongejan develop an extensive review of these cofactors for quinoprotein dehydrogenases which are important in enzymatic dissimilation of methanol, ethanol, and a number of other substrates.

G. D. AURBACH
DONALD B. McCORMICK

xi

VITAMINS AND HORMONES, VOL. 45

Experimental Obesity: A Homeostatic Failure due to Defective Nutrient Stimulation of the Sympathetic Nervous System

G. A. BRAY,* D. A. YORK,† AND J. S. FISLER*

*Department of Medicine
Section of Diabetes and Clinical Nutrition
School of Medicine
University of Southern California
Los Angeles, California

†Department of Nutrition
School of Biochemical and Physiological Sciences
University of Southampton
Southampton S09 3TU, England

I. INTRODUCTION

It has been nearly 10 years since we published our review on hypothalamic and genetic obesity (Bray and York, 1979). In the intervening years several major developments have occurred which provide new

insights for understanding the interactions of environment and genetics in the development of obesity. First, there have been major addi-
tions to the neuroanatomic basis for control of insulin secretion in
response to nutrient intake (Luiten *et al.*, 1987). Second, it has been
recognized that brain peptides act as both stimulators and inhibitors of
feeding (Leibowitz, 1986; Morley, 1987). Third, the response of the
autonomic nervous system to food intake and deprivation and the role
this plays in the regulation of obesity has become much clearer
(Landsberg *et al.*, 1984; Bray, 1987). Finally, adrenalectomy is now
known to attenuate the development of all types of experimental
obesity (Bray, 1982; Bruce *et al.*, 1982; Debons *et al.*, 1982; King *et al.*,
1983). These developments make the time ripe for a new review of the
field of experimental obesity. For additional reviews of this topic, the
reader is referred to papers by Powley (1977), Sclafani (1984), Bray
(1984b), Jeanrenaud (1985), Levin (1986), Sims (1986), Bernardis and
Bellinger (1986a), and Steffens and Strubbe (1987).

The regulation of body fat stores and the development of obesity can
be viewed as problems of disturbed nutrient ingestion, disturbed energy expenditure, or disturbed internal balancing of these two processes.
It is the thesis of this review that fat stores and the energy they
contain operate as a regulated system, as in the regulation of glycogen
and protein (Bray, 1987). Moreover, each of these regulated or homeostatic systems, one for fat, one for carbohydrate, and one for protein,
operate independently, although they must obviously be integrated
into the entire body economy. Failure of homeostasis and the ensuing
obesity, regardless of the model, represent defective nutrient stimulation of the sympathetic nervous system with a relative or absolute
decrease in the activity of this system. This inadequacy of the sympathetic nervous system does not occur after adrenalectomy and is
thus dependent on at least a permissive action of glucocorticoids.

There are three time domains over which this process of homeostasis
or regulation can be viewed. The first is the short-term regulation of
individual meals (Cannon and Washburn, 1912; Carlson, 1912; Smith
and Gibbs, 1984; Van Itallie and Kissileff, 1985; Woods *et al.*, 1980).
There is also a 24-hour time frame in which individual meals are
integrated, particularly in small rodents, to provide a reasonable balance of nutrient intake and requirements (Le Magnen, 1983; Collier,
1985; Woods *et al.*, 1980). The third domain is the longer-term regulation of nutrient stores, in which obesity or anorexia is the result of
disturbed homeostasis.

A meal begins at a point in time, continues usually at a decelerating
rate over a subsequent interval (Kissileff *et al.*, 1982), and then ceases.

Each meal is followed by an intermeal interval of variable length, after which the ingestive process begins again. Within a 24-hour daily cycle, there is a periodicity to meals with diurnal variability (Le Magnen, 1983). In rodents, for example, the most frequent and largest meals occur during the nighttime or shortly after lights go out, with smaller, less frequent meals during the daytime. Other animals reverse this cycle and eat predominantly in the daylight, with few meals at night. This diurnal cycle appears to be regulated by the suprachiasmatic nucleus (Nagai et al., 1978). If the suprachiasmatic nucleus is destroyed, this diurnal rhythm is lost (Nishio et al., 1979). The work of Collier (1985) has shown that, when the frequency of meals is limited, rodents increase the size of their meals so that the integrated 24-hour intake remains remarkably stable. This compensation also occurs when cholecystokinin (CCK), an eight-amino acid peptide suggested to be a satiety signal, is given intraperitoneally prior to each meal (West et al., 1987). The size of individual meals was reduced by 44% or more and the frequency of meals was increased to 160% of control, thus maintaining a constant 24-hour intake. In the discussion that follows, we attempt to distinguish between disturbances in short-term feeding and those in longer-term control of homeostasis in the development of obesity in the models to be described.

This review is divided into five sections. The three middle sections deal with specific types of experimental obesity: Section II, the obesity or weight loss associated with injury to the hypothalamus; Section III, the genetic types of obesity; and Section IV, obesity associated with altered dietary patterns. Following this, we attempt to provide a framework for conceptualizing the homeostatic problems leading to the development of different types of experimental obesity. The organization of the discussion within each of the sections is based on the model of a regulated system shown in Fig. 1. This figure shows a controller located in the central nervous system. The controlled system represents the ingestive and digestive processes, the absorbed and postingestional nutrient pools, and finally the storage and metabolic processes by which nutrients are oxidized for various purposes. The controller receives afferent signals from the controlled system which reflect its functional state. These can be sensory signals such as smell, taste, or sight. These signals can also arise from gastric or intestinal distension related to the presence of food in the mouth, esophagus, or stomach. They may also be neural signals generated by nutrient or hormonal responses to these nutrients. And finally, they may represent the nutrients in the circulating pool themselves. The controlled system is modulated by the controller through efferent controls which

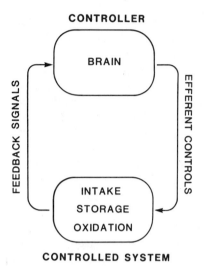

CONTROLLER

FIG. 1. Feedback model for the regulation of nutrient intake. The brain is depicted as the central controller; the intake, storage, and oxidation of food represent the controlled system; the afferent and efferent signals connect these components of the system.

include the autonomic nervous system, the endocrine system, and the motor nervous system.

II. HYPOTHALAMIC OBESITY

Hypothalamic obesity has been known for more than 150 years (Mohr, 1840; Rayer, 1823). The initial clinical descriptions were published by Rayer in 1823 and by Mohr in 1840, but the primary clinical impetus to study this problem was provided by the case reports by Babinski (1900) and by Frohlich (1901) at the beginning of the twentieth century. Although a variety of clinical studies on hypothalamic obesity in humans has been described (Bray and Gallagher, 1975; Bray, 1984a), the major developments in this field have resulted from studies on experimental animals (Bray and York, 1979; Bernardis, 1985a,b; Hetherington and Ranson, 1940; Brobeck, 1946; Mayer, 1960; Keesey and Powley, 1986; Sclafani, 1984).

Hypothalamic obesity can be produced by lesions which destroy the ventromedial part of the hypothalamus in humans and non-human primates, dogs, cats, rats, mice, ground squirrels, and chickens (Bray,

1984b; Bray and York, 1979; Mrosovsky, 1975). Table I provides a list of the variety of experimental maneuvers which have been associated with alterations in body weight. The largest weight gains have been associated with electrolytic lesions in the ventromedial hypothalamus (VMH) (Bray and York, 1979), with parasaggital hypothalamic knife cuts producing somewhat lesser effects (Sclafani and Grossman, 1969). The use of asymmetrical knife cuts has been helpful in localizing some of the fiber tracts involved. When a parasaggital knife cut is put on one side of the hypothalamus and coronal cuts are placed in the posterior hypothalamus, in the midbrain, in the pons, or in the medulla, the hyperphagic syndrome is produced (Sclafani and Kirchgessner, 1986a). These coronal knife cuts appear to divide descending pathways, since horseradish peroxidase applied to the cut ends of the axons is localized in parvocellular neurons of the paraventricular nucleus (PVN). Neither noradrenergic nor serotonergic fiber tracts appear to

TABLE I

MECHANISMS FOR PRODUCING HYPERPHAGIA
AND OBESITY BY HYPOTHALAMIC INJURY

Mechanical injury
  Electrolytic
    VMH
    PVN
    Dorsal tegmental
    Amygdala
  Knife cut
    Medial hypothalamic
    Midbrain
  Hypothalamic islands
  Thermal (radiofrequency)
Chemical injury
  6-Hydroxydopamine in VNB
  5,7-Dihydroxytryptamine
  Bipiperidyl mustard
  Gold thioglucose
  Monosodium glutamate
  Aspartate
  Kainic acid
Viral injury
Electrical stimulation of the LH
Chemical infusions
  Norepinephrine into the VMH
  Neuropeptide Y into the PVN

account for the pathway. Aravich and Sclafani (1983) have suggested that it may be an oxytocin pathway concerned with modulating afferent information from the vagal system in the nucleus of the tractus solitarius.

Substantial obesity has also been produced by electrolytic lesions in the PVN (Aravich and Sclafani, 1983; Leibowitz *et al.*, 1981; Tokunaga *et al.*, 1986b; Fukushima *et al.*, 1987). Lesions of the PVN in hamsters exaggerate the effects of dietary obesity and block the weight gain seen in these animals living in a short photoperiod (Bartness *et al.*, 1985). Dorsal tegmental lesions (Wellman *et al.*, 1984; Peters *et al.*, 1985) and hypothalamic islands made with the Halasz knife (Ohshima *et al.*, 1985) also produce obesity. Obesity can be produced with little or no hyperphagia following the injection of bipiperidyl mustard (Rutman *et al.*, 1966), monosodium glutamate (Olney, 1969; Kanarek *et al.*, 1979; Takasaki, 1978) and gold thioglucose (Brecher and Waxler, 1949), and aspartic acid (Burbach *et al.*, 1985). These various chemicals produce divergent lesions and provide some insight into the critical structures involved in hyperphagia and obesity. Bipiperidyl mustard damages the VMH and dorsal vagal complex (Laughton and Powley, 1981; Berthoud and Powley, 1985; Scallett and Olney, 1986), but produces little or no increase in food intake. Monosodium glutamate, on the other hand, damages the arcuate nucleus (Tanaka *et al.*, 1978; Scallett and Olney, 1986) and likewise produces obesity and hyperinsulinemia without hyperphagia. When monosodium glutamate and bipiperidyl mustard are administered together, the full-fledged syndrome of hyperphagia, obesity, and hyperinsulinemia appears. This suggests that damage to components of both the arcuate nucleus and the VMH may be needed for the full syndrome. It also makes it clear that hyperphagia and obesity and obesity without hyperphagia are separable syndromes. Injection of procaine, a topical anesthetic, into the VMH increases feeding and raises insulin, showing the importance of this region in metabolic regulation (Berthoud and Jeanrenaud, 1979b). Gold thioglucose produces hyperphagia and obesity by damage to the VMH.

Hypothalamic lesions can also produce weight loss. Lesions in the dorsomedial nucleus lead to a proportional reduction in body weight and fat stores (Bernardis, 1985a). Lesions in the nucleus of the tractus solitarius and area postrema (Hyde *et al.*, 1982; Hyde and Miselis, 1983) and in the lateral hypothalamus (LH) (Keesey *et al.*, 1976) are also associated with significant weight reduction (Yoshida *et al.*, 1983). For more details on these effects of these lesions, the reader is referred elsewhere (Keesey and Powley, 1986).

A. HYPOTHALAMIC CONTROLLER

1. *Neuroanatomic Structure of Hypothalamic Controller*

The application of methods for tracing neurons in either the retrograde or anterograde direction has provided important new insights into the neuroanatomic basis of hyperphagia and obesity (Luiten *et al.*, 1987). Microinjection of horseradish peroxidase is the principal technique for study of retrograde axonal transport. Horseradish peroxidase can be injected in the region of or into presynaptic boutons, where it will be transported back to the cell body from which that axon originated. Two principal techniques have been developed for tracing axons centrifugally from the cell body. The lectin from phaseolis vulgaris leucoagglutinin has been used with great success, as has the injection of radioactively labeled leucine ([^{3}H]leucine) (Luiten *et al.*, 1987).

Within the hypothalamus the ventromedial nucleus (VMN) is the recipient of information from two main limbic structures: the hippocampus and the amygdaloid body. The pathways from the amygdala to the VMN may involve the ventral amygdalofugal pathway or the bed nucleus of the stria terminalis. The descending limbic input into the LH is primarily influenced by information from the limbic–cortical areas and from the nucleus accumbens. The major input from the hippocampus to the hypothalamus is from the ventral subiculum, which sends fibers that terminate in the perinuclear fiber shell of the VMN. In contrast to the substantial innervation of the VMN from the limbic area, these investigations have failed to reveal any significant input into the PVN complex from the limbic area. In addition to these limbic inputs, there are inputs from noradrenergic fibers located in nuclear groups A_1 and A_2 which course via the ventral noradrenergic bundle to project to the LH and to the paraventricular and dorsomedial hypothalamic nuclei.

The projections within the hypothalamus described above provide a new understanding of the relationship between the VMH and the LH (Fig. 2). Studies with anterograde techniques have shown that there are important, direct, reciprocal connections between the ventromedial and dorsomedial nuclei. Similarly, there are important neural connections between the LH area and the dorsomedial nucleus. In addition, the LH area has efferent connections to the VMN and a minor direct connection to the PVN. Finally, there is a major, direct, and important connection between the dorsomedial nucleus and the magnocellular part of the PVN. The VMN also has at least two peptidergic pathways.

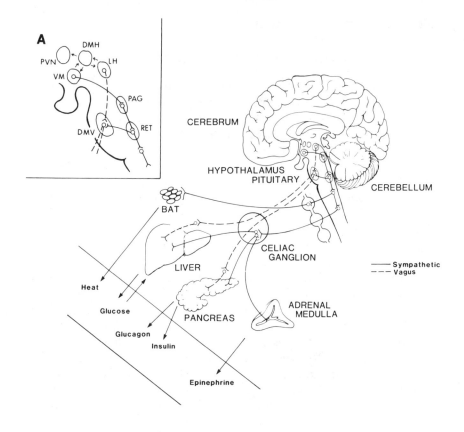

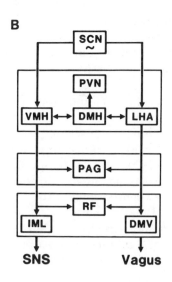

Inagaki *et al.* (1986) have described an enkephalin-containing pathway from the PVN to the VMN.

Studies of the efferent projections from the LH area and the VMN suggest that both of these areas exert primary efferent controls of metabolic functions through the autonomic nervous system. In relation to the changes in nutrient stores associated with destruction in each of these major areas, it is important to note that damage to the LH area reduces fat stores and initially lowers food intake, which then gradually returns to normal (Keesey *et al.*, 1976). Destruction of the VMN is associated with increased weight gain and fat stores, with or without an increase in food intake (Bray and York, 1979). Destruction of the PVN produces hyperphagia and obesity. If the hyperphagia is prevented, obesity does not develop (Weingarten *et al.*, 1985). In contrast, lesions in the VMH produce obesity with or without hyperphagia. Destruction of the dorsomedial hypothalamus, like an LH lesion, produces a significant reduction of a proportional nature in both fat and nonfat components (Bernardis, 1985a). The pathways leading from the VMN involve major fiber tracts passing to the periaqueductal gray (Fig. 2). A second major projection from the VMH is through the medial forebrain bundle. These fibers run caudally and appear to end primarily in the peripeduncular nucleus and adjacent mesencephalic tegmentum in the periaqueductal gray. From the periaqueductal gray, a large contingent of fibers course laterally to the various projections observed in the efferent sympathetic nervous system, as well as to the nucleus ambiguous and dorsomotor nuclei of the vagal efferent system (Luiten *et al.*, 1987).

From the LH area, the descending pathways are less complicated.

FIG. 2. (A) Sympathetic and parasympathetic controls of metabolic function. The ventromedial hypothalamus (VM) and lateral hypothalamus (LH) send direct pathways to the dorsomedial nucleus (DMH). The VM also sends direct sympathetic fiber tracts to the periaqueductal gray (PAG). The parasympathetic fiber tracts from the LH course to the dorsal motor nucleus of the vagus (DMV). Reticular (sympathetic) fibers also feed back on the vagal outflow. Sympathetic fibers travel from the reticular formation (RET) through the intermediolateral columns and then as preganglionic fibers to various organs. BAT, Brown adipose tissue. (B) Diagrammatic representation of the hypothalamic wiring shown anatomically in (A). The suprachiasmatic nucleus (SCN) is perceived to be the oscillator regulating diurnal patterns of feeding by modulating the ventromedial (VMH) and lateral hypothalamus (LHA). The LHA and VMH send fibers reciprocally to the dorsomedial nucleus of the hypothalamus (DMH), which provides the major input from these nuclei to the paraventricular nucleus (PVN). As noted in (A), the VMH and LHA send fiber tracts to the periaqueductal gray (PAG) and the reticular formation (RF) and then to the periphery through the intermediolateral columns (IML). SNS, Sympathetic nervous system. (Adapted from Oomura and Yoshimatsu, 1984.)

There are direct projections to the parasympathetic nuclei in the lower brain stem. There is a dorsal paraventricular bundle and a more ventral bundle that caudally takes a ventromedial position. From these bundles, there are major projections to the periaqueductal gray and the parabrachial nucleus. There are also direct connections to the vagal efferent system, including the ambiguous nucleus and the dorsomotor nucleus of the vagus.

The efferent pathways from the dorsomedial nucleus of the hypothalamus maintain projections similar to those of the LH area. The PVN, on the other hand, has a direct motor pathway to the dorsomotor nucleus of the vagus and is intimately involved with the modulation of endocrine factors, including the adrenal medullary system. These interconnections are presented schematically in Fig. 2.

2. *Physiological Function of the Hypothalamic Controller*

Food intake can be stimulated or inhibited by any of several peptides or monoamines. These are classified in Table II.

a. Monoaminergic Neurotransmitters. i. Norepinephrine. The norepinephrine-containing neuronal bodies are clustered in several groups. Two major ascending bundles of fibers from the A_1 and A_2 nuclei are involved in modulation of feeding. The dorsal noradrenergic bundle from the medullary reticular activating system courses anteriorly to the limbic system, the hippocampus and amygdala, and provides fibers to the medial hypothalamus (Ungerstedt, 1971). The second ascending system in the ventral noradrenergic bundle plays a critical role in feeding. It courses anteriorly to the LH area. Destruction of the ventral noradrenergic bundle by injection of 6-hydroxydopamine produces a modest hyperphagia and obesity without disturbance of diurnal

TABLE II
Peptides That Stimulate or Suppress Feeding

Increase food intake	Decrease food intake
Galanin	Serotonin (5-HT)
β-Endorphin	Anorectin (CTPG)
Norepinephrine	Neurotensin
Neuropeptide Y	Cholecystokinin-8
Dynorphin	Glucagon
Growth hormone-releasing hormone	Insulin
	Calcitonin
	Corticotropin-releasing factor
	Thyrotropin releasing hormone
	Cyclohispro

rhythms (Ahlskog and Hoebel, 1973; Ahlskog *et al.*, 1975). Amphetamine and related drugs may act on this system to inhibit feeding.

Injection of norepinephrine into the PVN produces feeding with preferential intake of carbohydrate (Leibowitz *et al.*, 1985). This effect can be attenuated by PVN lesions (Liebowitz *et al.*, 1983). This effect is mediated through α_2-noradrenergic receptors (Goldman *et al.*, 1985) which have a diurnal rhythm, peaking at dusk and having a nadir at dawn (Bhakthavatsalam and Leibowitz, 1986; Krauchi *et al.*, 1984; Leibowitz and Hor, 1982; Jhanwar-Uniyal *et al.*, 1986). This stimulation of food intake when norepinephrine is injected into the PVN is blocked by adrenalectomy (Leibowitz *et al.*, 1984; Roland *et al.*, 1986) and by a strong postingestional satiety signal (Gibson and Booth, 1986). Microinjection of norepinephrine into the VMH increases circulating concentrations of glucose, free fatty acids, and insulin (Steffens *et al.*, 1984). Injection of phentolamine, a drug which blocks α receptors, suppresses the norepinephrine-stimulated rise in glucose and exaggerates the rise in free fatty acids. This implies that α receptors mediate the rise in glucose and that β-receptors mediate the rise in free fatty acids. This is further supported by the fact that beta blockade with timolol prevents the rise in free fatty acids after microinjecting norepinephrine into the VMH. Norepinephrine in the VMH also stimulates the firing rate of sympathetic nerves to brown adipose tissue (BAT) (Sakaguchi and Bray, 1988).

Norepinephrine injected into the LH and perifornical areas depresses food intake through β receptors (Leibowitz, 1970). It also stimulates a rise in plasma insulin, but not in glucose or free fatty acids (Steffens *et al.*, 1984).

The metabolism of catecholamines in the hypothalamus can be enhanced by injecting insulin, which stimulates food intake. Within 10 minutes following the injection of insulin, the ratio of the metabolite of norepinephrine, 3-methoxy-4-hydroxyphenylglycol (MHPG), to norepinephrine in the hypothalamus of rats had declined, indicating increased norepinephrine release, whereas serotonin release had fallen, as indicated by a rise in the ratio of the metabolite 5-hydroxyindole-3-acetic acid (5-HIAA) to serotonin [5-hydroxytryptamine (5-HT)] (Grunstein *et al.*, 1985).

Chronic infusion of norepinephrine into the VMN produces obesity (Shimazu *et al.*, 1986). However, chronic infusion of norepinephrine into the PVN does not, and the acute effects of norepinephrine on meal ingestion appear to be located predominantly in the PVN. These anatomical differences in response to norepinephrine would suggest that the PVN may play a primary role in modulating meal-to-meal events, whereas the VMH may be more concerned with the homeostatic control of energy storage.

ii. Dopamine. Dopaminergic pathways originate from dopamine-containing neurons in the ventral tegmental area and ascend in the nigrostriatal bundle and mesolimbic pathway. This latter pathway activates the nucleus accumbens and is intimately involved in habituating behaviors. LH stimulation increase the release of dopamine in the nucleus accumbens, and animals will bar-press to deliver dopamine into this area. Dynorphin, an opioid peptide, and neurotensin are also rewarding in the nucleus accumbens. The potential role of dopamine in the development of hypothalamic obesity was suggested in studies in which 6-hydroxydopamine was injected into the raphe nuclei to deplete dopamine. When selective dopamine depletion occurred, radiofrequency VMH lesions did not produce obesity. If both norepinephrine and dopamine were depleted, obesity developed (Coscina and Nobrega, 1982).

iii. Serotonin. There is a wide variety of studies suggesting that enhanced concentration of serotonin under most circumstances is associated with reduced body fat stores (Blundell, 1986; Goudie *et al.*, 1976; Leibowitz, 1986). From nuclei located in the median raphe, serotonin fibers course anteriorly to provide inhibitory input into the medial hypothalamus. Both *p*-chlorophenylalanine, a serotonin antagonist, and 5,7-dihydroxytryptamine, a drug which destroys serotonin-containing neurons, will reduce food intake. Treatment with tryptophan and 5-hydroxytryptophan (5-HT), which are the precursors of serotonin, has been reported to reduce food intake in some but not all studies (Blundell, 1986). Drugs that release serotonin (e.g., fenfluramine) or block its reuptake (e.g., fluoxetine) also decrease feeding (Anderson *et al.*, 1979; Wong and Fuller, 1987).

Injection of serotonin into the PVN decreases total food intake, and this is blocked by drugs such as metergoline methysergide and ananserin, which block the action of serotonin (Weiss *et al.*, 1986; Shor-Posner *et al.*, 1986b).

iv. Histamine. Histamine appears to inhibit feeding by acting through H-1 receptors in the VMH. Chlorpheniramine, an H-1 antagonist, induces a large meal in the daylight, when hypothalamic histamine levels are high, but not at night, when hypothalamic levels of histamine are at their nadir. Antagonists of H-2 receptors do not affect food intake. Injection into the third cerebroventricle of a drug which blocks histidine decarboxylase (e.g., α-fluromethylhistidine) produces a prompt dose-related increase in food intake by shortening the latency to eat and increasing meal duration. This effect is specific for the

VMN and does not work in either the PVN or the LH (Sakata *et al.*, 1988).

In summary, monoamines appear to be involved in regulating both qualitative and quantitative aspects of single meals as well as modulating longer-term regulation of fat stores. Dopamine appears to be involved in the hedonistic or affective components of ingestion involving the nucleus accumbens and other limbic structures. Norepinephrine may initiate feeding and carbohydrate ingestion through the PVN, whereas in the VMN it seems to be involved in modulation of body fat stores. Serotonin reduces behavioral activity levels including feeding, with its locus of action in the PVN. Finally, histamine may be a diurnal inhibitor of feeding, acting on the VMH.

b. *Amino Acid Neurotransmitters.* Several amino acids have been suggested as potential neurotransmitters including γ-aminobutyric acid (GABA), aspartic acid, and glycine. These acids are of particular interest because injection of monosodium glutamate or aspartic acid into neonatal rats produces obesity (Olney, 1969). GABA is also of interest because it can both stimulate and inhibit feeding (Kelly *et al.*, 1979). GABA or its agonist, muscimol, given peripherally causes reduced food intake and body weight (Coscina and Nobrega, 1984). Injection of GABA into the medial hypothalamus, on the other hand, can increase food intake. Similar injections into the LH decrease food intake. Recent studies by Kamatchi *et al.* (1986) have shown that the stimulation of food intake by either insulin or 2-deoxy-D-glucose (2-DG) injections can be stopped by blocking the action of GABA at the VMN. Hypothalamic GABA levels are reduced in rats with VMH lesions (Orosco *et al.*, 1981). These data suggest that GABA may play a role in the modulation of feeding in the VMH syndrome.

c. *Peptidergic Neurotransmitters.* Many of the large and growing number of peptides isolated from the gut and the brain have been shown to have effects on feeding (see Table II) (Morley, 1987). β-Endorphin and dynorphin, from the opioid family, are among the most studied. The opioid antagonist, naloxone, has been shown to reduce food intake in rodents and a variety of other species (Holtzman, 1974; Morley, 1987). Dynorphin (Morley and Levine, 1981) or β-endorphin (Grandison and Guidotti, 1977; Leibowitz and Hor, 1982; McKay *et al.*, 1981), administered into the cerebral ventricular system or into medial hypothalamic nuclei, stimulates feeding, which appears to involve κ receptors. Further support for the role of endorphins was provided when antibodies to α-neoendorphin were shown to inhibit feeding when injected into the VMH (Schulz *et al.*, 1984). Lesions in the VMH do not block, and may have potentiated, the reduction in food intake induced by naloxone (King et al., 1979), but lesions in the dorsomedial hypothalamic nucleus have been reported to reduce the response to this drug (Bellinger et al., 1983). Electrolytic lesions in the PVN, but not depletion of norepinephrine by 70% following injection of 6-hydroxydopamine, have been shown to attenuate the effects of morphine (Shor-Posner et al., 1986a). The PVN appears to be among the most sensitive sites for stimulation of feeding by opioids. These data are consistent with the hypothesis that κ and possibly other opioid receptors in the dorsomedial and paraventricular hypothalamus are involved in modulating food intake through mechanisms which may involve GABA (Grandison and Guidotti, 1977; Morley, 1987). Although opiates and either paraventricular lesions or parasaggital knife cuts produce hyperphagia, they do so by different mechanisms (Gosnell et al., 1985). Just as endorphins have diffuse sites of action, so too does neuropeptide Y, a member of the family of pancreatic polypeptides (Stanley and Leibowitz, 1984, 1985; Clark et al., 1984, 1987; Levine and Morley, 1984; Gray and Morley, 1986; Gray et al., 1986). Multiple injections of neuropeptide have been shown to increase food intake and body weight (Stanley et al., 1986). Galanin, on the other hand, acts with much more specificity on the PVN (Kyrokouli et al., 1986).

A larger number of peptides inhibit food intake than stimulate it (Morley, 1987). In most cases these have only been tested with single injections into the ventricular system. Glucagon and insulin are among the most potent, although several other peptides also have a strong inhibitory effect on food intake. Concentrations of insulin in the cerebrospinal fluid have been proposed as a feedback signal for satiety. (For a more detailed discussion, see Sections III,B and V.) Most of these peptides have only been tested by acute injection, and demonstrations of chronic changes in weight by peptides which acutely increase or decrease food intake are limited. Chronic infusion of corticotropin-releasing factor (CRF) will lower food intake (Bray, 1987) and a peptide derived from growth hormone-releasing factor, called anorectin (CTPG), has been shown to reduce food intake and body weight in experimental animals (Arase et al., 1987).

d. Neuronal Responses. Functional characteristics of the neurons in the VMH and the LH area have been examined by a variety of techniques. Oomura and colleagues (1969) have suggested that there are "glucoreceptive" neurons located in the VMH and "glucosensitive" ones located in the LH area. Using multibarreled electrodes to record from isolated neurons in the ventromedial area, these workers found neuronal units whose electrical discharge rate was increased when glucose was iontophoretically applied and whose electrical discharge rate was reduced by insulin (Oomura *et al.,* 1969; Oomura, 1983). Neurons in the LH area show reciprocal changes to those in the VMH. The firing rate of these neurons is increased by insulin and reduced by glucose (Kow and Pfaff, 1985). Free fatty acids applied iontophoretically increase sodium as well as the firing rate, and antagonize the effects of glucose. The sodium pump may be involved in this action. During changes in blood levels of glucose and insulin, the simultaneous discharge rates in the VMH and the LH area vary inversely. Single neurons in the LH area recorded continuously show a diurnal rhythm in nearly 40% of the neurons. These same neurons undergo a significant reduction in firing rate when the animals take food (Ono *et al.,* 1986).

e. Metabolism of the Hypothalamus. Differential effects of applied nutrients into neurons of the hypothalamus suggest the possibility that nutritional states might modify the metabolic properties of neurons in these areas. With fasting, the transport of fatty acids (Kasser *et al.,* 1986) and ketones (Bray *et al.,* 1987) across the blood–brain barrier is increased relative to glucose. The oxidation of palmitate by the VMH was also increased, but the oxidation of glucose was not affected.

f. Effect of Hypothalamic Lesions on Neurotransmitters. Several approaches could be used to examine the changes in responsiveness to the neurotransmitter systems in animals with hypothalamic obesity. These would include measurements of neurotransmitter or peptide concentrations, turnover of neurotransmitters, concentration of the enzymes that are involved in the biosynthesis of these neurotransmitters, response to microinjections of neurotransmitters, or response to drugs that could modify neurotransmitter function. Orosco *et al.,* (1981) found similar levels of norepinephrine in the hypothalamus, the medulla, and the remainder of the brain and similar dopamine levels in the striatum and the rest of the brain. Norepinephrine turnover in the hypothalamus was significantly slower in VMH-lesioned rats, whereas dopamine turnover in the whole brain minus striatum was enhanced in the VMH-lesioned rats. Injections of monosodium glutamate reduced the hypothalamic content of dopamine, but not its metabolite, 3,4-dihydroxyphenylacetic acid (DOPAC) (Lorden and Caudle, 1986). Concentrations of CCK, bombesin, and neurotensin have been measured in the hypothalamus of fed and starved VMH-lesioned rats in comparison with normal rats, and no differences were found (Schneider *et al.,* 1979; Oku *et al.,* 1984c).

Effects of drugs likely operating through diverse central neurotransmitters have also been examined. Amphetamine-treated rats with VMH lesions suppressed food intake similarly to control rats (Bray and York, 1972), and rats with PVN lesions had an enhanced response to amphetamine (McCabe *et al.*, 1986). VMH-lesioned rats treated with fenfluramine also showed a drop in food intake similar to controls. Amphetamine is thought to act through noradrenergic systems, while fenfluramine is believed to release and block the reuptake of serotonin. Serotonin itself suppressed food intake in both VMH-lesioned and control rats (Bray and York, 1972). Thus, both of these neurotransmitters can be released and act when given to lesioned animals, but the sensitivity is increased. This would imply that the reduced neuronal mass after hypothalamic lesioning is more responsive or, alternatively, that the loss of inhibitory mass allows the effects of these released neurotransmitters to be more effective. Naloxone, a drug that blocks opioid receptors, produced a greater reduction in food intake in the VHM-lesioned rats than in the controls (King *et al.*, 1979). Levels of β-endorphin are also altered by VMH lesions. Jugular and portal vein concentrations have been reported to be increased along with those in the pituitary gland and the pancreas (Matsumura *et al.*, 1984), whereas duodenal levels of this peptide are reduced.

B. AFFERENT SYSTEMS

1. *Cephalic Sensory Systems*

A variety of evidence reviewed earlier suggests that animals with hypothalamic lesions and hyperphagia may be hyperresponsive to both rewarding and aversive afferent signals (Bray and York, 1972; Sclafani and Kirchgessner, 1986a; Kramer *et al.*, 1983). These would include taste aversions, reduced willingness to work for food, and exaggerated responses to palatable foods. This finickiness can be both positive, as when overeating a high-fat diet, and negative, as illustrated in the aversion to a quinine-adulterated diet. Attempts to dissociate hyperphagia and finickiness have been reported (McGinty *et al.*, 1965; Beven, 1973), but these results have not been replicated (Bauer, 1972; Sclafani and Kirchgessner, 1986a). Finickiness in the rat with both parasaggital knife cuts and obesity is not found in rats with obesity and hyperphagia due to ovariectomy, indicating that the finickiness is not secondary to obesity per se (Gale and Sclafani, 1977). The weight of evidence argues that the hyperphagia associated with parasaggital knife cuts and lesions in VMH is also associated with finickiness or, more properly stated, with disturbed feedback control by afferent sensory information. From the asymmetrical knife-cut studies of Sclafani and Kirchgessner (1986a), the hyperphagia and finickiness might be the result of impaired inhibitory signals from the PVN to the sensory input from vagal afferents to the nucleus of the tactus solitarius (solitary nucleus). Thus, larger meals of palatable items or smaller meals of unpalatable items would result from this partially impaired feedback circuit.

The enhanced preference for sweet taste has also been demonstrated by Sclafani (1978) and can be used as a test for assessing the effectiveness of the hypothalamic lesion. The addition of quinine, a bitter-tasting substance, to the diet will reduce food intake and restore body weight to normal (Sclafani et al., 1979; Oku et al., 1984a). Whether this is a taste aversion or a metabolic response to absorbed quinine is unclear. Dehydroepiandrosterone, as another dietary additive, produces aversion and can reduce the body weight of rats with parasaggital hypothalamic knife cuts (Gosnell, 1987). Whether this steroid, normally produced by the adrenal, acts by blocking endogenous corticosterone effects or through other mechanisms is currently unknown.

2. Gastrointestinal Satiety Signals

Gastrointestinal satiety has been examined in a variety of circumstances in animals with hypothalamic lesions producing hyperphagia and has been demonstrated to respond appropriately. Animals with hypothalamic hyperphagia tend to eat large meals, but this is characteristic of most types of experimental obesity. Meal size restriction leads to adaptation by these animals by eating more frequent, smaller meals. Rats with VMH lesions suppress oral intake proportionally when glucose, amino acids, or fat are infused into the duodenum (Novin et al., 1979). Stomach distension, the removal of food or its dilution, leads to appropriate alterations in intake in such animals (McHugh and Moran, 1978; Smutz et al., 1975; Smith et al., 1961). Dilution of the diet with cellulose, on the other hand, may not do so (Bray and York, 1972). The responses to CCK, a peptide requiring an intact afferent vagal system and a functional PVN, as well as bombesin have been shown to be intact in the animal with VMH lesions (Kulkosky et al., 1976; West et al., 1982). The role of hepatic signals has not been adequately examined. From the information available, it would appear that afferent signals are distorted from the oropharyngeal cavity and may play a role in the positive and negative finickiness and hyperphagia of animals with medial hypothalamic lesions. However, Cox and Powley (1981) have demonstrated that disturbances in the cephalic phase are not essential for the development of obesity in animals with VMH lesions. The alterations in hormonal signals in hypothalamic obese animals are probably secondary to the alterations in nutrient intake and energy storage, rather than primary driving factors.

Duggan and Booth (1986) have recently proposed that the mechanism for increased weight gain in hypothalamic obesity is the enhanced rate of gastric emptying. This implies that gastric distention is reduced, and that the animals may be increasing food intake to maintain their rate of gastric emptying (Brady *et al.*, 1986). The simplest explanation for this effect would be the enhanced vagal activity which has been associated with hypothalamic obesity and will be discussed below.

As found with obese human beings, in the rat with VMH lesions produced by parasaggital knife cuts jejunoileostomy surgery reverses obesity. This weight loss is associated with a reduction in food intake and in the volume of sucrose solution which the animals with bypass surgery would eat during a test period. Atkinson and Brent (1982) have found an appetite-suppressing activity in the serum of rats with an intestinal bypass, but its nature is not known. When the intestines of the animals are reconnected, they resume the hyperphagic status they had preoperatively and regain weight toward control levels (Sclafani *et al.*, 1978). Koopmans *et al.* (1982) have moved 5- and 10-cm segments of ileum to the duodenum (ileal transposition) and found a similar loss of body weight and a decrease in food intake of rats with knife cut-induced hyperphagia and obesity. Again, the simplest explanation for this response to ileal transposition may be the aversive nature of having a shorter small intestine.

3. *Circulating Afferent Satiety Signals*

a. Parabiosis. The use of parabiotic animals is one approach to testing the possibility that circulating factors may be involved in regulating nutrient stores of fat (Nishizawa and Bray, 1980; Hervey, 1959). When one member of a parabiotic pair of animals receives a VMH lesion, the lesioned animal becomes obese and the other member becomes less fat. Both electrolytic lesions and parasaggital knife cuts will produce this effect. The nature of the circulating signal generated by the fattening of one animal following a VMH lesion or other maneuver (Parameswaren *et al.*, 1977) that can lead to reduced food intake and body fat in the other is currently unknown.

b. Nutrient and Metabolic Signals. A number of nutrients and their metabolites as well as unknown circulating factors (Davis *et al.*, 1969; Atkinson and Brent, 1982; Koopmans, 1985) have been implicated in regulation of nutrient stores. The glucose concentration in rats with hypothalamic obesity may be low initially (Smith and Campfield, 1986). Changes in glucose may be a signal for initiation of a meal. Campfield *et al.* (1985) have shown that a 15% drop in glucose followed by a rise toward baseline is the signal for a meal in more than 60% of these transitions in glucose. In rats with VMH lesions the onset of meals may be delayed, but when they occur they are larger than in control rats. Changing blood glucose levels produce reciprocal changes in the afferent vagal firing rate (Niijima, 1983a,b, 1984a,b, 1986). These changes in vagal firing rate may provide part of the explanation for the afferent loop of a reflex arc that stimulates the efferent sympathetic nervous system (Glick and Raum, 1986; Sakaguchi *et al.*, 1988b). Fatty acids, on the other hand, are normal or increased in rats with VMH lesions (Nakai *et al.*, 1986), but their response to various stressful stimuli tends to be reduced (Nishizawa and Bray, 1978). The circulating levels of ketones are low in monosodium glutamate-treated mice without hyperphagia (Nakai *et al.*, 1986). The disturbances of insulin secretion appear to be the result of altered efferent systems in hypothalamic obesity (Inoue *et al.*, 1983; Campfield and Smith, 1983; Campfield *et al.*, 1986). There is increased sensitivity to norepinephrine and reduced sensitivity to acetylcholine. A number of glucose derivatives (Sakata *et al.*, 1980; Plata-Salaman *et al.*, 1986b; Puthuraya *et al.*, 1985; Shimizu *et al.*, 1984) and short-chain polyhydroxymonocarboxylic acids have been shown to modulate food intake (Arase *et al.*, 1984). It is possible that these metabolites may be involved in modulating normal feeding patterns through the medial hypothalamus. If so, VMH lesions would be expected to abolish these control signals. This hypothesis requires further testing.

c. Hormonal Signals. Many of the peptides located in the gastrointestinal tract are also located in the brain (Morley, 1987; Woods *et al.*, 1981; Baile *et al.*, 1986). This observation has led to testing the role of hormones that might be released from the gastrointestinal tract as potential signals for modifiers of food intake. A review of this literature is outside the scope of the current analysis. However, a few comments are germane.

Support for the hypothesis that long-term homeostasis of energy balance is regulated by the VMH, whereas short-term controls of food intake are located mainly in the PVN, is provided by the data on CCK. This peptide produces inhibition of food intake when injected peripherally into animals (Gibbs *et al.*, 1973) or humans (Kissileff *et al.*, 1981). The effect of low doses is mediated by an afferent system in the gastrointestinal tract and coursing through the gastric branch of the vagus nerve to the nucleus of the tractus solitarius (Crawley and

Schwaber, 1984; Smith *et al.*, 1981a) in the medulla oblongata and from there to the PVN. When cats are allowed to feed, an increase in CCK can be measured in the hypothalamus (Schick *et al.*, 1986). Truncal vagotomy (Smith *et al.*, 1981a; Lorenz and Goldman, 1982; Morley *et al.*, 1982) or selective hepatic vagotomy (Smith *et al.*, 1981a) and destruction of the nucleus of the tractus solitarius (Crawley and Schwaber, 1984) or the PVN (Crawley and Kiss, 1985) each abolish the satiety effects of CCK. VMH lesions, on the other hand, do not block the effects of CCK (Smith *et al.*, 1981a). Although CCK can induce satiety, long-term infusion of it does not produce a change in body weight (West *et al.*, 1984). Bombesin has similarly been shown to reduce food intake when given peripherally (Gibbs *et al.*, 1979). This effect is not blocked by VMH lesions (Gibbs and Smith, 1986; West *et al.*, 1982; Geary *et al.*, 1986), nor by vagotomy, although complete vagotomy plus high spinal cord transection abolishes the effect of bombesin (Smith *et al.*, 1981b; Stuckey *et al.*, 1985). Although a variety of other peptides has been tested centrally, we are unaware of other trials in which peripherally active peptides have been examined in animals with VMH lesions.

C. EFFERENT CONTROL

1. *Food Intake*

The fact that after hypothalamic injury obesity may occur with (Brobeck, 1946; Hansen *et al.*, 1983) or without hyperphagia (Han, 1967; Bray and York, 1979) suggests that there may be two types of "hypothalamic obesity" with different mechanisms (Bray *et al.*, 1982a). The lesion produced by localized damage to the PVN and after parasaggital knife cuts may be viewed as a primary disorder of food intake—a hyperphagic syndrome (Weingarten *et al.*, 1985; Shor-Posner *et al.*, 1985). Obesity without hyperphagia, on the other hand, appears to be associated with disturbed function of the autonomic nervous system and its metabolic control (Bray and York, 1979; Bray, 1987). In most cases of medial hypothalamic injury, however, both increased food intake *and* disturbed autonomic function are present, but from an analytical point of view we argue that they reflect separate mechanism for producing obesity. Hypothalamic lesions alter not only the quantity but the type of macronutrients that animals select (Sclafani and Aravich, 1983; Shor-Posner *et al.*, 1985). Following electrolytic lesions in either the PVN or the VMH or parasaggital knife cuts, rats primarily increased their intake of carbohydrate (Aravich and Sclafani, 1983; Shor-Posner *et al.*, 1985). Both the VMH-lesioned and para-saggital knife-cut rats increased their protein intake sufficiently to maintain the preoperative percentage of protein (Aravich and Sclafani, 1983). The PVH-lesioned rats, however, did not increase protein and thus had a smaller percentage of protein intake (Shor-Posner *et al.*, 1985). Interestingly, the PVH-lesioned rats that did not become hyperphagic still showed the increase in carbohydrate intake observed in those PVN-lesioned animals that did develop hyperphagia.

These increased intakes of carbohydrate are similar to the effect produced when norepinephrine is microinjected into the PVN (Leibo-witz *et al.*, 1985). Animals with PVN lesions also have impaired compensation. After fasting for 5 or 24 hours, they do not increase their food intake as much as control rats (Shor-Posner *et al.*, 1985). However, these animals do respond appropriately with an increase in food intake after injection of insulin or 2-DG. One report has suggested that the diurnal rhythm is impaired by PVN lesions (Shor-Posner *et al.*, 1985), but we have not found any significant impairment (Toku-naga *et al.*, 1986b; Fukushima *et al.*, 1987).

2. *Autonomic Nervous System*

The function of the autonomic nervous system is altered in the syndrome of VMH obesity produced by damage to the VMN (Bray and York, 1979). This involves increased activity of the vagus nerve but is almost universally associated with reduced activity of the sympathetic nervous system (Bray, 1987). Obesity produced by lesions in the PVN, on the other hand, produces either small or negligible changes in the function of the autonomic nervous system.

a. Parasympathetic (Vagal) Nervous System. Brooks *et al.* (1946) were the first to suggest that VMH lesions produced increased vagal activity. They demonstrated increased gastric acid secretion after VMH lesions, and this was subsequently confirmed (Inoue and Bray, 1977; Weingarten and Powley, 1980), but is not observed in rats with PVN lesions (Weingarten *et al.*, 1985). Powley and Opsahl (1974) carried this observation further by showing that the obesity of animals with hypothalamic lesions could be reversed by truncal vagotomy. This was confirmed by Inoue and Bray (1977), who suggested that impaired gastric emptying might be a major component of this effect. Additional studies have demonstrated that the effects of vagotomy performed prior to the introduction of VMH lesions attenuate the weight gain but do not completely block it (King and Frohman, 1982). King and Frohman (1982) showed that vagotomized rats with VMH lesions gained approximately 60% as much weight as VMH-lesioned rats with sham vagotomy. Using scopolamine to block vagal function reduced the weight of VMH-lesioned rats by about 40% (Carpenter *et al.,* 1979). Finally, selective celiac vagotomy reduced the weight gain of VMH-lesioned rats by 40% (Sawchenko *et al.,* 1981). Thus, vagotomy attenuates but does not eliminate VMH-lesioned obesity. Moreover, vagotomy that eliminates the hyperphagia of rats with VMH lesions when they are eating a chow diet may not eliminate the overeating when they have very palatable diets (Sclafani *et al.,* 1981).

b. Sympathetic Nervous System. Most evidence would argue that there is decreased sympathetic activity in rats with VMN lesions but not in animals with PVN lesions. The activity of the sympathetic nervous system can be assessed in one of four ways. The first involves histochemical staining of tissues containing catecholamines. The second involves measurement of physiological changes in sympathetically innervated tissues. An increase in heart rate, lipolysis, and increased thermogenic activity of mitochondria from BAT can all be used as physiological responses to estimate sympathetic activity. A third and more direct measure is provided by norepinephrine turnover in the nerve endings of sympathetically innervated tissues. Norepinephrine pools labeled with radioactive norepinephrine ([³H]norepinephrine) can be followed over time, with the decline in specific activity of the pool providing a measure of the rate of norepinephrine production. Blockade of tyrosine hydroxylase, the rate-limiting enzyme in norepinephrine production, with α-methyl-*p*-tyrosine leads to a decline in tissue norepinephrine concentration, which is related to its rate of secretion. Dopamine accumulation after blockade of dopamine-β-hydroxylase can also be used to measure the synthetic rate of norepinephrine in sympathetically innervated tissues. Finally, the electrical firing rate of sympathetic nerves can provide a direct measure of sympathetic activity.

The hypothesis that VMH lesions reduced sympathetic activity was originally suggested by Inoue *et al.* (1977b), who observed enlarged salivary glands and reduced glucagon levels in rats with hypothalamic lesions. Subsequently, the mobilization of fatty acids in animals with VMH lesions was shown to be impaired (Nishizawa and Bray, 1978; Bray and Nishizawa, 1978). A summary of the more recent data for various types of lesions using different techniques to assess sympathetic activity is presented in Table III. Thermogenic activity of BAT (Seydoux *et al.,* 1981, 1982b; Fukushima *et al.,* 1987; Saito *et al.,* 1985) and its responsiveness to diet (Rohner-Jeanrenaud *et al.,* 1983a; Hogan *et al.,* 1985) were impaired in animals with electrolytic lesions and were reduced to a lesser degree in animals with parasaggital hypo-

TABLE III
SYMPATHETIC ACTIVITY AFTER HYPOTHALAMIC LESIONS

Method of measurement	Change compared to control			
	VMN lesion	Parasaggital knife cut	PVN lesion	LH lesion
Physiological				
Salivary gland weight	↓	N[a]		
Free fatty acid mobilization	↓			
Thermogenic activity in brown fat (GDP binding)	↓	N	N	↑
Norepinephrine turnover				
Specific activity				
Weanling	↓			
Adult	N or ↑			
Block tyrosine hydroxylase	N or ↑		N	↑
Block dopamine-β-hydroxylase				
Electrical firing rate				
Nerves to innervating brown adipose tissue	↓		N	↑
Splanchnic nerve	↓		↓	

[a] N, Normal.

thalamic knife cuts (Coscina et al., 1985). This impaired sympathetic activity may account for the impaired thermoregulation in rats with hypothalamic obesity (Vander Tuig et al., 1986), although impaired response to cold has not been reported by others (Hogan et al., 1982; Rohner-Jeanrenaud et al., 1983a). It may also explain increased metabolic efficiency (Walgren and Powley, 1985). Norepinephrine turnover in weanling rats (Vander Tuig et al., 1982) was likewise reduced. However, norepinephrine turnover in adult animals is not reduced and may even be increased (Young and Landsberg, 1980; Yoshida and Bray, 1984; Vander Tuig et al., 1985; Romsos, 1985). The electrical firing rate of sympathetic nerves to BAT is consistently reduced following hypothalamic lesions (Yoshimatsu et al., 1984; Niijima et al., 1984; Sakaguchi and Bray, 1987a,b).

This apparent paradox of normal or increased norepinephrine turnover in adult rats appears to contradict the other types of measurements in rats with VMH lesions. One explanation for the discrepancy in norepinephrine turnover is that the hyperphagia and hyperinsulinemia of adult rats with VMH lesions may change the metabolism of norepinephrine. The low rate of electrical activity in sympathetic nerves and the increased concentration of insulin may enhance the leak of norepinephrine out of its storage granule, which would then be metabolized by the monoamine oxidase in the mitochondria of the nerve ending rather than being secreted into the neuroeffector cleft. This increased catabolism within the nerve ending of norepinephrine could account for the apparent increase in norepinephrine turnover at a time when electrical firing rate is reduced. Sympathetic control of the adrenal nerve seems to be opposite of that in BAT (Katafuchi et al., 1985a,b, 1986). Yoshimatsu et al. (1985) have reported that VMH lesions increase sympathoadrenal nerve activity. These same investigators (Yoshimatsu et al., 1984) have reported that splanchnic sympathetic activity is reduced.

Impaired norepinephrine turnover has also been reported in obese mice with VMH lesions due to monosodium glutamate (Yoshida et al., 1984, 1985b). In the mice with gold thioglucose-induced obesity, the responsiveness of BAT as an index of sympathetic activity is also reduced when the animals are given a cafeteria-type diet, but not when they are exposed to the cold (Hogan and Himms-Hagen, 1983).

On the other hand, three experiments suggest that the reduced activity of the sympathetic nervous system following VMH lesions is not involved in the development of obesity. In these studies sympathectomy was induced with guanethidine, which did not block the obesity produced by VMH lesions (Tordoff et al., 1984; Powley et al., 1983). Acceptance of these findings rests on the assumption that treatment with guanethidine has completely removed sympathetic innervation. Since catecholamines still persist in some tissues, the effects of VMH lesions on sympathetic activity would still be present (Seydoux et al., 1981; Levin and Sullivan, 1984).

3. Efferent Hormonal System

A variety of endocrine systems are disturbed by VMH lesions. These include the release of growth hormone, the secretion of insulin, and the control of the reproductive cycle. In addition, the presence of adrenal corticosterone appears to be essential for the expression of obesity following both VMN and PVN lesions.

a. Growth Hormone. Hypothalamic lesions in weanling and adult rats are associated with the stunting of growth (Bray and York, 1979; Bernardis, 1985b; Frohman et al., 1969). The detailed studies by Frohman and Bernardis (1971) showed that there was an acute secretion of growth hormone after a VMH lesion, followed by a blunted release of growth hormone (Martin et al., 1974). Administration of growth hormone has been reported to reduce the development of VMH lesion obesity by some (York and Bray, 1972) but not by others (Goldman et al., 1972). It is clear, however, that the pituitary gland is not essential for the development of hypothalamic obesity which occurs in animals that have had a complete hypophysectomy (Bray, 1974).

b. *Insulin.* Hales and Kennedy (1964) were the first to show that there was hyperinsulinemia following VMH lesions, and this was readily confirmed (Han and Frohman, 1970; Frohman et al., 1969; York and Bray, 1972; Bray and York, 1979; Jeanrenaud, 1985). Perfused pancreata (Rohner-Jeanrenaud and Jeanrenaud, 1980) and isolated pancreatic islets (Campfield et al., 1986; Caterson and Taylor, 1982) likewise show enhanced insulin secretion. The rise in insulin after such hypothalamic lesions developed in animals that did not overeat and in weanling rats, indicating that it could not simply be explained by hyperphagia. The fact that insulin injections can lead to obesity suggested that the hyperphagia and obesity of the VMH-lesioned rat might be the result of hyperinsulinemia (Inoue and Bray, 1977). This hypothesis was initially supported by the fact that vagotomy could reverse hypothalamic obesity (Powley and Opsahl, 1974). One explanation for this observation could be the role of the vagus nerve in controlling insulin secretion. When anesthetized rats being infused with glucose are given an acute VMH lesion, there is an early increase in insulin without an additional rise in glucose. This acute hyperinsulinemia is prevented by bilateral truncal vagotomy (Berthoud and Jeanrenaud, 1979a; Tokunaga et al., 1986a). Moreover, direct stimulation of the vagus nerve increases insulin release (Kaneto et al., 1974). VMH lesions also increase the firing rate of the vagus nerve (Yoshimatsu et al., 1984). Additional support for this hypothesis is provided by the fact that disconnection of the vagus from the islet, following pancreatic transplantation of fetal islets beneath the renal capsule of diabetic rats treated with streptozotocin, reduces the hyperphagia and the rise of insulin by 80% following a VMH lesion (Inoue et al., 1977a, 1978). Selective transection of the celiac branch of the vagus nerve attenuates the hyperphagia of VMH-lesioned rats, as noted above (Sawchenko et al., 1981), but other vagal branches may also be involved (Berthoud et al., 1983).

It is now clear, however, that basal hyperinsulinemia is not essential for the development of hypothalamic obesity. After VMH lesions in rats with prior vagotomy, the initial rise in insulin secretion following a meal is impaired, and the basal levels of insulin are not increased (King and Frohman, 1982). Moreover, vagotomy may have aversive effects (Bernstein and Goehler, 1983; Sclafani and Kramer, 1985). In addition, insulin is controlled by both the gastric and the celiac

branches of the vagus nerve. More convincing, however, are the observations that several varieties of hypothalamic hyperphagia and
obesity are not associated with hyperinsulinemia: Bray et al.
(1982a) found no rise in basal insulin in the knife-cut rats, and Sclafani (1981)
has also reported that animals with obesity due to hypothalamic parasaggital knife cuts do not show hyperinsulinemia. A more recent report from that laboratory, however, found an increase of insulin in
knife-cut rats (Sclafani and Aravich, 1983). Lesions made with plati-
num electrodes which are "nonirritative" also do not increase plasma
insulin (King and Frohman, 1985). Studies with PVN lesions that
produce obesity likewise do not show basal hyperinsulinemia in the
afternoon, but may have increased insulin in the morning following
the nocturnal food intake (Sclafani and Aravich, 1983; Tokunaga et
al., 1986b; Fukushima et al., 1987). Acute PVN lesions cause both
glucose and insulin to rise, in contrast to the hyperinsulinemia alone
found in VMH-lesioned rats (Tokunaga et al., 1986a, 1987). Acute
PVN lesions also produce increased serum glucagon, an effect dependent on an intact vagus nerve (Tokunaga et al., 1987). This suggests
that there may be a pathway from the PVN to the dorsal motor nucleus of the vagus which mediates the vagal activity of glucagon-
secreting cells from the pancreas. Finally, rats with hypothalamic islands produced by the severance of connections to the hypothalamus,
with a circular knife motion above the hypothalamus, produced
obesity without hyperinsulinemia (Ohshima et al., 1985).

Hypothalamic lesions also affect glucagon, but the effect is unclear.
In two reports (Inoue et al., 1977a; Chikamori et al., 1980) plasma
glucagon was reduced after hypothalamic lesions, but in another report it was increased (Karakesh et al., 1977). There is no obvious explanation for this difference, but differences are also reported in glucagon
secretion. In vivo, the injection of arginine intraperitoneally produced
a greater response in the rats with hypothalamic lesions than in the
controls. Moreover, in this report there was a significant inverse relationship between plasma glucagon levels and body weight (Chikamori
et al., 1980). Using perfused pancreas in vitro, however, glucagon secretion was enhanced when arginine was used (Rohner-Jeanrenaud
and Jeanrenaud, 1980). One difference between the in vitro and in vivo
studies may be the glucose concentration. In vitro glucose was not
added. In vivo, of course, glucose is circulating during arginine infusion. The intravenous administration of glucose after the hypothalamic lesion produced a smaller suppression of glucagon than in the
control rats, indicating that the control of this system was different
following hypothalamic lesions.

c. *Reproductive Function.* Among the earliest observations in animals with hypothalamic obesity was a deranged estrus cycle. Since the presence of such impairment was associated with lesions that are now known to damage sexually dimorphic components of the VMH, it is not surprising that this occurred (Bray and York, 1979).

d. *Adrenal Steroids.* The effects of adrenal steroids deserve special comment. Animals with lesions in the VMH show a blunted diurnal rhythm for corticosterone (Krieger, 1979; Tokunaga *et al.*, 1986b). This disturbance can be partially corrected by limiting food intake (Krieger, 1979). Animals with lesions in the PVN have been reported to have a blunted diurnal rhythm for corticosterone (Shor-Posner *et al.*, 1985; Tokunaga *et al.*, 1986b; Fukushima *et al.*, 1987). As noted in the introduction, adrenalectomy reverses all forms of obesity including obesity associated with ventromedial (King and Smith, 1985; Bruce *et al.*, 1982) and paraventricular (Shimizu *et al.*, 1989) lesions and the injection of gold thioglucose (Debons *et al.*, 1983, 1986). This reversal of hypothalamic obesity is associated with a restoration of food intake to normal and with increased energy expenditure. Administration of small doses of corticosterone will reinitiate hyperphagia in VMH-lesioned rats (King *et al.*, 1984). One explanation for the effects of adrenalectomy may be enhanced CRF produced when the feedback signal of corticosterone is removed (Sawchenko *et al.*, 1984; Bray, 1987; Arase *et al.*, 1989a).

To test the hypothesis that CRF might be involved, this peptide was infused into the third ventricle of normal rats. Food intake was reduced (Morley and Levine, 1982), as was body weight, but the reduction in body weight was greater than could be accounted for by the reduction in food intake, suggesting that there was enhanced thermogenesis resulting from this peptide (Arase *et al.*, 1989a). This is consistent with data from other laboratories, showing that the circulating concentration of norepinephrine is significantly increased when CRF is injected into the lateral cerebral ventricle (Brown *et al.*, 1982; Brown and Fisher, 1985). When CRF was injected into the third ventricle of rats with hypothalamic obesity, it likewise reduced their food intake and produced a modest reduction in body weight (Arase *et al.*, 1989b), suggesting that enhanced levels of CRF might play a role in the reversal of obesity associated with adrenalectomy (Bray, 1987).

An alternative hypothesis has been suggested by Leibowitz *et al.* (1984). Norepinephrine microinjected into the PVN increases food intake (Leibowitz, 1970), and this effect is abolished by adrenalectomy (Roland *et al.*, 1986). Replacement with corticosterone restores the sensitivity to norepinephrine and raises the concentration of α_2 receptors in the PVN, through which norepinephrine acts (Roland *et al.*, 1986).

D. CONTROLLED SYSTEM

There are functional changes in several components of the controlled system following a VMH lesion. Insulin hypersection develops rapidly (Berthoud and Jeanrenaud, 1979a; Tokunaga et al., 1986a) and reflects both increased vagal and reduced sympathetic activities (Inoue et al., 1983). Insulin secretion by isolated islets or perfused pancreas rises by 2-fold or more within 7 days after VMH lesions (Smith and Campfield, 1986; Rohner-Jeanrenaud and Jeanrenaud, 1980). The neurotransmitter acetylcholine is less effective in stimulating insulin from islets of VMH-lesioned rats than from control rats and there is a shift in the log dose response curve. This is the effect one might expect from a tissue exposed to increased tonic stimulation. On the other hand, the suppression of insulin release from islets by norepinephrine is more responsive. In vivo, the effect of bethanechol, an analog of acetylcholine, on insulin release is smaller in VMH lesioned than in control animals. Norepinephrine, on the other hand, has a more suppressive effect on insulin secretion from isolated islets of VMH-lesioned rats. These effects in islets from VMH-lesioned rats persist for more than 100 days in vivo and in tissue culture (Campfield et al., 1986).

Changes in adipose tissue metabolism after VMH lesions are also well known (Bray and York, 1979; Enser et al., 1985). By 14 days after VMH lesions, there is an impairment in norepinephrine-stimulated lipolysis. In a recent longitudinal study of this problem, Penicaud et al. (1986) found that, by 1 week after a VMH lesion, adipose tissue, muscle, and liver were overresponsive to insulin. By 6 weeks, however, the characteristic insulin resistance had appeared. Suppression of hepatic glucose output by insulin is found with a dose of 550 μU/ml in control rats, but 6 weeks after a VMH lesion even a dose of 16,000 μU/ml is unable to suppress hepatic glucose output. Jeanrenaud and colleagues (Penicaud et al., 1986) attribute this to the effects of the higher glucagon levels.

The increases in body fat stores in animals with hypothalamic obesity are largely produced by an increase in fat cell size. This was first demonstrated by the work of Hirsch and Han (1969). Recently, two studies in the diet-sensitive Osborne–Mendel rat have shown that, after hypothalamic obesity, when animals are fed a high-fat diet, there may indeed be an increase in the total number of fat cells (Stern and Keesey, 1981; Faust et al., 1984). Gold thioglucose-treated mice also show hypertrophy and hyperplasia of their adipocytes as they become obese (Enser et al., 1985). Circulating triglycerides are increased in rats with VMH lesions (Goldman *et al.*, 1972; Bray and York, 1979; Inui *et al.*, 1987). This results from increased hepatic synthesis (Inui *et al.*, 1987) and secretion of lipoproteins (Karakash *et al.*, 1977; Nordby *et al.*, 1979). Heparin-releasable lipoprotein lipase also is increased (Murase and Inoue, 1985). The heart adapts with hypertrophy and there is a tendency for blood pressure to rise (Reisin *et al.*, 1980).

III. GENETIC OBESITY

In this section we shall concentrate on the genetically inherited forms of obesity. Since our last review of this area (Bray and York, 1979), a number of new models of obesity, e.g., the corpulent rat (*LA/Cp* or *SR/Cp*) and the diabetes (*db pas*) mouse (Aubert *et al.*, 1985), have been introduced, and these are summarized in Table IV. These new models differ in a number of ways from the existing known models. However, as this review is directed toward understanding the basic mechanisms contributing to the development of obesity, it does not aim to offer a comprehensive review of the literature, but rather a selection of the literature which helps us to formulate possible etiologies for the obese syndromes. Further, it should be recognized that

TABLE IV
GENETIC OBESITY

Single gene
  Dominant
    Yellow mouse (A^{vy}/a; A^{iy}/a)
    Adipose mouse (Ad)
  Recessive
    Obese mouse (*ob*)
    Diabetes mouse (*db*)
    Fat mouse (*Fat*)
    Tubby mouse (*tu*)
    PAS mouse
    Fatty rat (*fa*)
    Corpulent rat (*SHR/N–cp*)
Polygenic
  New Zealand obese mouse (*NZO*)
  Japanese KK mouse (*KK*)
  Paul Bailey black mouse (*PBB/Ld*)
  NH mouse
  Wellesley mouse

while the final pathway(s) responsible for generating the energy imbalance and the obesity may have many similarities between the various species, the precise genetic biochemical defects, located on a range of different chromosomes (Bray and York, 1979), may be varied and multiple. Interpretation of experimental data on the genetically obese models must also be viewed with qualification because, in the great majority of the studies, heterozygotes, which do not phenotypically express the obesity, are used as control animals. It is possible that the use of these controls rather than the homozygous lean strains may mask some important gene–dose changes in the obese strains.

A. ENERGY IMBALANCE

Obesity may result from either excessive energy intake not matched by a compensatory increase in energy expenditure or a reduction in energy expenditure not matched by a compensatory reduction in energy intake.

1. *Energy Intake*

All of the genetically obese rodents show some degree of hyperphagia (Bray and York, 1971, 1979), but the obesity is independent of the excess food intake since it occurs even with yoked feeding, which eliminates excess food intake. Moreover, the excess adiposity of the recessive strains precedes the appearance of hyperphagia. There are thus defects in both the control of energy intake and energy expenditure which any hypotheses for the various obesities must explain.

2. *Energy Expenditure*

As a reduction in physical activity is not important for the early development of obesity but may result as a consequence of the increasing adiposity, the major focus for research has been on adaptive thermogenesis. Low oxygen consumption and low body temperatures have been described in the first few days of life of *ob/ob* mice and *fa/fa* rats (Bray and York, 1979; Planche *et al.*, 1983; Lavau *et al.* 1985; Bazin *et al.*, 1984), before development of the ability to regulate body temperature by nonshivering thermogenesis. However, as laboratory animals are routinely housed at temperatures below thermoneutrality and as body temperatures of the obese genotypes are depressed, the capacity of these animals for nonshivering thermogenesis has been of natural interest. A normal adaptive response to cold acclimation, involving hypertrophy and hyperplasia of BAT and production of mitochondrial uncoupling protein after an increase in sympathetic stimulation of this tissue, has been described in a number of the genetically obese rodents, including the Zucker (*fa/fa*) and corpulent (*LA/N–cp*) rats and the obese (*ob/ob*) and diabetes (*db/db*) mice (Holt *et al.*, 1983; Lee *et al.*, 1987; Knehans and Romsos, 1983; Zaror-Behrens and Himms-Hagen, 1983; York *et al.*, 1985b; Armitage *et al.*, 1984).

Unfortunately, there is no unanimity in the research literature, since a majority of research groups have also demonstrated severe impairments in thermogenic response to cold, which may even lead to death in the same obese strains, particularly the *ob/ob* mouse (Saito and Bray, 1984; Himms-Hagen and Desautels, 1978; Trayhurn and James, 1978). The differences in these studies may be a reflection of the varying background genome on which the mutant obese genes are maintained or may be an effect of age. Indeed, the defective metabolic response to cold has been observed in suckling preobese *ob/ob* mice (Trayhurn, 1977). Further, the chronic impairment in sympathetic drive to brown fat may lead to the loss of response to nerve stimulation, noradrenaline, and subsequent severe cold exposure (Seydoux *et al.*, 1982a). However, it is now clear from a series of studies by Carlisle and colleagues that the lower body temperatures maintained by both the *ob/ob* mouse and the *fa/fa* rat are not the result of a lower thermoregulatory "set-point" in these animals (Carlisle and Dubuc, 1982, 1984; Kaul *et al.*, 1985).

BAT thermogenesis is also of central importance in rodent species for the regulation of energetic efficiency in response to changes in dietary composition and energy intake (see Rothwell and Stock, 1984a). Genetically obese animals are characterized by an impairment in diet-related BAT thermogenesis. This has been most clearly illustrated in the *fa/fa* rat and the *ob/ob* mouse, in which the failure to show the normal increase in oxygen consumption after feeding has been associated with the lack of response in the thermogenic function of BAT to changes in energy intake and diet composition (Holt *et al.*, 1983; Triandafillou and Himms-Hagen, 1983; Rothwell *et al.*, 1983a; Vander Tuig *et al.*, 1979; Knehans and Romsos, 1984; Trayhurn and James, 1978; Marchington *et al.*, 1983). While the obese rat appears to be insensitive to a range of nutrients, there is some evidence to suggest that the *ob/ob* mouse may show differential responses toward high-carbohydrate and high-fat diets (Himms-Hagen *et al.*, 1986; Smith and Romsos, 1985).

The brown adipose tissue of ad libitum-fed obese rodents (*fa/fa, LA/N–cp, ob/ob, db/db*) housed at normal environmental temperatures has the characteristics of a tissue of low thermogenic activity, i.e., low blood flow, increased lipid deposits, low levels of mitochondrial guanosine diphosphate (GDP) binding, and often low levels of uncoupling protein (Hogan and Himms-Hagen, 1981; Goodbody and Trayhurn, 1981; Holt *et al.*, 1983; Wickler *et al.*, 1986; Lee *et al.*, 1987; Allars *et al.*, 1987; Thurlbey and Trayhurn, 1980; Ashwell *et al.*, 1977, 1985; Ricquier *et al.*, 1986). As the BAT is responsive to exogenous noradrenaline and to activation of its sympathetic supply during cold acclimation, it has been surmised that a central defect is responsible for the failure of the obese mutants to respond normally to dietary signals (York, 1987). This could reflect a lack of afferent information, the failure to recognize afferent signals centrally, or the inability to couple signal recognition to efferent response (see Section V).

B. AFFERENT SIGNALS

1. *Sensory and Gastrointestinal Satiety Signals*

Unlike hypothalamic forms of obesity, the ability of genetically obese genotypes (*fa/fa*, A^Y/a) to respond normally to dietary dilution, to adulteration of food, and to an increase in their work rate in order to obtain food (Greenwood *et al.*, 1974) has been interpreted as showing a normal motivation to feeding.

2. *Circulating Afferent Satiety Signals*

a. Nutrient and Metabolic Signals. While it is clear that the diurnal pattern of feeding is changed in the obese *fa/fa* rat, an increased proportion of daily intake being consumed during the light period (Wangness *et al.*, 1978), there is considerable controversy over possible changes in meal patterns. This has probably resulted from the definitions of "intermeal interval" and "minimal meal size," which have been used to define a meal (Castonguay *et al.*, 1982) and to some extent from the type of meal provided. However, although meal frequency may not change in the *fa/fa* rat, its feeding is characterized by the incorporation of an occasional "super-meal" into the feeding pattern that is not observed in lean littermates (Castonguay *et al.*, 1982).

Enhanced cephalic responses to saccharin ingestion have been demonstrated recently (Ionesco *et al.*, 1988) in the *fa/fa* rat, but these do not appear to be essential since vagotomy fails to prevent the development of obesity (Opsahl and Powley, 1974). Enhanced cephalic stimulation of insulin secretion has also been reported in the *ob/ob* mouse (Flatt *et al.*, 1983). This may be attributed to enhanced activity of both the afferent parasympathetic system and the enteroinsular axis (see Section III,D,2).

Cholecystokinin (CCK) may have both peripheral and central actions in causing satiety (Baile *et al.*, 1986), the peripheral effects probably being mediated via the vagus and subsequent neural connections from the nucleus of the tractus solitarius to the PVN (Crawley and Kiss, 1985). Chronic treatments with either CCK-8 or trypsin inhibitor, which enhances endogenous release of CCK (McLaughlin *et al.*, 1983a,b) suppressed food intake and reduced the body weight of obese Zucker rats, while no effect was observed in lean rats in the latter experiment. The results indicate the potential for CCK therapy and suggest an increased responsiveness of the obese rat to endogenous CCK. In contrast, both the obese (*fa/fa*) rat and the obese (*ob/ob*) mouse exhibit a smaller acute suppression of feeding to low-threshold doses of CCK-8 than their lean controls, although the satiety effects of high doses are normal, indicative of a reduced sensitivity to exogenous hormone (McLaughlin and Baile, 1978, 1980b, 1981). This reduction in sensitivity is apparent at an early stage in the development of obesity in the Zucker rat (4–5 weeks) (McLaughlin and Baile, 1980a). The secretory responses of the exocrine pancreas to CCK stimulation are also reduced in the *fa/fa* rat (McLaughlin *et al.*, 1984; Praissman and Izzo, 1986), this impairment reflecting a reduction in receptor capacity possibly resulting from the hyperinsulinemia. Changes in brain CCK physiology have also been described in the genotypes (see Section III,C,4).

Parabiosis experiments with lean and genetically obese rodents have suggested that defects in either the production or the response to a circulating "satiety" factor might be responsible for the hyperphagia and impaired thermogenesis that lead to obesity. When obese animals (*db/db, ob/ob, fa/fa,* or A^Y/a) were parabiosed to their appropriate lean partners, the obese animals remained fat but the lean animals lost body fat and frequently died (see Bray and York, 1971, 1979; Harris *et al.*, 1987). However, when the *db/db* mouse was parabiosed to either a lean or an *ob/ob* mouse, the *db/db* mouse survived while the lean and *ob/ob* partners became hypophagic and died (Coleman, 1978). The hypotheses proposed from these data, that *db/db* mice and *fa/fa* rats produce excessive "satiety factor" but are insensitive to its actions and that *ob/ob* mice respond but do not produce the factor, require the identification of the satiety factor for their validation. Recently, Spiegelman and colleagues (Cook *et al.*, 1987; Flier *et al.*, 1987) have identified a serine protease homolog, adipsin, which may have the role of a feedback signal from adipose tissue. Adipsin is primarily produced and secreted by adipocytes but may also be secreted to a lesser extent by other tissues with highly active lipid metabolism. Adipsin mRNA synthesis and the secretion of the protein vary with nutritional state, increasing in situations when lipolysis is activated (e.g., starvation, streptozotocin-induced diabetes) and decreasing in lipogenic states (e.g., refeeding). Of particular interest are the observations that adipsin–mRNA and serum–adipsin concentrations were greatly reduced in both *ob/ob* and *db/db* mice and showed little variation with nutritional state. Adipsin–mRNA and circulating adipsin concentrations were also reduced in animals made obese by monosodium glutamate but not in cafeteria-fed rats. Thus, adipsin expression appears to be impaired in models of obesity associated with impaired sympathetic activity. The function of adipsin is at present unknown. The suggestion that its production is linked to thermogenesis (Flier *et al.*, 1987) is unlikely since thermogenesis is depressed in starvation and in the obese models when adipsin concentrations are increased and decreased, respectively. It is possible, however, that the protein is synthesized and released in response to sympathetic activation of white adipose tissue. One other possible role for adipsin is the regulation of lipoprotein lipase. As a serine protease, it might be involved in the cleavage of lipoprotein lipase from its binding to endothelial surfaces and thus terminate its action.

Basal glucose concentrations in the obese rats (*fa/fa* and *La/NCp*) are normal or slightly increased, although glucose intolerance develops progressively with age (see Bray and York, 1979). The obese mouse strains are hyperglycemic, this being most pronounced in the *db/db* and *ob/ob* mice, intermediate in KK and New Zealand obese (NZO) mice, and most moderate in the A^Y/a mouse (Bray and York, 1979). Fatty acids are increased in *fa/fa* rats but are normal in *ob/ob* mice (Martin *et al.*, 1978; Cuendot *et al.*, 1975). Ketone bodies are increased in the more severe diabetes of *ob/ob* and *db/db* mice, which depends in part on the genetic background on which the gene is expressed. Serum triacylglycerols and cholesterol are also increased, although the severity of the increase varies with the obese strain (Bray *et al.*, 1974).

b. Hormonal Signals. Insulin hypersection associated with hypertrophy and hyperplasia of islet tissue is a characteristic common to all of the genetic obesities, although the precise time of onset, its magnitude, and duration vary considerably in the different strains (see Bray and York, 1971, 1979). Although basal insulin levels appear to be normal during the preobese suckling stage of *fa/fa* rats (Rohner-Jeanrenaud *et al.*, 1983b; York *et al.*, 1981), glucose-induced secretion is greatly enhanced. In the genotypes that have been studied, the presence of adequate insulin secretion appears to be essential for hyperphagia, hyperlipogenesis, and obesity to develop, although it is not clear whether hypersecretion is an essential requirement or merely exaggerates the degree of obesity that develops (Stolz and Martin, 1982; York *et al.*, 1981). The hyperinsulinemia does, however, precede and appears to be essential for the development of the tissue insulin resistance that is common in all forms of obesity (Penicaud *et al.*, 1987; Grundleger *et al.*, 1980).

Three main possibilities have been considered to explain the hypersecretion of insulin: altered control by the autonomic nervous system or by circulating factors, or defects within the pancreas and enteroinsular axis (see Section III,C,2). The levels of serum glucagon in the genetic obesities have not been so clearly defined as in the case of insulin. Numerous conflicting reports have suggested normal, enhanced, or decreased glucagon secretion in *ob/ob*, *db/db*, and *fa/fa* mutants (see Bray and York, 1979), but all show an increase in the insulin–glucagon ratio. More recent work in the obese *fa/fa* rat, using a modified extraction procedure, has clearly demonstrated normal basal glucagon levels but an excessive secretory response to arginine stimulation, an effect which may also be modulated by the parasympathetic nervous system (Rohner-Jeanrenaud *et al.*, 1983b; Rohner-Jeanrenaud and Jeanrenaud, 1985). The relationship of this hyperglucagon secretory response to the excessive hepatic glucose production of obese rat awaits clarification, but the demonstration that a glucagon antiserum decreases serum glucose in *ob/ob* mice suggests a role for glucagon in promoting excess glucose production (Flatt *et al.*, 1984).

With the exception of the A^Y/a mouse, the linear growth of animals with genetic obesities is retarded, suggestive of a decrease in growth hormone secretion. In the genotypes in which this has been studied, a reduction in growth hormone and somatomedinlike activities has been shown (Martin and Jeanrenaud, 1985; Larson *et al.*, 1976; Sinha *et al.*, 1976; Finkelstein *et al.*, 1986), although the relatively late occurrence of this change in the *fa/fa* rat suggests it may be secondary to insulin resistance (Finkelstein *et al.*, 1986) and questions its relevance to the depression of muscle protein deposition.

Measurements of circulating thyroid hormones have not clarified the thyroid status of these animals. Some of this confusion may arise from the presence of an abnormal thyroid hormone-binding protein in the serum, in *ob/ob* mice at least, which interferes with the assay procedures (Kaplan *et al.*, 1985). However, evidence has been presented for defects in the hypothalamic control of thyroid-stimulating hormone production in both *ob/ob* mice and *fa/fa* rats, although the thyroid–pituitary axis appears to be essentially normal (York *et al.*, 1972; Ohtake *et al.*, 1977) (see also Section III,E).

The hypothalamohypophysial/adrenal axis is of central importance in controlling the development of the genetic obesities, although neither the precise mechanism nor the primary hormone responsible for this control has yet been clarified. In the mouse genotypes clear evidence of the excessive secretion of corticosterone has been reported by a number of laboratories, and the progressive rise in serum corticosterone has been related to the diminishing insulin sensitivity (see Bray and York, 1979). In the obese *fa/fa* rat there are reports of both normal serum corticosterone and normal diurnal rhythms (Shargill *et al.*, 1983; Yukimura *et al.*, 1978) and increased concentrations with loss of diurnal rhythm (Martin *et al.*, 1978; Fletcher, 1986; Gibson *et al.*, 1981). However, the increase in excretion of corticosterone despite normal plasma levels is indicative of excess secretion and turnover of glucocorticoid even in the obese rat (Cunningham *et al.*, 1986) and leads to dampened responses to CRF. Adrenocorticotropin (ACTH) levels appear to be normal (Yukimura *et al.*, 1978), as is the ratio of bound to free corticosterone (Shargill *et al.*, 1987).

Adrenal glucocorticoids are essential for the development of genetically inherited forms of obesity. Adrenalectomy prevents or suppresses the development of obesity in *ob/ob, db/db,* and *A^Y/a* mice and in the *fa/fa* rat (Yukimura and Bray, 1978; Saito and Bray, 1984; Freedman *et al.*, 1986a; Holt *et al.*, 1983). Detailed studies have shown that this response probably results from three major effects: the normalization of food intake, the restoration of normal sympathetic activity and thus BAT thermogenesis, and the suppression of insulin secretion (Saito and Bray, 1984; Ohshima *et al.*, 1984; Vander Tuig *et al.*, 1984; York *et al.*, 1985a; Fletcher, 1986). The net result of these changes is the restoration of energetic efficiency to levels seen in lean littermates (Marchington *et al.*, 1983; Vander Tuig *et al.*, 1984; Smith and Romsos, 1985). The restorative effects of adrenalectomy are wide ranging and encompass most of the abnormalities that have been associated with the development of obesity in these animal models: abnormal diurnal pattern of feeding, preference for fat macronutrient diets, insulin insensitivity, decreased basal glucose transport, low brain weight, adipocyte hyperplasia (according to one study but not another), and even fertility in male rats are all corrected after adrenalectomy (Saito and Bray, 1984; Freedman *et al.*, 1985, 1986a,b; Ohshima *et al.*, 1984). However, the excessive adipose tissue lipoprotein lipase activity remains unaltered in adrenalectomized *fa/fa* rats (Freedman *et al.*, 1986a), creating questions about the suggested relationship between this enzyme and the hyperphagia of these rats (see Section III,D,1).

Adrenalectomy may not restore body composition and serum insulin concentration precisely to normal. This may indicate the irreversibility of some of the changes. This is best illustrated by consideration of serum insulin, which falls to low levels after adrenalectomy but still remains somewhat elevated compared to the lean animals. This probably reflects the existing hyperplasia and hypertrophy of the islet tissue, since, if the adrenalectomy is performed prior to weaning, serum insulin levels of the weaned fa/fa rat remain at the lean levels (Fletcher, 1986). However, the fall in serum insulin after adrenalectomy of the obese strains implies a reduction in the activities of both the parasympathetic system and the enteroinsular axis. Thus, adrenalectomy appears to be associated with a normalization of the autonomic balance and with islet anatomy (Spear et al., 1987). At this time, it is not clear whether the responses to adrenalectomy are universal or diet dependent. Smith and Romsos (1985) were not able to demonstrate the effects of adrenalectomy when ob/ob mice were fed a high-fat diet, although the normal response was observed in fa/fa rats fed a more moderate high-fat diet (Allars et al., 1987).

The requirement for glucocorticoids for the expression of the obese genotypes is reflected in increased sensitivity and responsiveness to the effects of exogenous glucocorticoids. Studies with replacement doses of glucocorticoids given to adrenalectomized lean and obese animals have shown that food intake, serum insulin, lipogenesis and lipogenic enzyme activities, BAT function, weight gain, and fat deposition are all more responsive and more sensitive in the obese animals (Saito and Bray, 1984; Freedman et al., 1985, 1986a; Holt et al., 1983; Shimomura et al, 1987). This does not appear, in the fa/fa rat at least, to result from any changes in cytosolic or nuclear glucocorticoid receptor characteristics (Shargill et al., 1987). It is possible that the glucocorticoid dependence may represent an altered central control system. The possibility that either ACTH or CRF may regulate the glucocorticoid effects on feeding and autonomic balance in the obese animals is currently being considered. Although ACTH enhances BAT function in fa/fa rats, its action is not mediated via the sympathetic system but appears to be a direct effect on the tissue (York and Al-Baker, 1984; York et al., 1985b). Recent studies of the effects of corticosterone replacement to hypophysectomized fa/fa rats support this conclusion. The development of obesity is prevented by hypophysectomy but is completely restored by corticosterone (Holt et al., 1987a; Powley and Morton, 1976).

C. CENTRAL INTEGRATION

1. *Anatomy*

The similarity of the genetic obesities of a recessive origin to hypothalamic obesity has prompted studies of the role of the VMH and the
LH regions in these animals. Differences in brain size and brain morphology have been described in both *ob/ob* mice and *fa/fa* rats (Bereiter
and Jeanrenaud, 1980; Saito and Bray, 1984; Young and Grizard, 1985).
Studies of the effects of bilateral lesions of the VMN in *ob/ob* mice
(Chlouverakis *et al.*, 1973) and electrical stimulation of the VMN in
fa/fa rats (Holt *et al.*, 1987b) suggest that the VMN is functional.
Similarly, LH lesions of *ob/ob* mice and *fa/fa* rats produce the expected
acute aphagia, rapid weight loss, and maintenance of a lower body
weight (Chlouverakis and Bernardis, 1972; Milam *et al.*, 1980, 1982a,b).
However, the effects of these LH lesions on *fa/fa* rats cannot be attributed solely to the reduction in food intake and are associated with a
preferential loss of body fat, a relative gain in body protein, and a large
reduction in fat cell number (Milam *et al.*, 1982a,b). LH lesions of *fa/fa*
rats restore BAT function and presumably bring sympathetic activity
to normal (S. J. Holt and D. A. York, unpublished observations). The
data are consistent with a possible role for abnormal LH activity in
these animals.

2. *Insulin*

Insulin, the principal anabolic hormone, has a recognized peripheral
role in stimulating lipid deposition. More recently, evidence is ac-
cumulating to show a central role for insulin in the regulation of food
intake, sympathetic activity, and body weight. Insulin, injected intra-
cerebroventricularly into baboons and rats, reduces food intake and
body weight in a dose-dependent manner (Brief and Davis, 1984; Porte
and Woods, 1981). Similarly, insulin injection into the VMH has recently been shown to reduce the firing rate of sympathetic nerves
innervating BAT (Sakaguchi and Bray, 1987a). When insulin is injected into the LH, the firing rate of sympathetic nerves innervating
BAT is increased (Sakaguchi and Bray, 1988). All of the genetically
obese genotypes are characterized by hyperinsulinemia (Bray and
York, 1979). Since cerebrospinal fluid insulin concentration is thought
to reflect circulating insulin levels, the central actions of insulin in
these obese rodents are of particular interest. The majority of experimental evidence in this area has been obtained from studies of the
Zucker obese (*fa/fa*) rat. In these rats the cerebrospinal fluid insulin

concentrations are elevated, but the increase is less than expected from the peripheral hyperinsulinemia (Stein et al., 1983, 1985).

Despite serum and cerebrospinal fluid hyperinsulinemia, the insulin concentrations in various brain regions, including the hypothalamus, hippocampus, cortex, and olfactory bulb, are reduced in the obese rat (Figlewicz et al., 1985). Receptor-binding studies have produced some conflicting data (Figlewicz et al., 1985; Melynk, 1987), but evidence for a reduction in the number of receptors in both the hypothalamus and the olfactory bulb has been reported, whereas the receptor population in the cortex is normal (Figlewicz et al., 1985; Melynk, 1987). However, this attenuation of receptor population does not appear to represent down-regulation of receptors and cannot explain the reduction in brain insulin concentration. It is also observed in the Wistar fatty rat (Figlewicz et al., 1986). It may represent a physiological change associated with the expression of the fa gene which is responsible for the abnormality in the transport of insulin into the central nervous system. These alterations in the brain insulin system may be implicated in the changes in food intake and energy balance in the fa/fa rat. Acute and chronic intracerebroventricular injections of insulin produce little or no effect on the food intake and body weight of obese fa/fa rats, in contrast to the marked hypophagia and cessation of weight gain induced in lean rats (Ikeda et al., 1980, 1986b). The low brain content of insulin may explain the impaired response of obese rats to CCK, since insulin enhances the satiety response to CCK (Figlewicz et al., 1986). However, the defective central insulin action may be restricted to the food intake regulatory pathways, since S. J. Holt and D. A. York (unpublished observations) have recently observed a normal suppression of sympathetic firing rate after intracerebroventricular insulin injections into the fa/fa rat.

It is also possible that the described defects in the brain insulin system are a secondary reflection of the developing obesity and insulin insensitivity that are characteristic of peripheral tissues at this stage. The reduction in the hypothalamic insulin receptor population has been observed in 6-week-old fa/fa rats (Melynk, 1987), but at this age considerable insulin insensitivity is already evident in some peripheral tissues (Penicaud et al., 1987). However, since the defect in brain insulin uptake is not present in the ob/ob mouse, another genetic obesity (Havrankova et al., 1979; Agardh et al., 1986), it is unlikely to be secondary to the hyperinsulinemia. However, it should be noted that even in the ob/ob mouse brain insulin content does not respond to starvation in the manner observed in the lean genotype (Agardh et al., 1986).

3. *Glucoprivic Feeding*

The interrelationship of these changes in brain insulin status with central glucose metabolism is of clear relevance to our understanding of the control of energy balance in the genetic obesities. The presence of glucose- and insulin-responsive areas of the brain which are known to regulate feeding and autonomic function is recognized (Oomura, 1983) and has been described in more detail in Section II, A, 2, d. There are a number of reports which suggest that central nervous system responses to changes in glucose homeostasis might be abnormal in some obese genotypes.

The feeding response to intracerebroventricular 2-DG (Ikeda *et al.*, 1980), the reduction in metabolic rate (Rothwell and Stock, 1981a), and the inhibition of BAT function after peripheral 2-DG administration (Allars and York, 1986) are all absent in the obese *fa/fa* rat. This inhibition of BAT function by 2-DG observed in lean rats is thought to represent a central response to glucoprivation, since it is mimicked by both intracerebroventricular injection (Arase *et al.*, 1987) and carotid, but not hepatic portal, infusions of 2-DG (J. Allars and D. A. York, unpublished observations) and is specific to diet-induced changes in BAT function. These data, together with the normal satiating effect of intragastric glucose (Maggio *et al.*, 1983) and the normal response to the anorectic AD124 (Ikeda *et al.*, 1986a), which acts on glucostatic feeding mechanisms, might suggest that the hyperphagia of *fa/fa* rats is a response to existing central glucoprivation.

The loss of response to the glucoprivic actions of 2-DG in the *fa/fa* rat is dependent on glucocorticoids. Both the BAT and feeding responses are restored after adrenalectomy (Allars and York, 1986; Table V) and the feeding, hyperglycemic, and BAT inhibition responses to intracerebroventricular 2-DG are inhibited by corticosterone. Since the various peripheral responses to central 2-DG are thought to reflect the effects of glucoprivation at multiple central sites, the consistent suppression of these effects by corticosterone suggest that glucocorticoids must also act at multiple central loci, possibly through a common mechanism.

4. *Peptides*

A wide range of effects of glucocorticoids on the central nervous system have been described (Meyer, 1985). While the evidence to date implicates an interaction between glucocorticoids and glucose-initiated responses, it is not clear whether this a direct interaction. Among the possible alternatives is the development of a glucocorticoid-depen-

TABLE V
EFFECT OF ADRENALECTOMY ON THE RESPONSE OF LEAN AND OBESE (fa/fa)
RATS TO THE STIMULATION OF FEEDING BY 2-DG[a]

| | Food intake (g/3 h) | | | |
| | Intact | | Adrenalectomy | |
Rat	Saline	2-DG	Saline	2-DG
Lean ($Fa/?$)	1.2 ± 0.1	2.5 ± 0.2[b]	1.4 ± 0.2	2.5 ± 0.3[c]
Obese (fa/fa)	2.9 ± 0.1	2.9 ± 0.4	1.5 ± 0.3	2.6 ± 0.2[c]

[a] Values represent means ± SE for five rats in each group. Food intake was measured over the 3-hour period following intraperitoneal injection of 2-DG (360 mg/kg body weight) of ad libitum-fed rats. Adrenalectomies were performed 7 days prior to the experiment. Data are from J. Allars and D. A. York (unpublished observations).
[b] $p < 0.01$; significant effect of 2-DG.
[c] $p < 0.05$.

dent central insulin insensitivity, as is observed in the skeletal muscle of the obese ob/ob mouse (Ohshima et al., 1984). Glucocorticoids reduce insulin receptor populations of rat glial cells maintained in culture (Montiel et al., 1987). Alternatively, the corticosterone effects may be mediated through the induced reciprocal changes in either CRF or ACTH production and release. The wide distribution of CRF in the central nervous system and its broad range of biological effects are consistent with its mediation of centrally sensitive glucocorticoid responses (Brown and Fisher, 1985; Tache and Gunion, 1985; Levine et al., 1983). Further support for the suggestion is provided by our recent observations that intracerebroventricular CRF actually stimulates BAT function despite inhibiting feeding (Arase et al, 1988a). The ability of CRF to inhibit feeding and parasympathetic activity and to stimulate sympathetic activity is consistent with the hypothesis that the suppression of CRF synthesis, secretion, or actions may be of fundamental importance to the development of the genetic obesities. Recent observations on hypophysectomized fa/fa rats replaced with corticosterone would also implicate CRF rather than ACTH as the mediator of the corticosterone effect (Holt et al., 1987a).

The concentration of CCK in the brain is reduced in fasted animals (McLaughlin et al., 1985, 1986) but CCK receptor numbers are increased (Saito et al, 1981; Finkelstein et al., 1983). Strauss and Yallow (1979) initially reported that brain CCK content was reduced in ob/ob mice, but more recent studies, using extraction procedures which would yield predominantly CCK-8 (rather than CCK-33), were unable to demonstrate any differences in various brain regions of *ob/ob* or A^Y/a mice or *fa/fa* rats compared to their lean controls over a wide span of ages (see Table VI) (Oku *et al.*, 1984c; Schneider *et al.* 1979; Finkelstein and Steggles, 1981). However, using more localized regions, McLaughlin *et al.* (1985) identified increased CCK concentrations in the ventromedial, anterior, and dorsal hypothalami of obese rats, which would be consistent with the increase in potassium-stimulated CCK release from the superfused hypothalamus, but not the frontal cortex, of this genotype (Micevych *et al.*, 1985). However, the opiate control of CCK release was normal in *fa/fa* rats.

Alterations in CCK physiology in obesity are also exhibited as changes in receptor binding. CCK binding in the hypothalamus is normal in *ob/ob* mice and *fa/fa* rats; it is increased in the cortex of both genotypes and in the hippocampus and the midbrain of *fa/fa* rats (Finkelstein *et al.*, 1984; Hays *et al.*, 1981). In contrast, CCK binding to pancreatic acini is decreased (McLaughlin *et al.*, 1984). It is not yet clear whether the changes described in CCK physiology in the *fa/fa* rat and *ob/ob* mouse contribute to the development of obesity or are a consequence of the obese state which is already actively progressing at 4–5 weeks of age, the youngest age of any reported study. The differential effects of peripherally injected CCK on regional brain CCK

TABLE VI

NEUROPEPTIDE CONCENTRATIONS IN RODENT OBESITY[a]

Neuropeptide	Tissue	*ob/ob*	*fa/fa*	VMH
β-Endorphin	Pituitary	↑	↑	—
	Hypothalamus	—	↓	
	Plasma	↑	↑↓	↑
Dynorphin	Hypothalamus	—		
Leu-Enkephalin	Brain	—	—	
	Pituitary	↑		
Cholecystokinin	Brain	↓	—	—
			↑↓	
Somatostatin	Hypothalamus			
	Pituitary		↑	
Bombesin	Brain	—	—	—
Neurotensin	Brain	—	—	—
Insulin	Brain	—	↓	
	Hypothalamus		↓	
β-Cell tropin	Pituitary	↑		

[a] ↑, increased; ↓, decreased; —, no change compared to lean controls (see text for appropriate references).

concentrations in lean and obese rats clearly illustrate the altered functional relationships of the peripheral CCK afferent pathways (McLaughlin *et al.*, 1986). It is possible to speculate that the reduced sensitivity to exogenous CCK and the changes in local CCK concentration and CCK receptor numbers in the brain reflect an increase in afferent vagal information, and consequent down-regulation.

Margules *et al.* (1978) initially suggested that excessive production and secretion of β-endorphin induced hyperphagia after reporting increased pituitary and serum β-endorphin concentrations in *ob/ob* mice and *fa/fa* rats and showing that naloxone selectively prevented their hyperphagia. However, subsequent research has failed to correlate changes in serum β-endorphin with the changes in feeding behavior observed in the obese rodents (York, 1987). Conflicting reports have described increased, normal, or decreased pituitary and hypothalamic β-endorphin concentrations in *ob/ob* mice and *fa/fa* rats, the conflict possibly a result of the differing ages and sexes of the animals used in these studies (Govani and Yang, 1981; McLaughlin and Baile, 1985; Recant *et al.*, 1980, 1983; Rossier *et al.*, 1979; York, 1987). Both hypophysectomy and adrenalectomy abolish the hyperphagia of obese *fa/fa* rats yet have opposite effects on serum β-endorphin concentrations which decrease and increase, respectively. Glucocorticoid replacement to adrenalectomized *fa/fa* rats, which would be expected to suppress serum β-endorphin, restored the hyperphagia (Freedman *et al.*, 1986a). Finally, lesions of the ventral tegmental area increased hypothalamic β-endorphin concentrations in lean and obese rats without affecting food intake (Deutch and Martin, 1983).

Despite this inability to show a causal relationship between food intake and β-endorphin tissue concentrations and secretion in the genetic obesities, an increase in sensitivity to μ- and κ-opiate receptor antagonists has been reported consistently and may be of particular significance, since it has been demonstrated at an early stage of the development of obesity in the obese *fa/fa* rat (McLaughlin and Baile, 1984b). In acute experiments, both obese *fa/fa* rats and obese *ob/ob* mice were more responsive to the inhibitory actions of κ-opiate receptor antagonists on food intake (Ferguson-Segall *et al.*, 1982; McLaughlin and Baile, 1984a), the reduction reflecting a decrease in meal size without any effect on meal frequency. Chronic treatment of *ob/ob* mice with naloxone suppressed food intake, insulin secretion, and weight gain (Recant *et al.*, 1980), whereas in schedule-fed mice naloxone treatment actually increased food intake (Shimomura *et al.*, 1982). Decreased food intake of obese Zucker rats treated with Nalmefene has been reported (McLaughlin and Baile, 1983), but the response was even greater in *obese/SHR* rats in which a massive weight loss resulted from chronic naltrexone treatment (Wexler and McMurtry, 1985).

While a central site of action of opioid antagonists has been proposed, neither the precise locus of their effects on feeding behavior nor the reason for the increased sensitivity in the obese animals is clear (Baile *et al.*, 1986). Hyperinsulinemia may, however, be an important prerequisite for the sensitivity to these antagonists. As naltrexone selectivity inhibited insulin secretion from isolated pancreatic islets of *ob/ob* mice (Recant *et al.*, 1980), it is possible that the efficacy of opioid antagonists in preventing weight gain and hyperphagia in the obese rodents may partially be mediated through the suppression of insulin release.

There are few data on other opioid peptides. Increased concentrations of Leu^5-enkephalin in the neurophypophysis of *ob/ob* mice have been reported from an early age (Rossier *et al.*, 1979), while elevated levels of Met-enkephalin have been described in the pituitary, but not other tissues, of the diabetes (*db/db*) mouse (Greenberg *et al.*, 1985). Likewise, dynorphin concentrations in the neurophypophysis of *ob/ob* mice were increased, although concentrations in the hypothalamus and other brain regions were unaltered (Ferguson-Segall *et al.*, 1982; Morley *et al.*, 1983). Obese mice (*ob/ob*) are also more responsive to the insulin secretory effects of enkephalin analogs (Bailey and Flatt, 1987).

It has thus been impossible to establish any clear relationship between feeding behavior and tissue opioid peptide concentrations in the obese genotypes that have been studied. However, it should be emphasized that the interpretation of data on tissue concentrations in these genotypes is complicated by the lower tissue weight of the pituitary, hypothalamus, and other brain regions, and the data obtained with antagonists and agonists may give a more reliable indication of the involvement of opioid peptides in the development of obesity. It is possible that increased responsiveness to opioid peptides might contribute to the hyperphagia, hyperinsulinemia (directly and through stimulation of growth hormone release), and sterility (through suppression of luteinizing hormone and follicle-stimulating hormone) that are characteristic of a number of these obesities.

Other neuropeptides associated with proopiomelanocortin might be implicated in other genetic obesities. The various forms of yellow obese mouse are characterized by a close association between the obesity and the degree of coat color (Bray and York, 1971, 1979). Normal coat color can be restored by injections of α-melanocyte-stimulating hormone (MSH) (Geshwind *et al.*, 1972), the acetylated form being far more effective than desacetylated MSH (H. Shimizu and G. A. Bray unpublished observations). The apparent lack of MSH stimulation (i.e., yellow color) may result from the reduced pituitary levels of α-MSH relative to desacetyl-MSH. In the normal pituitary α-MSH accounts for 85% of total MSH. In A^Y/a (yellow) mice the proportion is reduced to nearly 50%. Pituitary secretion by the yellow mouse would thus release more desacetyl-MSH than normal. Desacetyl-MSH stimulates weight gain but little pigmentation, whereas α-MSH enhances pigmentation but does not increase the body weight of yellow obese mice (Fig. 3). Thus, one explanation for the biochemical defect in the yellow mouse may be the reduced acetylation of MSH (Bray *et al.,* 1989). The secreted desacetyl-MSH would stimulate food intake and obesity rather than darken the coat color (Shimizu *et al.,* 1989). As in other obesities, adrenalectomy prevents the excessive weight gain of A^Y/a obese mice (H. Shimizu and G. A. Bray, unpublished observations). This suggests that desacetyl-MSH may stimulate the adrenal and this has been documented in yellow mice treated with desacetyl-MSH (Shimizu *et al.,* 1989).

β-Cell tropin has been identified as the active insulin secretagogue

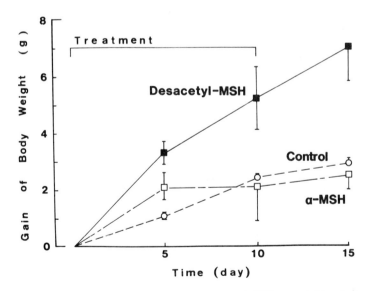

FIG. 3. Effects of desacetyl-MSH and acetyl-MSH (α-MSH) on weight gain in yellow mice. Animals were treated for 10 days with 150 μg of desacetyl-MSH or α-MSH per day, and body weights were determined at 5, 10, and 15 days. The animals treated with deacetyl-MSH gained significantly more weight than either of the other two groups (unpublished observations from this laboratory.)

derived from corticotropinlike intermediate lobe peptide (CLIP) by tryptic cleavage (Beloff-Chain *et al.*, 1983). The presence of high concentrations of CLIP in the pituitary of obese (*ob/ob*) mice (Dunmore and Beloff-Chain, 1982) and the demonstration of β-cell tropin in the plasma of *ob/ob* mice (Billingham *et al.*, 1982) have raised questions both of the role of this peptide in the development of hyperinsulinemia and of the cause of the excessive production of the peptide. Neither question can be answered at the moment. The absence of hypersecretion of β-cell tropin in another form of obesity, the sand rat, implies that changes in β-cell tropin secretion may be specific to *ob/ob* mice. The observation that β-cell tropin and CLIP secretion increase after adrenalectomy of *ob/ob* mice, a maneuver that reduces insulin secretion, raises questions about any possible role for these peptides in the genesis of hyperinsulinemia (Dunmore *et al.*, 1988). Likewise, the importance of the greatly enhanced insulin secretory response to ACTH in *ob/ob* mice (Bailey and Flatt, 1987) is unclear.

A number of laboratories have assayed concentrations of other brain neuropeptides, but the interpretation of such data is difficult since both the size and regional anatomy of the brain and brain regions may be altered in the obese genotypes (Bereiter and Jeanrenaud, 1979, 1980). Bombesin and neurotensin concentrations and regional distribution appear to be unaltered in the *ob/ob* mouse and the *fa/fa* rat, although a reduction in receptor numbers was described in two regions known to influence thermoregulatory behavior in the *ob/ob* mouse (Rostene *et al.*, 1985; Sheppard *et al.*, 1985; Oku *et al.*, 1984c). Changes in the concentrations of bombesin and neurotensin after adrenalectomy could not be related to the reduction in food intake. A reduction in nerve growth factor has been described in the submandibular glands of *ob/ob* mice in one study (Yamashita *et al.*, 1986) but not in another (Bray *et al.*, 1982b). Epidermal growth factor was likewise not reduced (Bray *et al.*, 1982b).

The considerable literature on the concentrations of the various neurotransmitters associated with the control of feeding and energy balance in the genetic obesities provides little insight into any functional abnormalities. In the *ob/ob* mouse, the general consensus is of little change in central noradrenergic systems (see York, 1987). The changes in norepinephrine concentration in the PVN and median eminence of *fa/fa* rats, together with evidence for increased norepinephrine biosynthesis, while consistent with increased activity of the PVN noradrenergic system inducing hyperphagia (Cruce *et al.*, 1976; Levin and Sullivan, 1979a,b), are not consistent with their preference for dietary fat, while the localized nature and the age dependence of the changes suggest they are secondary to the obesity (Orosco *et al.*, 1986). Obese (*fa/fa*) rats show a normal feeding response to intracerebroventricular norepinephrine (Ikeda *et al.*, 1980). No changes have been observed in brain dopamine concentrations in *ob/ob* mice or *fa/fa* rats but the demonstration of a 2-fold increase in hypothalamic dopamine-D_3 receptors has suggested a possible role for the dopaminergic pathway in the thermoregulatory defect of *db/db* mice (El-Refai and Chan, 1986).

The increase in brain 5-HT in *ob/ob* mice might reflect the elevated serum tryptophan (Garthwaite *et al.*, 1980), but without further evidence on turnover and functional response it is impossible to assess the significance of this observation. GABA synthesis is increased in the hypothalamus of *fa/fa* rats, while raising brain GABA concentrations will block the hyperphagia of both *fa/fa* rats and *ob/ob* mice (Coscina and Nobrega, 1984; Tews, 1981). Since GABA may stimulate or inhibit feeding behavior in normal rats (Garratini, 1986), a more detailed study of regional GABA response is required to obtain insight into the role of GABA-responsive neurons in the hyperphagia.

The normal discriminative behavior of *fa/fa* rats to amphetamine and fenfluramine would support the normality of noradrenergic and serotoninergic pathways (Schechter and Finkelstein, 1985), although attenuated responses to a 5-HT receptor antagonist and to the anorectic effect of amphetamine have been described (Schechter, 1986; Bray and York, 1972). An increase in specific amphetamine receptors in the hypothalamus of *ob/ob* mice might be a response to their hyperglycemia (Hauger *et al.*, 1986a), but the function of these receptors and their possible relationship to the dopamine-D_3 receptors described above require clarification. Thus, at this time there is little evidence to suggest that the hyperphagia characteristic of the genetic obesities can be related to any functional abnormality of the monaminergic pathways.

D. Efferent Systems

1. *Food Intake*

Both a protein basis and a lipid basis for the hyperphagia of *fa/fa* rats have been proposed. Radcliffe and Webster (1976, 1978, 1979) suggested that a reduction in the efficiency of utilizing dietary protein, also observed by Deb *et al.* (1976), necessitates a higher protein intake to sustain normal rates of protein deposition. However, a primary need for increased protein intake seems unlikely. When the *fa/fa* rat is given a choice of macronutrients, the obese rat has an enhanced preference for fat over protein (Castonguay *et al.*, 1982). Moreover, they reduce protein intake when given a choice of macronutrients (Castonguay *et al.*, 1984), they eat less of a high- rather than a low-protein diet (Anderson *et al.*, 1979), and hyperphagia is still evident in obese rats fed very high protein diets (Jenkins and Hershberger, 1978).

In contrast to the protein-drive hypothesis, Greenwood and colleagues have suggested that it is a primary drive to fat deposition, reflected in the early and sustained increase in adipose tissue lipoprotein lipase activity, which leads to the hyperphagia and/or impairment of protein deposition in the obese Zucker rat (Greenwood *et al.*, 1981; Greenwood, 1985). The increases in adipose tissue lipoprotein lipase and body fat, evident initially before weaning (Lavau *et al.*, 1985), are not secondary to either the hyperphagia or the reduction in physical activity and are resistant to pharmacological intervention (Bray *et al.*, 1973; Greenwood *et al.*, 1981). Similarly, the obese body composition of *ob/ob* mice is also retained in the face of the combined effects of exercise and food restriction (Dubuc *et al.*, 1984). The excess fat deposition achieved at the expense of protein deposition when hyperphagia is prevented (Bray *et al.*, 1973; Greenwood, 1985), the preference for the fat rather than protein or carbohydrate components of the diet (Maggio *et al.*, 1984), and the reduction in the satiety effect of intragastric lipid, but not carbohydrate or protein (Maggio *et al.*, 1983), are all consistent with a defect in control of the lipid component of nutrient balance. However, when related to the increasing adipocyte cell size, no genotype effect on lipoprotein lipase could be demonstrated (Chan and Stern, 1982) raising questions about the role of this enzyme as a primary signal. Further, the similar preference for dietary fat in *ob/ob* mice is not apparent in young animals, and the development of this preference has been related to the developing insulin resistance (Romsos and Ferguson, 1982).

2. Autonomic Nervous System

a. Parasympathetic (Vagal) Nervous System. Unlike the hypothalamic obese rat, vagotomy does not prevent the development of obesity in the Zucker *fa/fa* rat (Opsahl and Powley, 1974). Although gastric acid secretion is also normal in the Zucker rat, implying normal vagal activity, it is clear that increased vagal stimulation of the pancreas does play a role in the hypersecretion of both insulin and glucagon. In the adult *fa/fa* rat subdiaphragmatic vagotomy partially prevents the insulin hypersecretory response to glucose, while the secretory response to electrical stimulation of the vagus was enhanced (Rohner-

Jeanrenaud *et al.*, 1983b). *In vitro* studies with perfused pancreas also showed an atropine-sensitive excess insulin secretion from *fa/fa* rats. Similarly, in the preobese suckling *fa/fa* rat the excessive arginine-induced secretion of insulin and glucagon was partially prevented by atropine. From these data, Jeanrenaud and colleagues have suggested that the hyperinsulinemia of obese rats may result from the combined effects of an enhanced sensitivity to vagal stimulation and an increased parasympathetic tone to the pancreatic acini (Rohner-Jeanrenaud *et al.*, 1983b). The inability to completely restore normal insulin and glucagon secretory capacity may reflect a coincident reduction in sympathetic stimulation of the pancreas (Levin *et al.*, 1982). Whether there is any direct interrelationship between the increased vagal and reduced sympathetic activities in the obese rat is, at this stage, unclear. However, it is of interest to note that the impaired response of Zucker *fa/fa* rats to feeding (increase in oxygen consumption), thought to reflect the lack of sympathetic activation, was abolished by atropine pretreatment (Rothwell and Stock, 1981a). Further, it would appear that the abnormal autonomic control of pancreatic function may be present in the prenatal stage of development (Turkenkopf *et al.*, 1983), suggesting a close relationship between the *fa* gene and the control of autonomic imbalance.

The effects of atropine and pilocarpine on insulin secretion from islets of *ob/ob* mice suggest that an increased parasympathetic drive and response may also underlie the excess insulin secretory response of these mice. The hyperinsulinemia is associated with hypertrophy and hyperplasia of islet tissue, but the maintenance of high levels of insulin secretion is dependent upon the genetic background of the strain (Baetins *et al.*, 1978). The altered tissue morphology makes the interpretation of the many *in vitro* and *in vivo* studies on insulin secretion and tissue hormone concentrations difficult, but there is now considerable evidence to suggest that enhanced activity of the enteroinsular axis may help to maintain and potentiate the hyperinsulinemia (Flatt *et al.*, 1983, 1984). Whereas insulin secretion to parenteral glucose is impaired in *ob/ob* mice, basal insulin secretion and the secretion to oral glucose are greatly exaggerated (Flatt and Bailey, 1981). The concentrations of a wide range of neuropeptides, including gastrin, gastric inhibitory peptide, secretin, CCK, neurotensin, and glucagonlike immunoreactive peptide, are elevated in the intestines and the plasma of *ob/ob* mice (Bailey *et al.*, 1986; Flatt *et al.*, 1984; C. J. Bailey, personal communication) and both the secretory response of gastric inhibitory peptide to feeding and the insulin secretory response to gastric inhibitory peptide are elevated (Flatt *et al.* 1983, 1984). In the obese *fa/fa* rat, Chan *et al.*, (1984b) have related the increase in basal insulin secretion to an exaggerated effect of gastric inhibitory peptide on insulin secretion at low glucose levels, and the excessive secretion of insulin in response to low glucose levels has been suggested as a major stimulus of feeding (Curry and Stern, 1985). Developmental studies are required to elucidate the importance of these changes to the initial onset of hyperinsulinemia, but such changes are consistent with an exaggerated cephalic control of insulin secretion that has been observed in the *fa/fa* rat (Ionescu *et al.*, 1988).

The hyperinsulinemia of the NZO mouse, which can be prevented by transplantation of islet tissue from lean mice, has been attributed to a lack of pancreatic polypeptide secretion from NZO islet tissue (Gates *et al.*, 1974; Gates and Lazarus, 1977). Restoration of normal insulin and glycemia by pancreatic polypeptide treatment is also associated with a return to normal rates of weight gain. In contrast to these syndromes, parasympathetic stimulation of the pancreas of spiny mice initiates only a weak insulin secretory response that appears to be mediated via the endocrine–exocrine intermediate cells rather than as a direct effect on the β-cell (E. Ionescu and B. Jeanrenaud, personal communication). Other potential circulating factors, e.g., β-cell tropin, with a potential role in mediating hyperinsulinemia are discussed in Section III,C,4.

b. *Sympathetic Nervous System.* The state of sympathetic tone may be assessed by several methods (see Section II,C,2,b). The obese mutants show a very depressed level of sympathetic activity in BAT and other peripheral organs and a normal or near-normal increase in sympathetic activity after cold exposure but the absence of sympathetic response to diet (Young and Landsberg, 1983; Zaror-Behrens and Himms-Hagen, 1983; Triandafillou and Himms-Hagen, 1983; Levin *et al.*, 1981, 1982, 1983a; Marchington *et al.*, 1983; Knehans and Romsos, 1982, 1983, 1984; Ashwell and Dunnett, 1985). Using direct recording of the electrical activity of sympathetic nerves innervating the interscapular BAT pad, we have recently confirmed the low level of sympathetic drive to the tissue in young (6-week-old) Zucker (*fa/fa*) rats and the normal response of increased firing rate when body temperature is allowed to fall (Table VII).

In addition, by using electrical stimulation of various hypothalamic centers, it has been shown that the connections between these centers and BAT and other sympathetically innervated tissues are intact in the obese Zucker rat (Levin *et al.*, 1984a; Holt *et al.*, 1987b). These data confirm that the lack of diet-related sympathetic drive to BAT in this obese mutant results from the failure to activate the appropriate path-

TABLE VII

FIRING RATE OF SYMPATHETIC NERVES INNERVATING
INTERSCAPULAR BROWN ADIPOSE TISSUE OF LEAN AND OBESE
ZUCKER RATS AT DIFFERENT BODY TEMPERATURES[a]

| | Firing rate (impulses/sec) | |
Body temperature (°C)	Lean	fa/fa
37.50 ± 0.10	2.02 ± 0.21	0.92 ± 0.14
36.90 ± 0.05	4.06 ± 0.14	1.69 ± 0.17

[a] Values represent means ± SEM for four animals in each group.

This table was adapted from Holt and York, 1989.

way(s) centrally and not from a defect in the efferent connections. As the defect in BAT function has been demonstrated at 2 days of age (Bazin *et al.,* 1984), it is likely that the regulatory defect is fundamental to the development of the obesity in this species. A similar conclusion has been reached after studies of suckling *ob/ob* mice (Goodbody and Trayhurn, 1982). It is also apparent that the attenuation of sympathetic activity may not be universal but may be restricted to a number of specific tissues, e.g., pancreas, in addition to BAT, but again there is considerable conflict of evidence in this area (Levin *et al.,* 1983a; Marchington *et al.,* 1983; Knehans and Romsos, 1982, 1983). Administration of sympathomimetics impairs the development of obesity in a number of species (Bailey *et al.,* 1986; Dulloo and Miller, 1987) and improves insulin sensitivity (Challis *et al.,* 1985). As this latter effect was not related to the antiobesity effect, it is possible that the impaired sympathetic system may directly contribute to the development of insulin insensitivity.

E. CONTROLLED SYSTEM

Functional changes have been described in a number of peripheral tissues. Insulin hypersecretion is evident in the first few postnatal days or even prenatally in the recessively inherited forms of obesity. This hypersecretion of insulin appears to reflect the alteration in autonomic balance between parasympathetic and sympathetic nervous systems and also an overactivity of the enteroinsular axis, which may involve a number of neuropeptides. In the other forms of genetically inherited obesity, the hypersecretion of insulin does not appear at such an early age. In one model, the NZO mouse, hypersecretion of insulin may result from the lack of pancreatic polypeptide secretion. In some, but not all, species the abnormal regulation of pancreatic function is also reflected in changes in glucagon secretion.

Hyperinsulinemia is followed by the progressive development of insulin resistance, which is not uniform among the various target tissues or the individual metabolic pathways. For instance, the early development of insulin resistance in the muscle of obese (fa/fa) rats at a time of normal insulin sensitivity of white adipose tissue (Penicaud et al., 1987) has an important role in the preferential channeling of glucose carbon into adipose tissue stores. Such a situation would be exacerbated by the large increase in hepatic glucose production in these animals, probably resulting from a combination of hyperglucagonemia and insulin resistance (Terrettaz et al., 1986; Rohner-Jeanrenaud et al., 1986).

The distribution of the body fat between the various depots differ among the various genetic obesities. The increased adiposity is accommodated by hypertrophy of adipocytes in all species and by additional hyperplasia in the recessive obesities. However, this distinction may be obscured when the animals are fed a highly palatable diet and when hyperplasia is also evident, for instance, the polygenically inherited NZO obesity (Herberg et al., 1974). Many alterations in the control of lipolysis and lipogenesis have been described in the adipose tissue of these genetic obesities. However, these appear to reflect the changes in neural and endocrine environments since, upon transplantation, adipocytes from an obese animal assume the characteristics of the host lean animal and vice versa (Ashwell et al., 1977). A similar conclusion may be drawn from the many studies showing a reduction in BAT function, i.e., the impaired thermogenic function reflects in particular the reduced sympathetic drive to the tissue in the various obese genotypes. This conclusion is again supported by recent reports of transplantation studies with brown adipocytes (Ashwell et al., 1986) and by studies of blood flow in brown adipocytes of obese Zucker rats (West et al., 1987).

The low levels of thyroid hormones reported in some studies in ob/ob and db/db mice and fa/fa rats, together with low activities of thyroid-sensitive tissue enzymes, point to an effective tissue hypothyroidism (York et al., 1978a,b, 1985b; Kaplan et al., 1985; Bray and York, 1979). This may arise not only from lack of thyroid hormone uptake, but also from the lack of T_4 deiodination to T_3 at the tissue level (Kaplan and Young, 1987; Young et al., 1984). The low levels of tissue 5'-deiodinase activity and the low serum T_3 levels may be greatly enhanced or normalized when sympathetic activity is improved (Kaplan and Young, 1987; York et al., 1985b; Kates and Himms-Hagen, 1985). Nevertheless, it is clearly difficult to generalize on the thyroid status in these animals since the changes appear to be tissue specific. The changes in deiodination of T_4 may be related to the reduced sympathetic drive to the tissue or may reflect changes either in T_4 tissue uptake, e.g., brain (Kaplan and Young, 1987), or in the adrenergic receptor population, e.g., the reduced α_1 receptor population of BAT of obese *fa/fa* rats (Raasmaja and York, 1987) where type II 5'-deiodinase is regulated through the α_1-adrenergic system (Silva and Larsen, 1986).

In light of the described changes in tissue thyroid hormone metabolism, it is not surprising that exogenous thyroid hormones will not prevent the obesity and will only improve some of the defective thyroid-sensitive systems (for examples, see Hogan and Himms-Hagen, 1981; York *et al.*, 1978a,b; Ohtake *et al.*, 1977; van der Kroon *et al.*, 1981, 1982). Nevertheless, as in the *ob/ob* mouse, the functional hypothyroidism appears to be expressed in the first few days of life (Khan *et al.*, 1986; van der Kroon *et al.*, 1982) and is clearly important in the phenotypic expression of the defective *ob* gene. Indeed, van der Kroon *et al.* (1981) have shown that when thyroxine treatment was combined with the prevention of hyperphagia, body temperature, serum insulin, and body weight gain were all normalized. Hypothyroidism and hyperphagia, both of which are prevented by adrenalectomy (Saito and Bray, 1984; Shimomura *et al.*, 1981), are thus two factors closely associated with the *ob* gene.

IV. Dietary Obesity

A. Characterization of the Diet-Induced Obesities

Several animal models have been used to study dietary obesity (Table VIII). Obesity has been produced in experimental animals by feeding high-fat diets, by providing sucrose solutions to drink, by adding sucrose to moderate- or high-fat diets, or by providing a varied and palatable "cafeteria" diet. There are, in addition, two other types of experimental obesity which can be classified as to nutritional origin, tube or meal feeding, and perinatal overnutrition. This section will focus primarily on the types of obesity that result from altering the nutrient components of the diet.

1. High-Fat Diets

When animals eat a standard, low-fat, laboratory chow diet (10% kcal fat), they grow and accumulate fat at a steady rate. However, when given a diet in which fat comprises 30% or more of the calories,

TABLE VIII

CLASSIFICATION OF DIETARY OBESITIES

Obesity induced by diet composition or pal-
    atability factors
  High-fat diets
  Sucrose drinking solutions
  High-sucrose diets
  Combined high-fat, high-sucrose diets
  Cafeteria or supermarket diets
Obesity induced by a few large meals
  Meal feeding
  Tube feeding

most animals initially increase their energy intake, are more efficient
in energy utilization (Rattigan *et al.*, 1986; Robeson *et al.*, 1981; Rothwell *et al.*, 1985b), and become markedly obese (Schemmel, 1976;
Schemmel *et al.*, 1970).

In careful studies of the genetics of this phenomenon, Fenton and
Chase (1951) showed that high-fat diets promote weight gain in genetically susceptible mice, but not in all strains of mice. Schemmel and
colleagues (1970) have shown that feeding rats a diet containing 60% of
its calories as fat produces the greatest increase in body fat in Osborne–
Mendel rats, an intermediate level of increase in body fat in animals of
most other strains, and only a very small weight gain in rats of the S
5B/Pl strain. From this, a useful model for the study of dietary fat-
induced obesity has been developed. When eating a high-fat diet, Osborne–Mendel rats show a striking increase in the percentage of body
fat as well as having increased body weight, organ weights, DNA, and
protein (Stone *et al.*, 1980). The larger fat depots in Osborne–Mendel
rats are composed of a larger number of fat cells, which are also
increased in size (Obst *et al.*, 1981). When S 5B/Pl rats eat a high-fat
diet, on the other hand, there is little or no effect on growth (Stone *et al.*,
1980) and little effect on fat cell size and number (Obst *et al.*, 1981).

The effect of a high-fat diet is related to the percentage and the type
of fat in the diet, to the sex of the animal, and to the age at which the
diet is offered. The incidence of obesity increases progressively as the
fat content of the diet is increased (Salmon and Flatt, 1985). A diet
high in saturated fat (i.e., beef tallow) is associated with higher gross
efficiency and greater weight gain than is an equivalent diet high in
polyunsaturated fat (i.e., corn oil) (Mercer and Trayhurn, 1987).
Females sometimes (Sinha *et al.*, 1977), but not consistently (Schemmel *et al.*, 1970), achieve greater obesity than males with high-fat

feeding. In young rats at or just after weaning the effect of a high-fat diet is less than when fed to older animals.

When the animals are returned to the standard chow diet after becoming obese by eating a high-fat diet, food intake is reduced, weight is lost and the adipocytes decrease to the same size as those of the chow-fed group (Faust *et al.*, 1976, 1978). If the animals eat the high-fat diet long enough, the total number of fat cells is increased and the total body fat remains elevated even though food intake returns to normal.

Since most dietary triglycerides are composed primarily of long-chain fatty acids, studies of high-fat diets have dealt mainly with the effect of triglycerides of long-chain fatty acids on obesity. Substitution of a diet equivalent in the amount of lipid but composed of medium-chain triglycerides (eight- to ten-carbon fatty acids) produces little or no obesity (Bray *et al.*, 1980; Schemmel, 1976; Leveille *et al.*, 1967). Food intake is lower for rats fed a medium-chain triglyceride diet than for rats fed corn oil or lard (Bray *et al.*, 1980; Schemmel, 1976; Wiley and Leveille, 1973). However, reduced food intake cannot totally account for the lack of weight gain. Food efficiency is also reduced in rats fed medium-chain triglycerides (Schemmel, 1976; Rothwell and Stock, 1987a).

2. High-Sucrose Diet

Giving sucrose as a drinking solution increases energy intake by 10–20% and there is a gradual increase in body weight and body fat (Kanarek and Hirsch, 1977; Kanarek and Orthen-Gambill, 1982; Schemmel *et al.*, 1982b; Sclafani, 1987a). There is little difference in the supplementation of sucrose, glucose, fructose, or polysaccharide solutions on the development of obesity (Kanarek and Orthen-Gambill, 1982). Sclafani (1987b) found that, although rats consumed slightly increased calories when powdered saccharide was available in addition to chow, the degree of hyperphagia was proportional to the hydration of the saccharide. Ramirez (1987b) also demonstrated that feeding a liquid diet produces greater hyperphagia and adiposity than does feeding a dry diet, regardless of sugar or polysaccharide content. Sclafani (1987a) has recently reviewed the literature on the substitution of sugar for starch in the diet of rats. In the 13 studies reviewed, there was considerable variability in food intake, weight gain, and body fat. Generally, however, body weight and fat showed no change or increased, even if food intake decreased, suggesting that the high-sugar diets may have enhanced food efficiency in these studies. There are age, sex, and strain differences in the susceptibility to high-

sucrose-induced obesity just as there are among rats with susceptibility to fat-induced obesity: Weanling rats overeat but tend not to gain
weight with sucrose solutions (Hirsch et al., 1982; Kanarek and Marks-
Kaufman, 1979); females more consistently become obese than males
(Sclafani, 1987a); and animals of the S 5B/P1 strain actually decrease
their body weight when drinking sucrose solutions (Schemmel et al.,
1982b).

3. Combined High-Fat, High-Sucrose Diets

A model of dietary obesity which incorporates both increased fat and
high sucrose in the diet has been described by Levin and associates
(1983b, 1984b,c, 1985). The diet is composed of chow (47%), corn oil
(8%), and sweetened condensed milk (44%). With this feeding paradigm, genetic variability also exists in the expression of obesity (Levin
et al., 1983b): Between one third and two thirds of the Sprague–
Dawley rats are resistant (Levin et al., 1983b, 1985, 1986a,b, 1987). In
the Sprague–Dawley strain, animals with the highest food intake also
show the highest efficiency of weight gain and become the most obese
(Levin et al., 1985). Rats chronically fed the high-fat, high-sucrose diet
eventually reduce food intake to below control levels (Levin et al.,
1985).

4. Cafeteria or Supermarket Diets

Sclafani and associates (Gale and Sclafani, 1977; Sclafani and
Springer, 1976) noted that rats allowed a variety of palatable snack
foods in addition to standard laboratory chow readily gained weight.
The foods that have been used in the cafeteria or supermarket diets
include cookies, salami, cheese, bananas, marshmallows, candy, pea-
nut butter, and sweetened condensed milk. Rats and mice given a
choice of a variety of foods increase energy intake by as much as 60%
(Hill et al., 1984; Rothwell et al., 1982b; Cunningham et al., 1983;
Armitage et al., 1983; Flatt et al., 1985) and gain 50–200% more
weight than control animals fed only laboratory chow (Cunningham et
al., 1983; Flatt et al., 1985; Sclafani and Gorman, 1977; Hill et al.,
1984; Sclafani and Springer, 1976). The weight increase is due to an
increase in both fat cell size and fat cell number (Mandenoff et al.,
1982). Allowing rats access to a running wheel resulted in a 27% lower
weight gain than observed in sedentary rats eating the cafeteria diet
(Sclafani and Springer, 1976). The weight gain of animals on a cafeteria diet is greater in females than in males (Sclafani and Gorman,
1977), is enhanced in older rats (Gillian-Barr and McCracken, 1984;
Armitage et al., 1983; Sclafani and Gorman, 1977), and is greatly

decreased in weanling rats (Rothwell and Stock, 1982). As with the high-fat diet, access to a cafeteria diet increases both mean body weight and the variability of the body weight. Also, like the animals fed a high-fat diet, when laboratory chow becomes the only available form of calories, food intake initially falls below then returns to control levels over the next 2–3 weeks (Armitage *et al.*, 1983). Although weight gain is attenuated, body weight generally remains above that of control (Hill *et al.*, 1984; Rowe and Rolls, 1977; Armitage *et al.*, 1983), and this elevated body weight appears to be defended (Rolls *et al.*, 1980).

B. Afferent Systems

1. *Cephalic Sensory Systems*

Palatability has been implicated in the overeating of high-fat or cafeteria diets (Mickelsen *et al.*, 1955; Rolls *et al.*, 1983; Sclafani and Springer, 1976). Palatability refers to the hedonistic response to foods due to the stimulus properties of a food such as taste, smell, texture, and temperature (Young and Green, 1953). In the model shown earlier (Fig. 1) this would be a positive afferent feedback signal acting on the controller to increase food intake or to suppress negative feedback signals. A major problem in studying the effect of palatability on food intake has been to separate the postingestional consequences of the diet from the diet's hedonistic properties, i.e., determining how much the animal would eat if only taste factors were operative. Rats made obese with either the high-fat (Maller, 1964) or the cafeteria (Sclafani and Springer, 1976) diet have been reported to have dietary finickiness, with increased rejection of unpalatable foods compared with controls.

In a study using a semisynthetic high-fat diet, to which strong food flavors and desirable textures were added, however, there was only a slight increase in food intake and weight gain in rats eating the more palatable diet (Naim *et al.*, 1985), suggesting that weight gain with high-fat diets is due primarily to the fat content of the diet, not to taste or texture. Variety and high palatability of the diet in one study were sufficient to overcome regulatory mechanisms and to increase food intake (Louis-Sylvestre *et al.*, 1984). Ramirez (1987a) has recently suggested that diet palatability for rats is more a function of diet moisture than diet texture. Using a semisynthetic diet made with corn starch containing 0–75% water, he found that weight gain and carcass fat were increased with increasing water content 0–50% in the diet.

Sham feeding is one paradigm which permits the isolation of the oropharyngeal stimulus of food from ingestive signals by opening up the feedback system (eliminating other feedback signals). In sham feeding the food is ingested orally but drains out of the alimentary tract through a fistula placed in the nonglandular part of the stomach (Weingarten and Watson, 1982). Sham feeding thus eliminates the confounding effects of the oropharyngeal stimulation by food with postingestional effects of food intake. Sham feeding does not, however, bypass the oral and cephalic phases of hormonal release. Experiments using sham feeding in dogs (Diamond *et al.*, 1985) and humans (Le-Blanc *et al.*, 1984) revealed that diet-induced thermogenesis is biphasic; the first phase is due to palatability factors and the second phase is due to postabsorptive factors. LeBlanc *et al.* (1984) suggest that the sensory-stimulated increase in thermogenesis was mediated through activation of the sympathetic nervous system. A palatable meal also results in a higher thermogenic response than a nonpalatable meal of the same energy and nutrient composition in humans (LeBlanc and Blondel, 1985).

2. *Gastrointestinal Satiety Signals*

Several studies have shown that signals arising from the stomach respond to both nutrient content and volume to help regulate short-term food intake. In particular, meal size, as an index of satiety, appears to be governed to a large extent by pregastric and gastric signals (Bach and Babayan, 1982; Baile *et al.*, 1971; Deutsch and Wang, 1977; Deutsch, 1978; Kraly and Smith, 1978; Young *et al.*, 1974). Food in the stomach appears to be the primary requirement for satiety. Removal of food from the stomach through a gastric fistula leads to exaggerated eating (Davis and Campbell, 1973; Young *et al.*, 1974). Filling the stomach with food, then withdrawing it, induces animals to eat additional food to compensate for the calories, but not the volume, withdrawn (Deutsch, 1978; Vanderweele *et al.*, 1974). Both neural (Deutsch, 1978) and hormonal (Koopmans, 1983) signals from the stomach have been proposed for termination of a meal. Mechanical distention is also an important satiety signal, with attenuation of feeding resulting from mechanical distension of the stomach or intestine independent of nutrient load (Janowitz and Grossman, 1949; McHugh and Moran, 1978; Davis and Collins, 1978).

Rats given 34–75% of their usual intake by gastric tube are able to compensate precisely for the load by reducing voluntary food intake (Rothwell and Stock, 1978a, 1984b). Despite this compensation, the tube-fed rats become fatter. Rothwell and Stock (1984b) have shown that this enhanced energetic efficiency of tube-fed rats is due, at least in part, to lower levels of thermogenesis, and LeBlanc and colleagues (1984) have demonstrated this also in humans. Whether this reduction in thermogenesis results from bypassing oral and cephalic signals is in question, however. For practical reasons, tube-fed animals receive several large meals per day, a feeding paradigm which is known to increase energetic efficiency and body energy gain (Fabry, 1973; Cohn and Joseph, 1959).

Intestinal factors are also involved in satiety. McHugh and Moran (1978) showed that gastric emptying of nutrients in monkeys is tightly regulated, with nutrient delivery through the pylorus occurring at a constant rate. Nutrients delivered not through the pylorus but infused instead into the duodenum in feeding animals suppresses meal size (Baile *et al.*, 1971; Booth, 1972; Novin *et al.*, 1974; Vanderweele *et al.*, 1974). Experiments in rats with crossed intestines have shown that the upper 30 cm of the small intestine does not generate signals for the short-term control of food intake (Koopmans, 1985; Koopmans *et al.*, 1984) but that the terminal ileum does. Transposition of a 5- to 10-cm section of the terminal ileum to the mid-duodenum with the remainder of the gastrointestinal tract intact results in the correction of the obesity of VMH rats primarily due to reduced food intake (Koopmans *et al.*, 1982). Koopmans and associates (1982) have proposed that the release of ileal hormones may have mediated the effect on food intake.

3. Circulating Afferent Satiety Signals

a. Nutrient and Metabolic Signals. Numerous gut peptides, including CCK, bombesin, pancreatic glucagon, and somatostatin, have been tested as potential controllers of food intake (Smith and Gibbs, 1984; Morley, 1987) (also see Sections II,A,2,c and III,B,2,a). CCK, bombesin, and glucagon act to terminate feeding and thus are considered to affect satiety (Antin *et al.*, 1975; Bernz *et al.*, 1983). The site of action of CCK and somatostatin is the afferent vagal fibers (Morley *et al.*, 1982; Niijima, 1981). Levels of CCK in the blood can be dissociated from the state of satiety in the rat. In crossed-intestine experiments the presence of CCK in the bloodstream did not inhibit food intake in the hungry rat and was not necessary for satiation in the fed rat (Koopmans and Heird, 1977). Whether CCK function is normal in models of dietary obesity has not been examined.

Postabsorptive nutrient stimuli do not appear to regulate meal size (Novin *et al.*, 1974) but do suppress feeding in hungry animals (Novin *et al.*, 1974; Russek, 1970). There have been some conflicting results with respect to the suppression of food intake by nutrient infusion into the intestine or hepatic portal system. Novin et al. (1974) pointed out, in their own work as well as that of others, that in animals deprived of food nutrient infusions into the gastrointestinal tract have little or no influence on eating (Baile et al., 1971; Booth, 1972; Novin et al., 1974; Vanderweele et al., 1974). The reverse was true for hepatic portal infusions, which suppress eating in animals deprived of food (Booth, 1972; Novin et al., 1974) but have no effect in free-feeding animals (Novin et al., 1974).

An emulsion composed of long-chain triglycerides given to rats orally (Friedman et al., 1983), intragastrically (Friedman et al., 1983; Ramirez and Friedman, 1983), or intraintestinally (Glick and Modan, 1977) causes suppression of voluntary feeding. The effect on food intake of oral ingestion of fat develops after a latency of 2–4 hours (Glick and Modan, 1977), and chronic infusion into the intestine causes suppression of total 24-hour food intake. The intestinal infusion of soybean oil reduces food intake similarly to that produced by intraintestinal infusion of an equicaloric load of glucose (Glick and Modan, 1977).

As described above, when animals are made obese by high-fat or cafeteria diets and are then returned to a low-fat stock diet, food intake is reduced and body weight decreases. A study using sham feeding has shown that the anorexia noted upon removal of the palatable diet is not dependent upon stimuli derived from the gastrointestinal tract (Vanderweele and Van Itallie, 1983). Thus, some signal(s) past the absorptive phase must be controlling food intake during recovery from diet-induced obesity.

The concept that metabolic signals may participate in the regulation of body weight has been suggested by several authors (Bray and Campfield, 1975; McCaleb et al., 1979; Nishizawa and Bray, 1980; Carpenter and Grossman, 1983a). Cellular glucoprivation is a potent stimulator of feeding (Ritter, 1986). The possibility that metabolic products from fat or carbohydrate metabolism, such as glycerol, fatty acids, ketones, pyruvate, or lactate might also serve as signals has been proposed (Friedman and Granneman, 1983; Carpenter and Grossman, 1983a).

2-DG, an inhibitor of glucose utilization, tends to lower plasma fatty acid and ketone levels, apparently through increased utilization (Friedman and Tordoff, 1986), and, like insulin induced hypoglycemia, initiates feeding. Animals allowed free selection display an increase in calories solely due to increased carbohydrate intake (Kanarek et al., 1980). The feeding response to insulin-induced hypoglycemia can be reduced by most sugars including fructose, which does not cross the blood–brain barrier (Stricker *et al.*, 1977; Rowland *et al.*, 1985), suggesting a peripheral site of action of insulin in the induction of eating. On the other hand, fructose has no effect on 2-DG-induced feeding, whereas glucose abolishes this feeding response (Rowland *et al.*, 1985). Infusion of 3-hydroxybutyrate, which under certain conditions can be utilized by the brain, has been reported to suppress 2-DG-induced feeding in one study (Stricker *et al.*, 1977), but this has not been replicated (Friedman and Tordoff, 1986; Rowland *et al.*, 1985). Feeding a high-fat diet to diabetic animals prevents glucoprivic feeding because fat provides the animals with a metabolic fuel that they can oxidize (Friedman *et al.*, 1985; Koopmans and Pi-Sunyer, 1986), although rats made severely diabetic with streptozotocin may actually avoid a high-fat diet (Koopmans and Pi-Sunyer, 1986).

Studies with the S 5B/Pl/Osborne-Mendel rat model of dietary fat-induced obesity indicated that rats of the obesity-resistant S 5B/Pl strain show a greater response of food intake, with a shorter latency period to both insulin and 2-DG, than do the diet-sensitive Osborne–Mendel rats (Fisler and Bray, 1985). The sensitivity of S 5B/Pl rats to glucoprivation induced by insulin was further increased when these animals were eating a high-fat diet, whereas the stimulus to eat induced by insulin was, if anything, depressed by a high-fat diet in Osborne–Mendel rats (J. S. Fisler and G. A. Bray, unpublished observations). The high-fat diet, however, had little impact on 2-DG-induced eating in either strain.

The relationship between food intake and the fat content of the diet of diabetic rats is mediated through oxidation of the ingested fat. Inhibitors of fatty acid oxidation increase short-term food intake of rats fed a high-fat, but not a low-fat, diet, and this effect is more potent during the bright phase of the light cycle (Friedman and Tordoff, 1986; Langhans and Sharrer, 1987b) when the rate of fatty acid oxidation is higher (Le Magnen, 1983). Le Magnan (1983) has suggested that the increased flow of endogenous fuels, free fatty acids, glycerol, and 3-hydroxybutyrate, from enhanced lipolysis may be responsible for the low daytime food intake in rats. The hypophagia resulting from withdrawal of a high-fat diet may be due to a persistent increase in fat oxidation (Ramirez, 1986). Inhibitors of fatty acid oxidation and glucose utilization combined have a synergistic effect on food intake in the rat (Friedman and Tordoff, 1986). Since intramitochondrial oxidation of substrates to CO_2 is the common pathway for metabolism of both glucose and fatty acids, this pathway could provide the signal indicating energy deficit.

Peripheral injection of glycerol (Wirtshafter and Davis, 1977) results in reduced darktime food intake and a gradual decline in body weight, irrespective of the dietary fat intake. Likewise, peripheral injection of 3-hydroxybutyrate, but not acetoacetate, reduces food intake (Langhans et al., 1983, 1985a).

The fact that a diet supplemented with medium-chain triglycerides does not promote obesity is most likely due to the rapid oxidation of medium-chain fatty acids to ketone bodies. Medium-chain triglycerides are more rapidly hydrolyzed and absorbed than long-chain triglycerides, and the medium-chain fatty acids enter the liver via the portal vein, whereas long-chain triglycerides are repackaged into chylomicrons by the intestinal cells and enter the circulation through the thoracic duct (Bach and Babayan, 1982). Medium-chain triglycerides are not significantly incorporated into depot lipids in the liver but instead readily enter the mitochondria where they undergo β-oxidation with formation of acetyl-coenzyme A (Bach et al., 1976), much of which is directed toward the synthesis of ketone bodies (Bach and Babayan, 1982; Bach et al., 1977; Yeh and Zee, 1976).

That 3-hydroxybutyrate, but not acetoacetate, injections inhibit feeding suggests that the dehydrogenation of 3-hydroxybutyrate to acetoacetate is the crucial metabolic step contributing to the satiety effect of 3-hydroxybutyrate (Langhans et al., 1983). d-3-Hydroxybutyrate dehydrogenase oxidizes 3-hydroxybutyrate to acetoacetate, thereby producing reducing equivalents in the liver and the intestine. In a review on the effect of various redox pairs (glycerol/dihydroxyacetone, malate/oxaloacetate, 3-hydroxybutyrate/acetoacetate, lactate/pyruvate) on feeding, Langhans and associates (1985a) noted that the suppression of feeding seems to depend on the mitochondrial oxidation of the nutrients. The increased generation of reducing equivalents in the mitochondria may be the common signal generated by these redox pairs for inhibiting food intake. E. Scharrer (personal communication) has outlined a scheme whereby the oxidation of a metabolic fuel with the resultant increase in NADH [nicotinamide–adenine–dinucleotide (reduced form)] can elicit a sustained hyperpolarization of the cell membrane (Dambach and Friedmann, 1974; Fitz and Scharschmidt, 1987) and lead to satiety (see Fig. 4). The increased NADH would enter the respiratory chain yielding increased adenosine triphosphate (ATP). The ATP, in turn, would stimulate Na^+,K^+-ATPase activity (Langhans and Scharrer, 1987c), inducing hyperpolarization of the cell membrane which, Sharrer suggests, could reduce the spikes generated in the hepatic vagal afferents, thus increasing signals of satiety in the brain.

  b. Hormonal Signals. i. Insulin. Although hyperinsulinemia is not

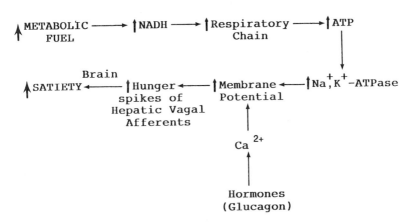

Fɪɢ. 4. Regulation of food intake by metabolic fuels. Metabolic fuels, such as glucose or 3-hydroxybutyrate, produce reducing equivalents in the mitochondria with the resultant generation of adenosine triphosphate (ATP). Scharrer has proposed that the ATP would stimulate Na^+,K^+-ATPase activity, leading to hyperpolarization of the cell membrane, which, via the vagus nerve, could increase the signals of satiety to the brain (Scharrer and Langhans, 1986; E. Scharrer, personal communication).

a prominent feature of diet-induced obesity (see Section IV,E), there are some abnormalities in insulin secretion and sensitivity. Rats with high intakes of sucrose have high insulin levels stimulated by the glucose load (Sundin and Nachad, 1983). Circulating insulin levels are modestly elevated in rats genetically susceptible to dietary obesity (Yoshida et al., 1987; Levin et al., 1985). A high-fat diet does not consistently alter insulin levels, but does decrease whole body glucose utilization in all animals studied (Kraegen et al., 1986; Storlien et al., 1986, 1987; Underberger et al., 1987).

ii. *Adrenal steroids.* As discussed earlier (see Sections II,C,3,d and III,B,2,d), adrenal steroids appear to be necessary for the expression of most, if not all, forms of obesity. However, few data are available regarding the importance of adrenal steroids in dietary obesity. Adrenalectomy reduces the fat intake of lean Zucker rats given free choice of separate macronutrient sources (Castonguay and Stern, 1983). Rothwell and associates (1984) have shown that adrenalectomy prevents the development of obesity in cafeteria-fed rats due to a depression of both food intake and energetic efficiency. There is increased energy expenditure following adrenalectomy in both stock diet- and cafeteria-fed animals, which is at least partly due to increased thermogenesis in brown fat (Rothwell and Stock, 1986; Rothwell et al., 1984). In Osborne–Mendel rats (J. S. Fisler, unpublished observations) and *ob/ob* mice (Smith and Romsos, 1985) fed a high-fat diet, on the other hand, adrenalectomy results in only slight reductions in energy gain or the efficiency of energy retention.

iii. Thyroid hormones. Thyroid hormones may directly influence diet-induced changes in thermogenesis. Triiodothyronine (T_3) levels in rats are increased by overfeeding and reduced by fasting (Rothwell *et al.*, 1982a). In humans the replacement of carbohydrate completely by fat in the diet results in a decrease in circulating T_3 levels equivalent to that seen in subjects fasted for 1 week (Danforth *et al*, 1979). Blanco and Silva (1987) have recently shown that intracellular conversion of thyroxine to T_3 by 5'-deiodinase in the brown fat is required for the production of uncoupling protein and optimal thermogenic function. A single low-protein, high-carbohydrate meal, which results in a significant increase in thermogenic activity of brown fat, is accompanied by significant increases in the activity of thyroxine 5'-deiodinase in brown fat (Glick *et al.*, 1985). The activity of brown fat 5'-deiodinase is elevated during norepinephrine treatment (Silva and Larsen, 1986), and norepinephrine turnover is increased in brown fat by overfeeding (Schwartz *et al.*, 1983; Rothwell *et al.*, 1981).

4. *Vagal Signals*

The hypophagic signal generated peripherally by oxidation of the metabolites, discussed in Section IV,B,3,a, is most likely mediated by hepatic vagal afferent nerves. Members of the redox pairs discussed above reduced food intake in sham-vagotomized rats but had no effect in rats which had the hepatic branch of the vagus nerve severed (Langhans *et al.*, 1985b), suggesting that vagal hepatic afferents were necessary for the hypophagic effect of these metabolites. Likewise, hepatic oxidation of fatty acids provides a satiety signal that is mediated by vagal afferents: Mercaptoacetate, an inhibitor of fatty acid oxidation, stimulates feeding to a much greater extent in sham-vagotomized than in vagotomized rats (Langhans and Sharrer, 1987a). In addition, the satiety effects of certain gut peptides are mediated by vagal afferent nerves. Bilateral abdominal or gastric vagotomies block the satiety effect of peripheral CCK-8 (Smith *et al*, 1981a), and hepatic vagotomy blocks the satiety effect of pancreatic glucagon in Sprague–Dawley rats (Geary and Smith, 1983).

Generally, no effect of vagotomy on basal food intake or feeding pattern has been observed (Langhans *et al.*, 1985b; Tordoff *et al.*, 1982; Louis-Sylvestre *et al.*, 1980; Bellinger *et al.*, 1984). However, in a detailed examination of meal patterns as predictors of short-term and 24-hour food intake in intact and vagotomized rabbits, Geiselman and associates (1982) found that vagotomy disrupted the interrelationships among meal size, meal frequency, and long-term food intake. Vagotomy in cafeteria-fed rats either had no effect on weight gain or only partially reduced the weight gain in these animals (Sclafani *et al.*, 1981; Gold *et al.*, 1980).

C. Central Integration

The most likely central site for integration of signals regarding the fat content of the diet is the medial hypothalamus. Rats with injury to the VMN (Corbit and Stellar, 1964) or PVN (Bartness *et al.*, 1985) are particularly responsive to a high-fat diet, whereas they respond to palatable diets with great hyperphagia and obesity when the dorsomedial nucleus of the hypothalamus is injured (Bernardis and Bellinger, 1986b). In experiments utilizing S 5B/P1 rats, which normally do not develop obesity when fed a high-fat diet (Schemmel *et al.*, 1970), the introduction of bilateral parasagittal hypothalamic knife cuts was followed by hyperphagia and obesity when the rats ate a 30% fat diet but not when they ate a 10% fat diet (Oku *et al.*, 1984b). The knife-cut lesions also disturbed the diurnal feeding pattern in these rats, causing them to shift from eating 96% of their food during the dark phase to eating only 59% of their food during the dark (Oku *et al.*, 1984b). The parasaggital knife cut produces an obesity similar to the PVN lesion. We interpret these results to indicate that the PVN has inhibitory effects on the afferent signals from taste receptors as they reach the solitary tract nucleus in the sensory vagal complex. Thus, the adaptive reduction in caloric intake when S 5B/P1 rats eat a high-fat diet involves a detector system for some component of the diet which is monitored through the PVN to inhibit taste factors in the sensory vagal system.

1. Ketones

The products of fat metabolism act in the brain to reduce food intake and/or body weight. Glycerol infusion into the third ventricle reduces both food intake and body weight (Davis *et al.*, 1981). The chronic infusion of 3-hydroxybutyrate into the third ventricle of the brain was found to reduce food intake in one study (Arase *et al.*, 1988a) but not in another (Davis *et al.*, 1981). Body weight, however, was reduced by 3-hydroxybutyrate in both of these studies (Davis *et al.*, 1981; Arase *et al*, 1988c). This reduction in food intake and body weight by intraventricular infusion of 3-hydroxybutyrate was not influenced by dietary fat content (Arase *et al.*, 1988a). In S 5B/P1 rats the intraventricular infusion of 3-hydroxybutyrate had no effect on either food intake or body weight (Arase *et al.*, 1988a). This strain of rats, which is resistant to obesity when eating a high-fat diet, has a higher blood concentration of ketones (Yoshida *et al.*, 1987; Arase *et al.*, 1988b; Fisler *et al.*, 1989) and a higher transport of 3-hydroxybutyrate across the blood–brain barrier under conditions of both low- and high-fat diets (Bray *et al.*, 1987), suggesting that the brain in this strain is habitually exposed to high ketone levels. In fact, whole-brain 3-hydroxybutyrate concentrations are higher in S 5B/P1 rats than in Osborne–Mendel rats, although circulating levels do not tightly reflect brain concentrations (Fisler *et al.*, 1989). A high-fat diet did not consistently increase the brain 3-hydroxybutyrate levels (Fisler *et al.*, 1989). Injection of 3-hydroxybutyrate into either the PVN or the VMN of the hypothalamus of Sprague–Dawley rats causes a significant increase in firing rate of the sympathetic nerves to BAT (Sakaguchi *et al.*, 1988b). The response in both regions to 3-hydroxybutyrate is dose dependent. Thus, 3-hydroxybutyrate can activate the sympathetic nervous system and may signal utilization of fat metabolites.

2. *Insulin*

Several lines of evidence indicate that insulin provides neuroendocrine signals that modulate food intake (see also Sections II,B,3,b and III,C,2). Specific receptor sites for insulin have been found in the hypothalamus and other brain sites (Havrankova *et al.*, 1983; Landau *et al.*, 1983). Insulin stimulates norepinephrine turnover in the hypothalamus (Bellin and Ritter, 1981; McCaleb and Myers, 1982; Sauter *et al.*, 1983) and affects responses of the central nervous system to taste (Giza and Scott, 1984) and odor (Cain, 1975). Acute and chronic infusions of insulin into the third ventricle of the brain reduce food intake in rats and baboons after a delay of about 3 hours, with the dark-period food intake primarily affected (Woods *et al.*, 1979; Plata-Salaman *et al.*, 1986a; Brief and Davis, 1984; Arase *et al.*, 1988c). Chronic infusion of insulin into the brain also reduces body weight (Woods *et al.*, 1979; Plata-Salaman *et al.*, 1986a; Brief and Davis, 1984; Arase *et al.*, 1988a).

Conversely, food intake is increased by the injection of insulin antibodies (Strubbe and Mein, 1977) into the VMH. These effects of insulin may operate through the glucosensitive neurons in the VMH which have been identified by Oomura (1976), and whose sensitivity may vary with the diet. That 2-DG does not completely block the effect of insulin (Rothwell *et al.*, 1983c) suggests that the action of insulin in the hypothalamus may involve mechanisms other than glucose uptake. However, since a high-fat diet completely abolishes the reduction of food intake and body weight by intracerebroventricular insulin (Arase *et al.*, 1988a), the suppression of feeding by insulin appears to be due to increased glucose utilization by the brain, a substrate perhaps superceded by ketones when fat intake is high.

3. *Glucoprivic Feeding*

Glucoprivation-induced feeding may be acting via the .hypothalamus, particularly the PVN, with GABA as the neurotransmitter (Kimura and Kuriyama, 1975; Leibowitz, 1980, Leibowitz and Stanley, 1986b). This amino acid transmitter either stimulates or inhibits feeding, depending on the site of injection and deprivation state of the animal (see Leibowitz and Stanley, 1985a,b). The levels of satiety of the animal alter glucose flux through the GABA shunt in the ventrolateral hypothalamus. The GABA shunt activity was lower in hungry rats and higher in force-fed rats, relative to controls (Kasser *et al.*, 1985b). With hypoglycemia, the levels of GABA in the medial hypothalamus increase, while GABA decreases in the LH (Kimura and Kuriyama, 1975). Under control diet conditions, S 5B/P1 and Osborne-Mendel rats have equivalent levels of whole-brain GABA. GABA concentration in whole brain increases with fat feeding in both strains, although the increase is much greater in brains of S 5B/P1 rats than those in Osborne–Mendel rats (Fisler *et al.*, 1989). Local brain regions were not analyzed and it is not known whether the increase in GABA attributed to eating high-fat diets is reflected in the medial hypothalamus. Since S 5B/P1 rats are more sensitive to glucoprivation-induced feeding (Fisler and Bray, 1985) and have higher blood and brain ketone levels (Yoshida *et al.*, 1987; Fisler *et al.*, 1989) than do Osborne–Mendel rats, it may be that S 5B/P1 rats eating a high-fat diet utilize less glucose in the hypothalamus than do Osborne–Mendel rats.

4. *Other Neurotransmitters and Peptides*

Another neurotransmitter which may be acting through the PVN to regulate feeding is serotonin (5-HT). Manipulations which increase central 5-HT suppress feeding, whereas those that deplete central 5-HT increase feeding (see Leibowitz and Stanley, 1986a,b). Consistent with this is the observation that in diet-sensitive Osborne–Mendel rats tryptophan metabolism is altered (Weekley *et al.*, 1982) and brainstem levels of 5-HT are reduced (Kimbrough and Weekley, 1984), which in one study were not altered by a high-fat diet, even though 5-HT was reduced by fat-feeding in Sprague–Dawley rats (Kimbrough and Weekley, 1984). As determined in cerebrospinal fluid dialysate from the VMN of conscious rats, 5-HT was depressed in Osborne–Mendel rats, relative to S 5B/P1 rats. In rats taking a high-fat diet, 5-HT from the VMN increased in Osborne–Mendel rats, whereas it decreased in S 5B/Pl rats (H. Shimizu, J. S. Fisler, and G. A. Bray unpublished observations). The metabolite of 5-HT, 5-HIAA, on the other hand, did not differ between strains but did increase in both when eating the high-fat diet.

Osborne–Mendel rats are more sensitive to both acute and chronic administration of fenfluramine, a serotonergic drug (Fisler and Bray, 1986), implying that they are more sensitive to serotonergic stimulation than are S 5B/Pl rats. Fenfluramine prevents the obesity induced by a high-fat diet in Osborne–Mendel rats largely by reducing food intake (Underberger *et al.*, 1987). Fenfluramine also causes a significant reduction in food intake and increased weight loss in cafeteria-fed rats, the effect being much greater in the plateau phase than in the dynamic phase of obesity (Blundell, 1986). Blundell (1986) has suggested that the greater effect in stable obesity is due to the reduction in meal size in animals eating large, less frequent meals. In addition to reducing food intake, fenfluramine stimulates the sympathetic nervous system. Fenfluramine apparently stimulates thermogenesis via central serotonergic mechanisms which modify sympathetic outflow to BAT since BAT temperature (Rothwell and Stock, 1987b) and GDP binding (Lupien and Bray, 1985) increase with central and peripheral injections of fenfluramine, respectively.

CRF is another hypothalamic neuropeptide that differs functionally between S 5B/Pl and Osborne–Mendel rats. The suppression of feeding by CRF infused into the third ventricle of the brain was greater in Osborne–Mendel rats than in S 5B/Pl rats eating a low-fat diet. A high-fat diet partially blocked the suppression of feeding by intracerebroventricular CRF in Osborne–Mendel rats (J. S. Fisler, K. Arase, and G. A. Gray, unpublished observations). As discussed earlier (see Section II,C,3,d), the effect of adrenalectomy on food intake may be mediated through increased secretion of CRF. Thus, the inhibition by high-fat diets of CRF action on feeding may explain why adrenalectomy causes only partial reductions of body weight gain in Osborne–Mendel rats eating a high-fat diet (see Section IV,B,3,b).

Several studies suggest that brain adrenergic systems are also affected by dietary obesity. Levin and associates (1986a) found that the moderate-fat, high-sucrose diet fed for 3 months led to accelerated brain norepinephrine and dopamine turnover in the PVN of the hypothalamus. When obesity developed, however, there was a decrease in dopamine turnover in several brain sites. Norepinephrine and DOPAC, a metabolite of dopamine, have also been measured in cerebrospinal fluid dialysate from the VMH of S 5B/Pl and Osborne–Mendel rats eating either high-fat or low-fat diets (H. Shimizu, J. S. Fisler, and G. A. Bray, unpublished observations). The norepinephrine and DOPAC levels followed a pattern very similar to that of 5-HT, being higher in S 5B/Pl rats but increasing with the fat content of the diet only in Osborne–Mendel rats. Studies with amphetamine in the S 5B/Pl–Osborne–Mendel model of dietary obesity suggest that Osborne–Mendel rats are more sensitive than S 5B/Pl rats (Fisler and Bray, 1985) to α-adrenergic stimulation of feeding (Leibowitz, 1970), since low-dose peripheral injections of d-amphetamine acutely stimulated food intake in Osborne–Mendel rats, while having no effect in S 5B/Pl rats. Moderate and high doses of amphetamine suppressed feeding in all animals. Leibowitz (1970) proposed the existence of both α- and β-adrenergic systems in the hypothalamus which function antagonistically in the regulation of food intake. d-Amphetamine can serve as an agonist for both of these systems. The β-receptor action of amphetamine in the suppression of food intake was found to be more potent than the α-receptor action which facilitated food intake. Thus, moderate or high doses of amphetamine would overpower the α-receptor response, resulting in suppression of feeding.

Finally, two studies have examined the effectiveness of opiate receptor antagonists to suppress feeding in dietary obesity. Rats eating a palatable cafeteria diet exhibit an enhanced suppression of feeding in response to naltrexone relative to chow-fed controls (Apfelbaum and Mandenoff, 1981). Tests on naloxone suppression of feeding in S 5B/Pl and Osborne/Mendel rats, however, showed no difference between strains (Fisler and Bray, 1985).

D. EFFERENT CONTROL

1. Food Intake

Total energy intake of Osborne–Mendel rats is usually increased when rats are switched from a low-fat to a high-fat diet but is then reduced to or below control levels within 2 weeks (Fisler et al., 1989). Osborne–Mendel rats eating a high-fat diet continue to gain excess weight, however, despite food intake returning to control levels. S 5B/P1 rats, on the other hand, do not increase caloric intake when eating a high-fat diet. With the moderate-fat, high-sucrose model of dietary obesity, absolute caloric intake is greater in rats fed the enriched diet. With intake expressed as kcal/100 g of body weight, however, food intake of the rats fed the high-energy diet was higher than that of chow-fed rats only during the first 17 days of the diet. Within 2 months the adjusted food intake was less in rats fed the high-energy diet than in those fed only chow (Levin et al., 1986b; Triscari et al., 1985). With this model of dietary obesity, approximately 50% of Sprague–Dawley rats resist the development of obesity. These animals reduce caloric intake to below control levels. Food efficiency is increased in all rats fed the high-energy diet, albeit more so in those animals that become obese (Levin et al., 1985, 1986b). On the other hand, energy intake (Rothwell and Stock, 1979, 1981b) and body weight gain (Rothwell and Stock, 1979; Sclafani and Springer, 1976) are consistently increased during feeding of a cafeteria diet.

2. Autonomic Nervous System

As with hypothalamic obesity, the syndrome of dietary obesity is associated with altered function of the autonomic nervous system.

a. Vagal Efferents. Few studies have examined the effect of dietary manipulations on vagal efferents. Rothwell and Stock (1983) have shown that the rise of oxygen consumption with diet-induced thermogenesis is enhanced by atropine, indicating that the parasympathetic nervous system inhibits this thermogenesis.

b. Sympathetic Activity. The literature on the effect of high-fat diets on the sympathetic nervous system is contradictory. Using norepinephrine turnover as a technique for estimating sympathetic activity, Schwartz and associates (1983) found that animals eating a high-fat diet for 4 days had an increased turnover of norepinephrine in the heart and brown fat, suggesting increased sympathetic activity. In other studies of animals eating a high-fat diet for either 2 or 4 weeks, there was no change in the level of sympathetic activity in the heart (Fisler et al., 1984; Yoshida et al., 1987). After 2 weeks of a high-fat diet, norepinephrine turnover in BAT was increased 3-fold in diet-resistant S 5B/Pl rats, and to a much lesser extent in diet-sensitive Osborne–Mendel rats (Yoshida et al., 1987). After 4 weeks of eating a high-fat diet, however, norepinephrine turnover in BAT was increased by only 40% in S 5B/Pl rats and not at all in Osborne–Mendel rats (Fisler et al., 1984). In contrast to these studies, GDP binding to mitochondria of BAT, which is regulated by the sympathetic nervous system, was decreased after 2–3 weeks and after 12 weeks in rats of either strain eating a high-fat diet (Fisler et al., 1987). Single meals acutely stimulate GDP binding to mitochondria of brown fat, with a high-fat meal producing less effect than a high-carbohydrate meal (Lupien et al., 1985). Whether a single meal would stimulate BAT thermogenesis in animals adapted to a high-fat diet is not known. The effect of a high-fat diet on the firing rate of sympathetic nerves to brown fat varies with the length of the diet. In Sprague–Dawley rats, after eating a high-fat diet for 1 week there was no effect of diet on the firing rate. After 3 weeks of ad libitum feeding, however, the animals eating the high-fat diet had a significantly depressed firing rate (T. Sakaguchi, J. S. Fisler, and G. A. Bray, unpublished observations). Thus, the data from direct measurement of sympathetic nerves to brown fat are consistent with the data from GDP-binding studies, showing decreased thermogenesis in BAT of animals chronically fed a high-fat diet.

The varying results among these studies may be caused by the differences in the length of time the animals were exposed to the high-fat diet, the methods of feeding the diets, the dietary fat composition, or the strains studied. The experiments of Schwartz *et al.* (1983) were short term (4 days), and fat was added to a standard diet, reducing the protein content of the diet, which itself will increase sympathetic activity (Rothwell *et al.*, 1982b, 1983d; Teague *et al.*, 1981). Yoshida and associates (1987) were examining the interaction of feeding and lighting and consequently were allowing the rats access to food for only 12 hours daily and were restricting the intake of the high-fat diet. Mercer and Trayhurn (1987) have reported that a high-corn oil diet induces higher cytochrome oxidase activity in BAT of both lean and obese (*ob/ob*) mice than does a high-beef tallow diet. These authors concluded that a diet rich in polyunsaturated fatty acids preferentially stimulates brown fat thermogenesis, especially in the *ob/ob* mouse (Mercer and Trayhurn, 1987). A difference in the saturation of the dietary fatty acids, however, cannot explain the discrepancy of results between norepinephrine turnover and GDP-binding studies from our laboratory, where vegetable shortening has regularly comprised the fat component of the diet. Data on norepinephrine turnover in VMH rats suggest that the metabolism of norepinephrine may be altered in the obese animal (see Section II,C,2,b). The increased norepinephrine turnover measurements, at a time when GDP binding and electric firing rate of nerves in BAT are decreased, lead us to conclude that norepinephrine turnover in BAT does not accurately reflect the sympathetic tone to that organ in dietary fat-induced obesity.

Levin and associates (1983b, 1987) fed Sprague–Dawley rats a moderate-fat, high-sucrose diet for 1–3 weeks and found consistent increases of norepinephrine turnover in brown fat, with variable effects on the heart and the pancreas. Given this diet for 4–5 months, approximately 50% of the rats became obese, whereas the remaining rats were able to reduce food intake sufficiently to prevent excess weight gain (Levin *et al.*, 1985; Levin and Sullivan, 1987). In the animals that became obese, norepinephrine turnover in the heart was reduced, whereas it was unchanged in animals that were resistant to dietary obesity. The turnover of norepinephrine in brown fat was reduced to undetectable levels in all animals eating the combined fat and sucrose diet regardless of their weight gain. Glucose-stimulated plasma norepinephrine levels actually decreased, however, in the rats that were resistant to obesity, a direct relationship being found between glucose-stimulated plasma norepinephrine concentration and weight gain in rats eating the high-energy diet (Levin and Sullivan, 1987). Whether this reflects an enhanced clearance of norepinephrine from plasma in the resistant rats is not clear. Tyrosine hydroxylase inhibition failed to increase the lipid content of the brown fat in either cold-exposed or control rats fed the moderate-fat, high-sucrose diets even when norepinephrine turnover was normal, suggesting a postsynaptic defect in basal norepinephrine-stimulated lipolysis (Levin *et al.*, 1983b,c). Feeding the same diet to 1-month-old Sprague–Dawley rats caused a sustained increase in basal norepinephrine turnover in the heart, the pancreas, and BAT. Despite this increased sympathetic activity, the rats began to develop obesity at 2 months of age (Levin *et al.*, 1986b).

Norepinephrine turnover is greater in rats fed cafeteria diets, relative to chow-fed controls. Rothwell and associates (1981) concluded that this increase in turnover was not due to alterations in reuptake nor metabolism of norepinephrine, but was due to an augmented release of norepinephrine from nerve terminals. Consistent with the data on norepinephrine turnover, feeding a cafeteria diet has been associated with increases of 50–200% in GDP binding to mitochondria of brown fat (Brooks *et al.*, 1982; Himms-Hagen, 1984; Fisler *et al.*, 1987). The capacity for diet-induced thermogenesis decreases with age (Rothwell and Stock, 1983; Fisler *et al.*, 1987), explaining the greater sensitivity of older rats to obesity produced by cafeteria feeding.

Direct assessment of changes in the function of the sympathetic nervous system in response to nutrients has been made by measuring the sympathetic firing rate of efferent nerves to BAT (Sakaguchi and Bray, 1987a,b; Sakaguchi *et al.*, 1988a). The microinjection of either glucose or 3-hydroxybutyrate into the hypothalamus will increase the sympathetic firing rate (Sakaguchi and Bray, 1987a; Sakaguchi *et al.*, 1988a), whereas injection of insulin will reduce (Sakaguchi and Bray, 1987a) the firing rate of sympathetic nerves to BAT.

E. Controlled System

A high-fat diet caused increased carcass fat and reduced lean tissue mass (Kraegen *et al.*, 1986; Storlien *et al.*, 1986). The increased fat mass reflects both increased fat cell size (Robeson *et al.*, 1981; Faust *et al.*, 1978, 1980; Applegate *et al.*, 1984) and number (Faust *et al.*, 1978, 1980; Applegate *et al.*, 1984). Sprague–Dawley rats eating the moderate-fat, high-sucrose diet also showed increased carcass fat, but even when the diet was instituted in 6-month-old rats, the increased fat cell mass reflected an increased number of fat cells with no change in size (Triscari *et al.*, 1985). The degree of obesity obtained with the cafeteria diet varies even though severe hyperphagia is induced. This is especially true in weanling rats which, due to increased thermogenesis, are quite resistant to obesity induced by a cafeteria diet.

These differences in weight gain with high energy intake with cafeteria feeding must be due to differences in energy expenditure (Rothwell and Stock, 1978b, 1979; Rothwell *et al.*, 1985b). Resting oxygen consumption is greater in animals eating a cafeteria diet than in those with either chow or high-fat diets (Rothwell *et al.*, 1985b). Rothwell and Stock (1979) proposed that this dietary thermogenesis involves increased sympathetic activity acting in part through BAT. Within 3 days of beginning a cafeteria diet in weanling rats there is a 2-fold increase in the mass of the brown fat depot and in the binding of purine nucleotide to mitochondria, changes which are maintained during at least 1 month on a cafeteria diet (Brooks *et al.*, 1982).

Rothwell and associates have extensively examined heat production upon oral ingestion of carbohydrate, fat, or cafeteria diets in laboratory rats. Cafeteria diets increase energy expenditure. Both carbohydrate and fat ingestion cause a rise in oxygen consumption, which can be blocked by propranolol, indicating that the increase in heat production is sympathetically mediated (Rothwell and Stock, 1983; Rothwell *et al.*, 1985b). Beta blockade with propranolol attenuated the increase due to glucose ingestion in cytochrome oxidase activity in brown fat but did not effect the specific binding of GDP to mitochondria (Sundin and Nachad, 1983). As previously mentioned, the rise in oxygen consumption is enhanced by atropine (Rothwell and Stock, 1983), indicating that parasympathetic inhibition is also involved in this dietary thermogenesis. The thermic effect of carbohydrate is insulin mediated, since it can be blocked by inhibition of insulin secretion, whereas that of fat cannot be (Rothwell *et al.*, 1985a). The size of the acute rise in metabolic rate after fat or carbohydrate feeding is dependent on the thermogenic capacity of the animal and most likely involves the same mechanisms as do the chronic changes observed in nonshivering thermogenesis (Rothwell and Stock, 1983).

Dietary obesity resulting in rats given high-fat diets is significantly different metabolically from other models of obesity. The hyperinsulinemia seen in hypothalamic and genetic obesity is much reduced or lacking in diet-induced obesity (Blazquez and Quijada, 1968; Malaisee *et al.*, 1975; Abumrad *et al.*, 1978; Carmel *et al.*, 1975; Zaragoza-Hermans and Felber, 1972; Eisenstein *et al.*, 1974; Robeson *et al.*, 1981; Grundleger and Thenen, 1982; Kraegen *et al.*, 1986; Burnol *et al.*, 1987; Yoshida *et al.*, 1987). Insulin levels are higher, however, in rats susceptible to diet-induced obesity (Yoshida *et al.*, 1987; Levin *et al.*, 1985). Animals eating high-fat diets do not show consistent hyperglycemia but do consistently exhibit an impaired response to glucose (Schemmel *et al.*, 1982a) and to insulin (Ogundipe and Bray, 1974; Grundleger and Thenen, 1982; Zaragoza-Hermans and Felber, 1972). Use of *in vitro* and *in vivo* techniques in rats eating a high-fat diet has shown widespread *in vivo* insulin resistance in peripheral tissues, with the effect being most pronounced in oxidative skeletal muscle, BAT, and the liver (Kraegen *et al.*, 1986; Storlien *et al.*, 1986, 1987; Susini and Lavau, 1978; Underberger *et al.*, 1987). Differences in insulin sensitivity, however, do not explain the discrepant weight gain patterns between Osborne–Mendel and S 5B/P1 rats eating a high-fat diet.

Although S 5B/Pl rats display higher insulin sensitivity than do Osborne–Mendel rats, perhaps because of the greater body fat of Osborne–Mendel rats, sensitivity is reduced in both strains upon feeding of high-fat diets (Underberger *et al.*, 1987). The impaired glucose uptake due to eating high-fat diets is associated with decreased levels of hexokinase (Bernstein *et al.*, 1977). The oxidation of glucose to CO_2 is spared (Lavau and Susini, 1975), with evidence of a decrease in the activity in other pathways of glucose metabolism as well (Lavau and Susini, 1975; Zaragosa-Hermans and Felber, 1970; Smith *et al.*, 1974). The moderate-fat, high-sucrose diet does cause hyperinsulinemia; Sprague–Dawley rats taking this diet for 3 months showed a 4- to 5-fold increase in insulin levels, relative to chow-fed controls (Levin *et al.*, 1987; Triscari *et al.*, 1985). Insulin is elevated but glucose and glucagon levels are unaffected by the high-energy diet (Triscari *et al.*, 1985). Rats drinking sucrose solutions are also hyperinsulinemic (Sundin and Nachad, 1983). Cafeteria diets are associated with hyperglycemia, hyperinsulinemia, and glucose intolerance (Rolls *et al.*, 1980; Cunningham *et al.*, 1983).

In addition to the changes in carbohydrate metabolism, there are several abnormalities in lipid metabolism in dietary obesity. There is a decrease in fatty acid synthesis from glucose (Lavau and Susini, 1975; Storlien *et al.*, 1986; Rothwell *et al.*, 1983b; Schemmel *et al.*, 1982a) associated with decreased insulin-stimulated lipogenesis in rats eating a high-fat diet. The activity of enzymes that generate NADPH [nicotinamide–adenine–dinucleotide phosphate (reduced form)] for fatty acid synthesis, specifically glucose-6-phosphate dehydrogenase and malic enzyme are reduced in these rats (Lavau *et al.*, 1979). The activity of fatty acid synthetase is also reduced (Robeson *et al.*, 1981), and there is decreased lipogenesis in response to norepinephrine (Bernstein *et al.*, 1977). Diets high in sucrose lead to increased capacity for fatty acid synthesis *in vitro,* but actual rates *in vivo* are unchanged (Triscari *et al.*, 1985). There are increased hepatic triglyceride and fatty acid levels (Eisenstein *et al.*, 1974), and β-oxidation of fatty acids is increased, resulting in increased ketone production (Triscari *et al.*, 1985) and blood ketone levels (Yoshida *et al.*, 1987; Friedman *et al.*, 1985).

The only reported alteration in protein metabolism in animals with dietary obesity is a decrease in urea synthesis in animals fed a cafeteria diet (Barber *et al.*, 1985).

V. Summary and Conclusions

A. Integrative Hypotheses

The basic hypothesis of this review is that studies on models of experimental obesity can provide insight into the control systems regulating body nutrient stores in humans. In this homeostatic or feedback approach to analysis of the nutrient control system, we have examined the afferent feedback signals, the central controller, and the efferent control elements regulating the controlled system of nutrient intake, storage, and oxidation. The mechanisms involved in the beginning and ending of single meals must clearly be related to the long-term changes in fat stores, although this relationship is far from clear. Changes in total nutrient storage in adipose tissue can arise as a consequence of changes in the quantity of nutrients ingested in one form or another or a decrease in the utilization of the ingested nutrients. A change in energy intake can be effected by increased size of individual meals, increased number of meals in a 24-hour period, or a combination of these events. Similarly, a decrease in utilization of these nutrients can develop through changes in resting metabolic energy expenditure which are associated with one of more of the biological cycles such as protein metabolism, triglyceride for glycogen synthesis and breakdown, or maintenance of ionic gradients for $Na^+ + K^+$ across cell walls. In addition, differences in energy expenditure related to the thermogenesis of eating or to the level of physical activity may account for differences in nutrient utilization.

1. *Afferent Signals*

Meal intake can be initiated by several kinds of signals. Positive sensory cues, which would include the visual sighting of food and the detection of food through its aroma or through various positive aspects of taste, including sweetness or characteristics of palatability, are of major importance in dietary obesity. Control of these sensory cues involves inhibitory signals from the PVN to the vagal taste centers in the nucleus of the tractus solitarius. There may also be a feedback loop between the LH and these same taste/pleasure centers which accounts for the reward system associated with bar-pressing for electrical current delivered into the LH. These relationships are diagrammed schematically in Fig. 5.

The second mechanism for initiating a meal is a dip in serum glucose concentration. A transient decline of 15% in glucose and a return to normal is followed within a short time by the onset of a meal. The mechanism for the fall in glucose may be a brief rise in insulin and the ensuing fall in hepatic glucose production. This transient fall in glucose may be similar to the effect from injecting 2-DG, with its attendant decrease in glucose availability, within the cell because of

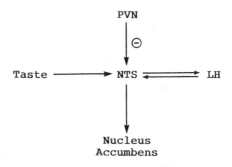

Fig. 5. Regulation of palatability factors. Taste provides information about food to the nucleus of the tractus solitarius (NTS). The positive input from this area can serve as a positive stimulus for activation of the lateral hypothalamus (LH). The paraventricular nucleus (PVN) acts as a tonic inhibitory influence on the NTS, thus limiting the effect of positive taste stimuli on feedings. There is also feedback from the NTS to the nucleus accumbens, which is activated by taste and which can be activated by electrical stimulation of the LH. It is this latter circuit which accounts for the self-stimulation of rats with electrodes in the LH.

competition for glucose metabolism. This sequence of events, along with the observation that insulin may directly act on the VMH to reduce sympathetic activity, is presented diagrammatically in Fig. 6.

Decreased oxidation of fatty acids in the liver will also enhance the likelihood of eating.

There are also several afferent signals which inhibit single meals. These include sensory factors related to aversive events, such as the sighting of a much larger animal than oneself or the presence of aversive odors or tastes. It is also clear that high glucose concentrations in the portal vein or duodenum can inhibit feeding, probably by a vagally mediated mechanism which is the reverse of that shown in Fig. 6. The release of CCK from the gastrointestinal tract and possibly other gastrointestinal peptides (e.g., bombesin or glucagon) also act on vagal mechanisms in the gut, the liver, or elsewhere in the subdiaphragmatic, vagally innervated area to generate afferent signals which can inhibit feeding. This too is presented in diagrammatic form in Fig. 7. Increased fatty acid oxidation by the liver may also be associated with a decrease in feeding. It is thus clear that changes in metabolism of both glucose and fatty acids provide afferent signals to initiate and inhibit feeding. This is consistent with the hypothesis that individual nutrients and their metabolism may be regulated separately in the control of nutrient balance. In reviewing the data on experimental models of obesity, we conclude that the afferent signals appear to be intact.

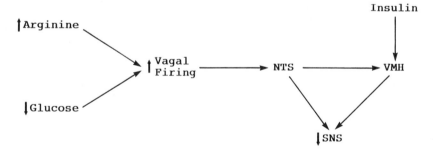

FIG. 6. Effects of glucoprivation on the sympathetic nervous system (SNS). Either lowered glucose or increased arginine will enhance the vagal firing rate of hepatic vagal afferents. These afferent fibers travel to the sensory part of the vagus (nucleus of the tractus solitarius [NTS]) and then can reduce activity of the SNS by acting directly on sympathetic pathways (see Fig. 2A and B) or indirectly through reducing the tonic effect of the ventromedial hypothalamus (VMH) on sympathetic activity. Insulin in this diagram is depicted as acting on the VMH to reduce the activity of the SNS.

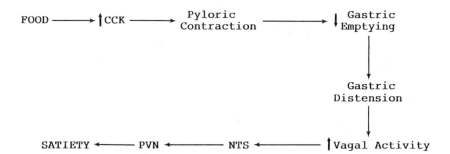

FIG. 7. Potential mechanisms for satiety induced by cholecystokinin (CCK). Food increases CCK release, which produces pyloric contraction and thus delays gastric emptying. The delayed gastric emptying increases tonic gastric distension and thus vagal activity. The increased afferent vagal activity is transmitted to the vagal afferent nucleus of the tractus solitarius (NTS) and thence to the paraventricular nucleus (PVN), which may be involved in the satiety.

2. *The Controller*

The controller for modulating food intake and nutrient stores involves the hypothalamus and other regions of the brain reviewed earlier. From a mechanistic point of view, this controller can be divided into a series of sensing elements, which transduce metabolic and neural messages, and into efferent signals involved with the selection of food and the peripheral modulation of neural and hormonal messages. The importance of altered neuronal activity in the medial hypothalamus for the development of obesity has been clearly demonstrated by several studies: (1) neuronal damage in the VMH with kanic acid or gold thioglucose produces obesity, (2) the infusion of norepinephrine into the VMH produces obesity, and (3) the intermittent injection of neuropeptide Y, a potent stimulator of feeding, will produce obesity. Of interest is the fact that infusion of norepinephrine into the PVN does not produce obesity.

The sensors or transducers directly and/or indirectly through neurally transmitted signals appear to respond to afferent information about glucose, fatty acid, and amino acid metabolism. Although amino acids have not been a focus of this review, it is quite clear that serotonin metabolism is one of the regulators of body fat stores. The existence of a central glucose-sensing system is suggested by several lines of evidence. Oomura and colleague (1969) have identified so-called glucosensitive neurons in the VMH whose discharge rate is accelerated by increasing the local concentration of glucose. Sakaguchi and Bray (1987b) have shown that injections of glucose into this region stimulate sympathetic outflow. 2-DG, which inhibits glucose utilization, increases food intake and decreases sympathetic activity. A failure of the glucoregulatory sensing system is postulated to be one mechanism for development of obesity. One formulation for the effects of 2-DG and glucoprivation is shown in Fig. 8. The glucoreceptive elements may well be in the hind brain (medulla), since 2-DG applied directly to the VMH is without effect. GABA appears to be involved at the level of the VMH since feeding is inhibited by drugs that block GABA receptors in the VMH (e.g., picrotoxin and bicucculine).

The development of obesity in animals fed a high-diet appears to involve a failure of the sensing systems for fatty acids or their metabolites to respond with adequate stimulation of the sympathetic nervous system. Oku *et al.,* (1984b) demonstrated that knife cuts in the parasaggital region at the hypothalamus were associated with the development of hyperphagia and obesity in animals normally resistant to dietary fat-induced obesity. This is schematically shown in Fig. 9.

3. *Efferent Signals*

In contrast with the impairment of the systems to transduce afferent information about nutrient status in obese animals, the efferent systems appear to be intact in all experimental models of obesity. Stimulation of the VMH in rats with genetic obesity increases sympathetic activity. From the studies on adrenalectomy, it is clear that the mechanisms for food seeking and visceral autonomic activity remain functional in all models of obesity and that, in the absence of

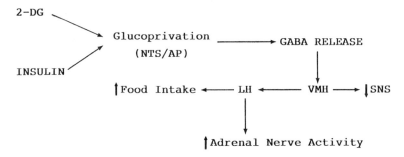

FIG. 8. Pathways through which glucoprivation may affect food intake and the sympathetic nervous system (SNS). Either 2-deoxy-D-glucose (2-DG) or insulin can initiate glucose deprivation, which may activate glucose-responsive systems in the nucleus of the tractus solitarius (NTS) or area postrema (AP). It is postulated that this increases the release of γ-aminobutyric acid (GABA), which interacts with receptors in the ventromedial hypothalamus (VMH) to reduce sympathetic activity and through fiber tracts in the lateral hypothalamus (LH) to increase food intake and adrenal nerve activity.

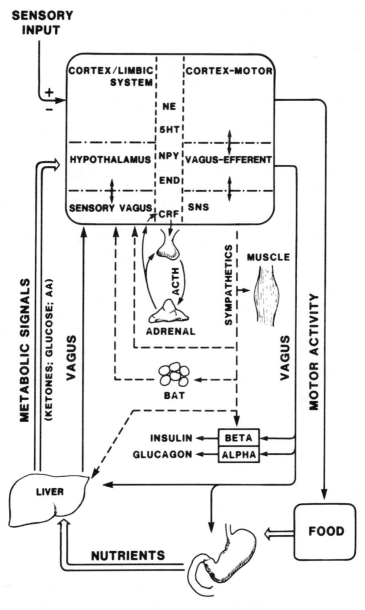

F IG. 9. Model of the feedback system. The same components are shown as in Fig. 1 except that the elements have been specified in more detail. The afferent signals consist of nutrients and vagal and sympathetic nervous inputs. The controller has been divided into the receivers (left), transduction messengers (middle), and efferent signal generators (right). The efferent components are the motor activity associated with food intake adrenal steroids, disturbance of the sensing or transducing mechanisms will not produce obesity. The one exception may be the failure of adrenalectomy to completely prevent the obesity induced by a high-fat diet. Food intake and sympathetic activity also revert to normal following adrenalectomy in the genetically transmitted forms of obesity, in animals with hypothalamic obesity, and in most animals with dietary obesity, indicating that neither the efferent food intake nor the efferent sympathetic systems are primarily deranged.

4. The Controlled System

Three elements of the controlled system also appear to modulate food intake. The first is exercise. It is clear that chronic levels of exercise can influence total overall metabolism and total fat stores. Second, food deprivation is associated with increased hunger. Experimental data suggest that the deprivation signal may be reflected by decreased activity of the sympathetic nervous system which, in turn, is a predictor of increased food intake. Similarly, acute changes in food intake, upward with overfeeding, also appear to activate compensatory systems which decrease food intake, and these may be associated with decreased sympathetic activity. However, chronic slow increases in fat stores do not appear to generate signals of sufficient magnitude for reducing their storage capacity.

B. HOMEOSTATIC MECHANISMS

1. The Autonomic Hypothesis

a. Sympathetic Activity. Ten years ago we proposed an autonomic hypothesis as an explanation for obesity caused by hypothalamic lesions. During the ensuing decade, many facets of this hypothesis have been examined, and the hypothesis stands buttressed by additional studies. Specifically, the essential role for reduced activity of thermogenic components of the sympathetic nervous system in the pathogenesis of obesity has been more firmly established. From the tentative proposal of reduced sympathetic activity 10 years ago, we would

---

and the sympathetic and vagal controls of metabolism. The controlled system represents the intake, digestion, storage, and metabolism of nutrients. The adrenal–pituitary corticotropin-releasing factor (CRF) system represents a key element of this system which modulates the operation of the other components. NE, Norepinephrine; 5-HT, 5-hydroxytryptamine; NPY, neuropeptide Y; END, endorphin; SNS, sympathetic nervous system; AA, amino acids; ACTH, adrenocorticotropic hormone; BAT, brown adipose tissue.

now conclude that a relative or absolute reduction in activity of the thermogenic component(s) of the sympathetic nervous system is the sine qua non for obesity. The data for reduced sympathetic activity have been reviewed for each model in Fig. 9. Obesity ensues upon reduction of sympathetic nervous system activity through impaired sensing or transduction of afferent signals.

Two important elements in the control of the thermogenic sympathetic nervous system deserve note. First, the VMH nucleus serves as a tonic stimulatory system for activating the sympathetic nervous system. Stimulation of the VMH increases sympathetic activity to BAT, whereas destruction of the VMH lowers the sympathetic electrical firing rate. Second, stimulation of the LH area inhibits the sympathetic nervous system and lesions of the LH area activate the sympathetic nervous system since the midbrain sympathetic structures through which the VMH acts are also innervated more by fibers from the LH area. This reciprocal control provides the potential for even greater changes in sympathetic thermogenic activity if the VMH is stimulated at the same time that the LH is lesioned, and vice versa.

The PVN, on the other hand, appears to have little effect on the autonomic nervous system. Stimulation of the PVN does not increase sympathetic activity, nor does lesion in this region reduce the sympathetic firing rate or increase insulin secretion secondary to the loss of tonic vagal inhibition.

b. The Vagal System. Ten years ago we viewed the increased activity of the vagus as the principal change in the autonomic nervous system. From the work reviewed above, increase vagal activity in VMH-lesioned rats may account for 40–50% of the syndrome. Vagal activity is also increased in rats treated with bipiperidyl mustard and in the genetically obese fatty rat. However, vagal activity shows little or no change after PVN lesions or hypothalamic islands or in animals with dietary obesity. It is in these groups of animals that insulin levels are essentially normal.

2. Adrenal Dependence of Obesity

Nearly 10 years ago we suggested that adrenal corticosteroids might be essential for the expression of genetically transmitted forms of obesity. We would now expand that hypothesis, based on data accumulated during the past decade, to argue that all obesities are dependent on minimal levels of adrenal glucocorticoids. Adrenalectomy prevents the further progression of all forms of recessively inherited obesity in animals eating a high-carbohydrate diet. This appears to be true for the fatty rat, the corpulent rat, the diabetes mouse, the obese mouse, and the yellow mouse. The yellow mouse is of particular interest because its obesity may be a reflection of disturbed acetylation of peptides in the pituitary, with the deacetylated form of MSH enhancing the adrenal secretion of corticosterone. The role of acetylation in modifying the activity of MSH and β-endorphin is shown in Fig. 10. Removal of the adrenal in the yellow mouse would thus prevent manifestations of the obesity associated with increased corticosterone secretion from the adrenal.

Ovariectomy produces obesity in female rats, and this is also reversed by adrenalectomy. The hypothalamic obesities associated with electrolytic lesions in the VMN, in the PVN, after parasaggital knife cuts, or after injection of gold thioglucose are all reversed by adrenalectomy. The effect of a high-fat diet, on the other hand, is only partially prevented by adrenalectomy. This observation suggests that the transfer of fat from dietary triglycerides into adipose tissue triglycerides is a process which is only partially influenced by adrenal steroids.

Adrenal glucocorticoids (i.e., corticosterone and related steroids) might affect the development of obesity by one of two general mechanisms. The first of these involves the effects of corticosteroids in the feedback system for the regulation of adrenal secretion. This feedback system involves the secretion of CRF from the PVN into the hypothalamic pituitary portal system, with secretion of ACTH from the pitui-

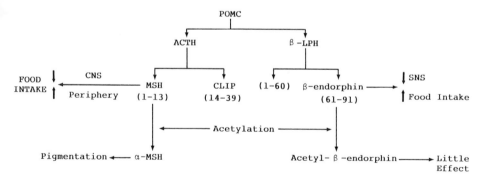

FIG. 10. Acetylation modifies action of opioid peptides. Proopiomelanocortin (POMC) is the precursor for several pituitary and hypothalamic peptides. During posttranslational processing, desacetyl-MSH is acetylated, with major changes in properties, including reduced effects on food intake and increased melanocyte activity. Acetylation of β-endorphin, on the other hand, eliminates effects on food intake. ACTH, Adrenocorticotropin; β-LPH, β-lipotropin; CNS, central nervous system; MSH, melanocyte-stimulating hormone; CLIP, corticotropinlike intermediate lobe peptide; SNS, sympathetic nervous system.

tary (Fig. 11). Corticosterone secretion from the adrenal rises, reflecting the increased level of circulating ACTH and feeds back on the central nervous system to suppress the secretion of CRF in a negative feedback manner. Removal of the adrenal gland lowers corticosterone levels and leads to an increase in CRF production in the hypothalamus. Studies by Sawchenko and colleagues (1984) have shown that CRF is distributed in three major systems. The first is in the PVN, concerned with control of ACTH secretion. CRF is also distributed along the efferent systems concerned with the LH, the periaqueductal gray, and the vagal system. Thus, increased amounts of CRF produced within the PVN by the removal of corticosterone might be secreted into the ventricular system and act at a more distal site in the food intake/sympathetic nervous system. It has been demonstrated that CRF is a potent inhibitor of food intake and that, with chronic treatment, body weight is reduced although food intake is depressed only slightly. These observations suggest that CRF might act both to inhibit food intake and to modulate sympathetic activity in the manner observed following adrenalectomy in species where it has been measured.

A second hypothesis for the effect of adrenalectomy is based on the work of Leibowitz (1986). Microinjection of norepinephrine into the PVN enhances food intake by interacting with α_2 receptors. Adrenalectomy reduces the concentration of α_2 receptors in the PVN and attenuates the effect of norepinephrine as a stimulator of feeding. The only difficulty with this mechanism for reversal of hypothalamic obesity is that adrenalectomy also reverses obesity resulting from

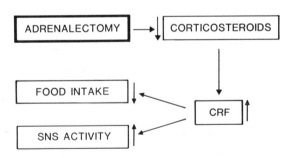

FIG. 11. Model of the effects of adrenalectomy in the control of sympathetic nervous system (SNS) activity and food intake. The central factor in this system is corticotropin-releasing factor (CRF), which can modulate the reciprocal changes in food intake and sympathetic activity.

damage to the PVN. Thus, changes in responsiveness of the PVN alone cannot explain the reversal of obesity by adrenalectomy when the PVN has been destroyed to produce the obesity.

A third proposal is that effects of glucocorticoids might be achieved through modulation of glucose transport. As already noted, glucose appears to be important in the systems which sense or monitor nutrient needs and status. Varying levels of corticosterone might modulate this system and thus modulate the responsiveness to other signals.

3. Hyperphagia

Almost all types of obesity are associated with increased food intake or hyperphagia. This hyperphagia, however, is usually not "essential" for the manifestation of obesity. Moreover, the hyperphagia may be dependent on the diet. Figure 12 shows the relative magnitude of dietary dependence and essentiality of hyperphagia in the development of several types of obesity.

Hypothalamic damage can produce obesity by one of two mechanisms. First, it may primarily increase food intake. Second, it may disturb energy balance by disrupting the autonomic nervous system. After damage to the PVN, hyperphagia is essential for the development of obesity in adult animals. Animals with parasaggital knife cuts, lesions in the ventral noradrenergic bundle, and hypothalamic

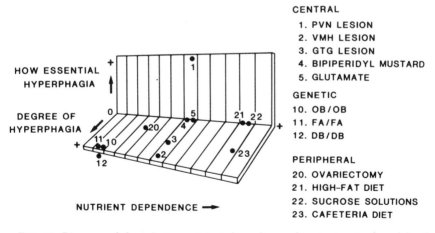

CENTRAL
1. PVN LESION
2. VMH LESION
3. GTG LESION
4. BIPIPERIDYL MUSTARD
5. GLUTAMATE

GENETIC
10. OB/OB
11. FA/FA
12. DB/DB

PERIPHERAL
20. OVARIECTOMY
21. HIGH–FAT DIET
22. SUCROSE SOLUTIONS
23. CAFETERIA DIET

FIG. 12. Diagram of the relative nutrient dependence of various animal models of obesity. Also shown are the dependence and presence of these models of hyperphagia for the appearance of obesity. PVN, Paraventricular nucleus; VMH, ventromedial hypothalamus; GTG, gold thioglucose; OB, obese; FA, fatty; DB, diabetic.

islands may also be in this category. Restriction of food intake in rats with PVN lesions will prevent the appearance of obesity or its manifestations and may do so in these other groups.

Sclafani and Kirchgessner (1986a) have presented evidence to suggest that the PVN may inhibit the nucleus of the tractus solitarious and thus serve to modulate feeding through a negative feedback system. The dietary types of obesity are obviously highly dependent on diet. Upon withdrawal of the high-fat, high-sucrose, or cafeteria diets, the animals return to normal weight. For the genetic types of obesity, on the other hand, obesity will develop in all, regardless of diet. In contrast, diet is of some importance in rats with medial hypothalamic lesions.

In obesity without hyperphagia, e.g., in weanling rats, the changes in the autonomic nervous system provide the principal mechanism for the development of obesity. The degree of obesity in those animals without hyperphagia is smaller than in animals with hyperphagia. The hyperphagia probably results from damage to fiber tracts originating in the PVN which modulate feeding behavior (see Fig. 5). In the absence of hyperphagia, however, obesity is usually associated with stunting of body size and hyperinsulinemia, and there may be a decline in body temperature.

4. *Sympathetic Nervous System*

The activity of the sympathetic nervous system appears to play an important, if not a pivotal, role in the development of experimental forms of obesity. Table IX shows some of the relationships between physiological variables and the sympathetic nervous system. An intriguing aspect is the inverse relationship between food intake and sympathetic activity in a variety of experimental settings. One of these is shown in Fig. 13. The basal firing rate of sympathetic nerves to BAT is plotted against the food intake in the preceding 4-hour period. This significant inverse relationship has been repeated in other experimental paradigms, suggesting that there may be a feedback relationship between sympathetic nervous system activity and BAT and food intake. At first, this appears to contradict the observations by Young and Landsberg (1977), who reported that starvation reduces sympathetic activity. These observations may be entirely consistent, however, if the level of sympathetic activity is a predictor of future food intake. Upon restoration of food to the starved animal, the initial meal is larger than usual, which is the prediction that would follow from the low level of sympathetic activity.

TABLE IX
FACTORS AFFECTING SYMPATHETIC ACTIVITY

Physiological variable	Sympathetic activity[a]		
	Low	Normal	High
Hypothalamic lesion	VMH	PVN	LH
Food intake (quality)	High fat diet	Mixed diet	High carbohydrate diet
Food intake (quantity)	Fasting	Average	Overeating
Genetic obesity	*fa/fa*	+/?	
	ob/ob	+/?	
	db/db	+/?	
Corticosterone level	High		Low (ADX)
Temperature	Hot	Neutral	Cold
Lactation	Lactating		

[a] VMH, Ventromedial hypothalamus; PVN, paraventricular nucleus; LH, lateral hypothalamus; *fa*, fatty; *ob*, obese; *db*, diabetic; ADX, adrenalectomy.

There are at least two mechanisms by which a change in the tonic level of sympathetic activity might influence food intake. The first is through changes in the release of free fatty acids from adipose tissue and the resulting increase in ketone levels. This might also be aided by the reduction in insulin secretion resulting from increased tonic sympathetic activity on the β cell of the islets of Langerhans. A second mechanism, also involving the sympathetic nervous system and adipose tissue, is the release of adenosine which accompanies lipolysis. Adenosine can act as an inhibitor of lipolysis directly, but can also act at a distance to reduce food intake. These concepts are presented schematically in Fig. 14.

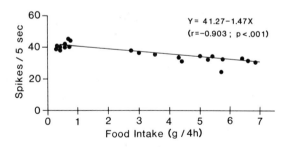

FIG. 13. Correlation between the firing rate of sympathetic nerves to brown adipose tissue and food intake. There is a highly significant negative correlation between the firing rate and sympathetic activity ($r = 0.903$; $p < 0.001$).

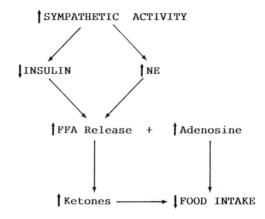

FIG. 14. Model for the effects of sympathetic activity on food intake. Increased levels of sympathetic activity would be expected to reduce insulin and increase norepinephrine (NE) levels. Collectively, these changes would increase lipolysis, which would release adenosine and free fatty acids (FFA). Ketone production in the liver is partially under substrate control, and an increased supply of fatty acids could increase ketone production. Both increased ketones and increased adenosine might be the signals to reduce food intake.

5. *Lipoprotein Lipase*

Lipoprotein lipase is a key enzyme involved in the mobilization from circulating lipoproteins of fatty acids prior to their entry into fat cells for storage as triglycerides. This enzyme thus acts as a gatekeeper for fat storage. It is elevated in genetic and hypothalamic forms of obesity, but not in dietary obesity. The obesities in which lipoprotein lipase is elevated are also those which have high levels of insulin and low levels of sympathetic activity. It may thus be that the high levels of lipoprotein lipase are reflecting the low levels of sympathetic activity along with the increased insulin levels. The recent report that adipsin, a serine protease which is synthesized in and secreted from adipocytes, is low in genetic and hypothalamic obesities may be consistent with this concept. If adipsin is viewed as a protease which cleaves lipoprotein lipase from its attachments to the endothelium, then low levels of sympathetic activity and high levels of insulin, states in which lipoprotein lipase is secreted, would be those in which adipsin would need to be reduced. Thus, adipsin levels may be inversely related to those of lipoprotein lipase through similar mechanisms of control, i.e., the sympathetic nervous system and insulin.

6. *Hyperinsulinemia*

Increased circulating insulin concentrations are prominent features of hypothalamic and genetic obesities, but are less apparent in animals with dietary obesity. In animals with hypothalamic forms of obesity, many of the features of these animals can be attributed to the high levels of insulin, and a similar conclusion is appropriate for the genetic forms of obesity. The mechanism for this increased insulin secretion has never been fully explained. Certainly the increased activity of the vagus nerve and the reduced activity of the sympathetic nerves may play a role. In addition, hypothalamic and pituitary factors have been identified which can stimulate insulin secretion. One of these factors, called β-cell tropin, is the product of the removal of two amino acids from CLIP (Fig. 10). This factor has been identified in genetically obese mice and in mice which become obese after treatment with gold thioglucose. Since proopiomelanocortin, the precursor molecule for CLIP, is found in both the pituitary and the hypothalamus, it is conceivable that the agents which stimulate the β cell from the pituitary and the hypothalamus are the same molecule. Since they are small peptides that might be acetylated (Fig. 10), this may be an important mechanism in their control. Increased CLIP and β-cell tropin production in genetic and hypothalamic forms of obesity would parallel the increased ACTH secretion needed to stimulate the adrenal gland to make the increased corticosteroids upon which obesity depends (see Section V,B,2). Thus, increased β-cell tropin secretion along with deranged function of the autonomic nervous system may provide the two mechanisms involved in the hyperinsulinemia of experimental obesity.

C. CONCLUDING REMARKS

From this review of the changes in the various components of the homeostatic model for the regulation of body fat, we would propose that the following are the essential elements of the controller, the afferent and efferent limbs, and the controlled system associated with the development of obesity. Although somewhat dogmatic, they reflect the sense and the direction of the data set forth in this review. Like all hypotheses, they are no better than the experimental work which they initiate.

1. Almost all experimental obesities result from derangements of the sensory elements of the controller.

2. Destruction of the VMH decreases the direct drive to the sympathetic nervous system, impairs growth hormone secretion, and removes inhibition from the vagus nerve.

3. Destruction of the PVN, parasaggital knife cuts, and lesions of the ventral noradrenergic bundle increase hyperphagia, possibly by removing inhibitory input to the vagal sensory nucleus (nucleus of the tractus solitarius). The autonomic nervous system is little impaired after these lesions.

4. Electrical stimulation of the LH produces hyperphagia and obesity.

5. All experimental obesity results from an absolute or relative decrease in the nutrient-stimulated activity of the thermogenic components of the sympathetic nervous system.

6. Defective nutrient-stimulated activation of the thermogenic sympathetic nervous system can result from abnormalities in a number of afferent sensing systems.

7. The thermogenic component of sympathetic activity is tonically activated by the VMH and is inhibited by the LH area, converging on common sympathetic pathways in the reticular formation.

8. The capacity of the sympathetic nervous system to stimulate thermogenesis appears to be intact in all experimental forms of obesity because it can be activated by cold, electrical stimulation, chemical infusion into the ventricular system, or adrenalectomy.

9. Sympathetic activity is inversely related to the adrenal corticosteroid level.

10. Sympathetic activity may serve as a feedback inhibitor of food intake as well as an activator of peripheral thermogenic mechanisms.

11. Vagal efferent activity is increased in some forms of experimental obesity and may be involved in the basal hyperinsulinemia as well as the exaggerated response of insulin to meals.

12. Basal hyperinsulinemia occurs in some forms of experimental obesity and, although not essential for development of obesity, may provide an explanation for many of the changes in some of the experimental models.

13. Most of the changes in the controlled system result from relative or absolute reduction in the thermogenic sympathetic nervous system or from hyperinsulinemia.

ACKNOWLEDGMENT

Supported in part by National Institutes of Health Grants DK 32018 and DK 31988.

REFERENCES

Abumrad, N. A., Stearns, S. B., Tepperman, H. M., and Tepperman, J. (1978). Studies on serum lipids, insulin, and glucagon and on muscle triglyceride in rats adapted to high-fat and high-carbohydrate diets. *J. Lipid Res.* **19**, 423–432.

Agardh, C.-D., Lesniak, M. A., Gerritsen, G. C., and Roth, J. (1986). The influence of plasma insulin on tissue insulin levels in rodents: A study of the diabetic hamster and the ob/ob mouse. *Metab., Clin. Exp.* **35**, 244–249.

Ahlskog, J. E., and Hoebel, B. G. (1973). Overeating and obesity from damage to a noradrenergic system in the brain. *Science* **182**, 166–169.

Ahlskog, J. E., Randall, P. K., and Hoebel, B. G. (1975). Hypothalamic hyperphagia: Dissociation from hyperphagia following destruction of noradrenergic neurons. *Science* **190**, 399–401.

Allars, J., and York, D. A. (1986). The effects of 2-deoxy-D-glucose on brown adipose tissue of lean and obese Zucker rats. *Int. J. Obes.* **10**, 147–158.

Allars, J., Holt, S. J., and York, D. A. (1987). Energetic efficiency and brown adipose tissue uncoupling protein of obese Zucker rats fed high carbohydrate and high fat diets: Effect of adrenalectomy. *Int. J. Obes.* **11**, 591–602.

Anderson, G. H., Leprohon, C., Chambers, J. W., and Coscina, D. V. (1979). Intact regulation of protein intake during the development of hypothalamic or genetic obesity in rats. *Physiol. Behav.* **23**, 751–755.

Antin, J., Gibbs, J., Holt, J., Young, R. C., and Smith, G. P. (1975). Cholecystokinin elicits the complete behavioral sequence of satiety in rats. *J. Comp. Physiol. Psychol.* **89**, 784–790.

Apfelbaum, M., and Mandenoff, A. (1981). Naltrexone suppresses hyperphagia induced by a highly palatable diet. *Pharmacol., Biochem. Behav.* **15**, 89–92.

Applegate, E. A., Upton, D. E., and Stern, J. S. (1984). Exercise and detraining: Effect on food intake, adiposity and lipogenesis in Osborne–Mendel rats made obese by a high fat diet. *J. Nutr.* **114**, 447–459.

Arase, K., Sakata, T., Oomura, Y., Fukushima, M., Fujimoto, K., and Terada, K. (1984). Short-chain polyhydroxymonocarboxylic acids as physiological signals for food intake. *Physiol. Behav.* **33**, 261–267.

Arase, K., Sakaguchi, T., Takahashi, M., Bray, G. A., and Ling, N. (1987). Effects on feeding-behavior of rats of a cryptic peptide from the C-terminal end of prepro-growth hormone-releasing factor. *Endocrinology (Baltimore)* **121**, 1960–1065.

Arase, K., Fisler, J. S., Shargill, N. S., York, D. A., and Bray, G. A. (1988a). Intracerebroventricular infusion of 3-OHB and insulin in a rat model of dietary obesity. *Am. J. Physiol.* **255**, R974–R981.

Arase, K., York, D. A., Shimizu, H., Shargill, N., and Bray, G. A. (1988b). Effects of corticotropin releasing factor on food intake and brown adipose tissue thermogenesis in rats. *Am. J. Physiol.* **255**, E255–E259.

Arase, K., Shargill, N., and Bray, G. A. (1989a). Effects of corticotropin releasing factor on genetically obese (fatty) rats. *Physiol. Behav.* **45**, 1–6.

Arase, K., Shargill, N., and Bray, G. A. (1989b). Effects of intraventricular infusion of corticotropin-releasing factor on VMH-lesioned obese rats. *Am. J. Physiol.* **256**, R751–R756.

Aravich, P. F., and Sclafani, A. (1983). Paraventricular hypothalamic lesions and medial hypothalamic knife cuts produce similar hyperphagia syndromes. *Behav. Neurosci.* **97**, 970–983.

Armitage, G., Hervey, G. R., Rolls, B. J., Rowe, E. A., and Tobin, G. (1983). The effects of supplementation of the diet with highly palatable foods upon energy balance in the rat. J. Physiol. (London) 342, 299–251.

Armitage, G., Harris, R. B., Harvey, G. R., and Tobin, G. (1984). The relationship between energy expenditure and environmental temperature in congenitally obese and non-obese Zucker rats. J. Physiol. (London) 350, 197–207.

Ashwell, M. A., and Dunnett, S. B. (1985). Fluorescent histochemical demonstration of catecholamines in brown adipose tissue from obese (ob/ob) and lean mice acclimated at different temperatures. J. Auton. Nerv. Syst. 14, 377–386.

Ashwell, M. A., Meade, C. J., Medawar, P., and Sowler, C. (1977). Adipose tissue: Contributions of nature and nurture to the obesity of an obese mutant mouse (ob/ob). Proc. R. Soc. London, Ser. B 195, 343–353.

Ashwell, M. A., Holts, S., Jennings, G., Stirling, D., Trayhurn, P., and York, D. A. (1985). Measurements by radioimmunoassay of the mitochondrial uncoupling protein from brown adipose tissue of obese (ob/ob) mice and Zucker (fa/fa) rats at different ages. FEBS Lett. 179, 233–237.

Ashwell, M. A., Wells, C., and Dunnett, S. B. (1986). Brown adipose tissue: Contributions of nature and nurture to the obesity of an obese mutant mouse (ob/ob). Int. J. Obes. 10, 355–373.

Atkinson, R. L., and Brent, E. L. (1982). Appetite suppressant activity in plasma of rats after intestinal bypass surgery. Am. J. Physiol. 243, R60–R64.

Aubert, R., Herzog, J., Camus, M.-C., Guenet, J.-L., and Lemonnier, D. (1985). Description of a new model of genetic obesity: The db^{Pas} mouse. J. Nutr. 115, 327–333.

Babinski, M. J. (1900). Tumeur du corps pituitaire sans acronmegalie et avec de dévelopement des organes génitaux. Rev. Neurol. 8, 531–533.

Bach, A. C., and Babayan, V. K. (1982). Medium-chain triglycerides: An update. Am. J. Clin. Nutr. 36, 950–962.

Bach, A. C., Phan, T., and Metais, P. (1976). Effect of fatty acid composition of ingested fats on rat liver intermediary metabolism. Horm. Metab. Res. 8, 375–379.

Bach, A. C., Schirardin, H., Bauer, M., and Weryha, A. (1977). Ketogenic response to a medium-chain triglyceride load in the rat. J. Nutr. 107, 1863–1870.

Baetins, D., Stefan, Y., Ravazzok, M., Malaise-lagase, F., Coleman, D., and Occi, L. (1978). Alteration of islet cell populations in spontaneously diabetic mice. Diabetes 27, 1–7.

Baile, C. A., Zinn, W., and Mayer, J. (1971). Feeding behavior of monkeys: Glucose utilization rate and site of glucose entry. Physiol. Behav. 6, 537–541.

Baile, C. A., McLaughlin, C. L., and Della-Fera, M. A. (1986). Role of cholecystokinin and opioid peptides in control of food intake. Physiol. Rev. 66, 172–234.

Bailey, C. J., and Flatt, P. R. (1987). Increased responsiveness to glucoregulatory effect of opiates in obese-diabetic ob/ob mice. Diabetologia 30, 33–37.

Bailey, C. J., Thornburn, C. C., and Flatt, P. R. (1986). Effects of ephedrine and atenolol on the development of obesity and diabetes in ob/ob mice. Gen. Pharmacol. 17, 243–246.

Barber, T., Vina, J. R., Vina, J., and Cabo, J. (1985). Decreased urea synthesis in cafeteria-diet-induced obesity in the rat. Biochem. J. 230, 675–681.

Bartness, T. J., Bittman, E. L., and Wade, G. N. (1985). Paraventricular nucleus lesions exaggerate dietary obesity but block photoperiod-induced weight gains and suspension of estrous cyclicity in Syrian hamsters. Brain Res. Bull. 14, 427–430.

Bauer, F. S. (1972). The role of affect in hypothalamic hyperphagia. Diss. Abstr. Int. B 32, 6067.

Bazin, R., Eteve, D., and Lavau, M. (1984). Evidence for decreased GDP binding to brown-adipose-tissue mitochondria of obese Zucker (fa/fa) rats in the very first days of life. *Biochem. J.* **221**, 241–245.

Bellin, S. I., and Ritter, S. (1981). Insulin-induced elevation of hypothalamic norepinephrine turnover persists after glucorestoration unless feeding occurs. *Brain Res.* **217**, 327–337.

Bellinger, L. L., Bernardis, L. L., and Williams, F. E. (1983). Naloxone suppression of food and water intake and cholecystokinin reduction of feeding is attenuated in weanling rats with dorsomedial hypothalamic lesions. *Physiol. Behav.* **31**, 839–846.

Bellinger, L. L., Mendel, V. E., Williams, F. E., and Castonguay, T. W. (1984). The effect of liver denervation on meal patterns, body weight and body composition of rats. *Physiol Behav.* **33**, *661–667.*

Beloff-Chain, A., Morton, A., and Dunmore, S. (1983). Evidence that B-cell tropin is ACTH. *Nature (London)* **301**, 255–258.

Bereiter, D. A., and Jeanrenaud, B. (1979). Altered neuroanatomical organization in the central nervous system of the genetically obese (ob/ob) mouse. *Brain Res.* **165**, 249–260.

Bereiter, D. A., and Jeanrenaud, B. (1980). Altered dendritic orientation of hypothalamic neurons from genetically obese (ob/ob) mice. *Brain Res.* **202**, 201–206.

Bernardis, L. L. (1985a). Body weight and fat regulatory "centers" in the medial hypothalamus of the weanling rat: Neurovisceral, neuroendocrine, metabolic, and anatomical correlates of ventromedial and dorsomedial hypothalamic lesions. *J. Obes. Weight Regul.* **4**, 61–86.

Bernardis, L. L. (1985b). Ventromedial and dorsomedial hypothalamic syndrome in the weanling rat: Is the "center" concept really outmoded? *Brain Res. Bull.* **14**, 537–549.

Bernardis, L. L., and Bellinger, L. L. (1986a). The dorsomedial hypothalamic nucleus revisited: 1986 update. *Brain Res.* **434**, 321–381.

Bernardis, L. L., and Bellinger, L. L. (1986b). Effect of palatable diet on growth, caloric intake and endocrine-metabolic profile in weanling rats with dorsomedial hypothalamic lesions. *Appetite (London)* 7, 219–230.

Bernstein, L. L., and Goehler, L. E. (1983). Vagotomy produces learned food aversions in the rat. *Behav. Neurosci.* **97**, 585–594.

Bernstein, R. S., Merville, M. D., Marshall, M. C., and Carney, A. L. (1977). Effects of dietary composition on adipose tissue hexokenase II and glucose utilization normal and streptozotocin-diabetic rats. *Diabetes* 26, 770–779.

Bernz, J. A., Smith, G. P., and Gibbs, J. (1983). A comparison of the effectiveness of intraperitoneal injections of bombesin (BBS) and cholecystokinin (CCK-8) to reduce sham feeding of different sucrose solutions. *Proc. East. Psychol. Assoc.* p. 95.

Berthoud, H.-R., and Jeanrenaud, B. (1979a). Acute hyperinsulinemia and its reversal by vagotomy after lesions of the ventromedial hypothalamus in anesthetized rats. *Endocrinology (Baltimore)* **105**, 146–151.

Berthoud, H.-R., and Jeanrenaud, B. (1979b). Changes of insulinemia, glycemia and feeding behavior induced by VMH-procainization in the rat. *Brain Res.* **174**, 184–187.

Berthoud, H.-R., and Powley, T. E. (1985). Altered plasma insulin and glucose after obesity-producing bipiperidyl brain lesions. *Am. J. Physiol.* **248**, R46–R53.

Berthoud, H.-R., Niijima, A., Sauter, J.-F., and Jeanrenaud, B. (1983). Evidence for a role of the gastric, coeliac and hepatic branches in vagally stimulated insulin secretion in the rat. *J. Auton. Nerv. Syst.* **7**, 97–110.

Beven, T. E. (1973). "Experimental Dissociation of Hypothalamic Finickiness and Motivational Deficits from Hyperphagia and from Hyperemotionality," Univ. Microfilms, No. 74-9665. University of Michigan, Ann Arbor.

Bhakthavatsalam, P., and Leibowitz, S. F. (1986). Alpha-2-noradrenergic feeding rhythm in the paraventricular nucleus: Relation to corticosterone. *Am. J. Physiol.* **250**, R83–R88.

Billingham, N., Beloff-Chain, A., and Cawthorne, M. A. (1982). Identification of B-cell tropin, a peptide of the pituitary pars intermedia which stimulates insulin secretion in plasma from genetically obese (ob/ob) mice. *J. Endocrinol.* **94**, 125–130.

Blanco, A. C., and Silva, J. E. (1987). Intracellular conversion of thyroxine to triiodothyronine is required for the optimal thermogenic function of brown adipose tissue. *J. Clin. Invest.* **79**, 295–300.

Blazquez, E., and Quijada, C. L. (1968). The effect of a high fat diet on glucose, insulin sensitivity and plasma insulin in rats. *J. Endocrinol.* **92**, 489–494.

Blundell, J. E. (1986). Serotonin manipulations and the structure of feeding behavior. *Appetite (London)* **7**, 39–56.

Booth, D. A. (1972). Postabsorptively induced suppression of appetite and the energostatic control of feeding. *Physiol. Behav.* **9**, 199–202.

Brady, L. J., Hoppel, C. L., and Brady, P. S. (1986). Obesity, overeating, and rapid gastric-emptying in rats with ventromedial hypothalamic-lesions. *Science* **231**, 609–611.

Bray, G. A. (1974). Endocrine factors in the control of food intake. *Fed. Proc., Fed. Am. Soc. Exp. Biol.* **33**, 1140–1145.

Bray, G. A. (1982). Regulation of energy balance: Studies on genetic, hypothalamic and dietary obesity. *Proc. Nutr. Soc.* **41**, 95–108.

Bray, G. A. (1984a). Syndromes of hypothalamic obesity in man. *Pediatr. Ann.* **13**(7), 525–536.

Bray, G. A. (1984b). Hypothalamic and genetic obesity: An appraisal of the autonomic hypothesis and the endocrine hypothesis. *Int. J. Obes.* **8**, 119–137.

Bray, G. A. (1987). Obesity—A disease of nutrient or energy balance? *Nutr. Rev.* **45**, 33–43.

Bray, G. A., and Campfield, L. A. (1975). Metabolic factors in the control of energy stores. *Metab., Clin. Exp.* **24**, 99–117.

Bray, G. A., and Gallagher, T. F., Jr. (1975) Manifestations of hypothalamic obesity in man: A comprehensive investigation of eight patients and a review of the literature. *Medicine (Baltimore)* **54**, 301–330.

Bray, G. A., and Nishizawa, Y. (1978). Ventromedial hypothalamus modulates fat mobilization during fasting. *Nature (London)* **274**, 900–902.

Bray, G. A., and York, D. A. (1971). Genetically transmitted obesity in rodents. *Physiol. Rev.* **51**, 598–646.

Bray, G. A., and York, D. A. (1972). Studies on food intake of genetically obese rats. *Am. J. Physiol.* **223**(1), 176–179.

Bray, G. A., and York, D. A. (1979). Hypothalamic and genetic obesity in experimental animals: An autonomic and endocrine hypothesis. *Physiol. Rev.* **59**, 719–809.

Bray, G. A., York, D. A., and Swerdloff, R. W. (1973). Genetic obesity in rats. I. The effects of food restriction on body composition and hypothalamic function. *Metab., Clin. Exp.* **2**, 435–442.

Bray, G. A., Luong, D., and York, D. A. (1974). Regulation of adipose tissue mass in genetically obese rodents. *In* "The Regulation of Adipose Tissue Mass" (J. Vague and J. Bryer, eds.), pp. 111–121. Excerpta Medica, Amsterdam.

Bray, G. A., Lee, M., and Bray, T. (1980). Weight gain of rats fed medium-chain triglycerides is less than rats fed long-chain triglycerides. *Int. J. Obes.* **4**, 27–32.

Bray, G. A., Sclafani, A., and Novin, D. (1982a). Obesity-inducing hypothalamic knife cuts: Effects on lipolysis and blood insulin levels. *Am. J. Physiol.* **243**, R445–R449.

Bray, G. A., Shimomura, Y., Ohtake, M., and Walker, P. (1982b). Salivary gland weight and nerve growth factor in the genetically obese (ob/ob) mouse. *Endocrinology (Baltimore)* **110**, 47–50.

Bray, G. A., Teague, R. J., and Lee, C. K. (1987). Brain uptake of ketones in rats with differing susceptibility to dietary obesity. *Metab., Clin. Exp.* **36**, 27–30.

Bray, G. A., Shimizu, H., Retzias, A. D., Shargill, N. S., and York, D. A. (1989). Reduced acetylation of MSH: A biochemical explanation for the yellow obese mouse. *In* "Obesity in Europe 88" (P. Bjorntorp and S. Rossner, eds.), pp. 259–270. Libbey.

Brecher, G., and Waxler, S. H. (1949). Obesity in albino mice due to single injections of gold thioglucose. *Proc. Soc. Exp. Biol. Med.* **70**, 498–501.

Brief, D. J., and Davis, J. D. (1984). Reduction of food intake and body weight by chronic intraventricular insulin infusion. *Brain Res. Bull.* **12**, 571–575.

Brobeck, J. R. (1946). Mechanism of development of obesity in animals with hypothalamic lesions. *Physiol. Rev.* **26**, 541–559.

Brooks, C. M., Lockwood, R. A., and Wiggins, M. I. (1946). A study of the effect of hypothalamic lesions on the eating habits of the albino rat. *Am. J. Physiol.* **147**, 735–741.

Brooks, S. L., Rothwell, N. J., and Stock, M. J. (1982). Effects of diet and acute noradrenaline treatment on brown adipose tissue development and mitochondria purine-nucleotide binding. *Q. J. Exp. Physiol. Cogn. Med. Sci.* **67**, 259–268.

Brown, M. R., and Fisher, L. A. (1985). Corticotropin-releasing factor: Effects on autonomic nervous system and visceral systems. *Fed. Proc., Fed. Am. Soc. Exp. Biol.* **44**, 243–248.

Brown, M. R., Fisher, L. A., Spiess, J., Rivier, J., Rivier, C., and Vale, W. (1982). Corticotropin releasing factor: Actions on the sympathetic nervous system and metabolism. *Endocrinology (Baltimore)* **111**, 928–931.

Bruce, B. K., King, B. M., Phelps, G. R., and Veitia, M. C. (1982). Effects of adrenalectomy and corticosterone administration on hypothalamic obesity in rats. *Am. J. Physiol.* **243**, E152–E157.

Burbach, J. A., Schlenker, E. H., and Goldman, M. (1985). Characterization of muscles from aspartic acid obese rats. *Am. J. Physiol.* **249**, R106–R110.

Brunol, A.-F., Leturque, A., de Saintaurin, M.-A., Penicaud, L., and Girard, J. (1987). Glucose turnover rate in the lactating rat: Effect of feeding a high fat diet. *J. Nutr.* **117**, 1275–1279.

Cain, D. P. (1975). Effects of insulin injection on responses of olfactory bulb and amygdala single units to doors. *Brain Res.* **99**, 69–83.

Campfield, L. A., and Smith, F. J. (1983). Alteration of islet neurotransmitter sensitivity following ventromedial hypothalamic lesion. *Am. J. Physiol.* **244**, R635–R640.

Campfield, L. A., Brandon, P., and Smith, F. J. (1985). On-line continuous measurement of blood glucose and meal pattern in free-feeding rats: The role of glucose in meal initiation. *Brain Res. Bull.* **14**(6), 605–616.

Campfield, L. A., Smith, F. J., and Larue-Achagiotis, C. (1986). Temporal evolution of altered islet neurotransmitter sensitivity after VMH lesion. *Am. J. Physiol.* **251**, R63–R69.

Cannon, W. B., and Washburn, A. L. (1912). An explanation of hunger. *Am. J. Physiol.* **29**, 441–454.

Carlisle, H. J., and Dubuc, P. U. (1982). Unchanged thermoregulatory set-point in the obese mouse. *Nature (London)* **297**, 678–679.

Carlisle, H. J., and Dubuc, P. U. (1984). Temperature preference of genetically obese (ob/ob) mice. *Physiol. Behav.* **33**, 899–902.

Carlson, A. J. (1912). "The Control of Hunger in Health and Disease." Univ. of Chicago Press, Chicago, Illinois.

Carmel, N., Konijn, A. M., Kaufmann, N. A., and Guggenheim, K. (1975). Effects of carbohydrate-free diets on the insulin-carbohydrate relationships in rats. *J. Nutr.* **105**, 1141–1149.

Carpenter, R. G., and Grossman, S. P. (1983a). Reversible obesity and plasma fat metabolites. *Physiol. Behav.* **30**, 51–55.

Carpenter, R. G., and Grossman, S. P. (1983b). Early streptozotocin diabetes and hunger. *Physiol. Behav.* **31**(2), 175–178.

Carpenter, R. G., Stamoutsos, B. A., Dalton, L. D., Frohman, L. A., and Grossman, S. P. (1979). VMH obesity reduced but not reversed by scopolamine methyl nitrate. *Physiol. Behav.* **23**, 955–959.

Castonguay, T. W., and Stern, J. S. (1983). The effect of adrenalectomy on dietary component selection by the genetically obese Zucker rat. *Nutr. Rep. Int.* **28**, 725–730.

Castonguay, T. W., Upton, D. E., Leung, P. M. B., and Stern, J. S. (1982). Meal patterns in the genetically obese Zucker rat: A reexamination. *Physiol. Behav.* **28**, 911–916.

Castonguay, T. W., Burdick, S. L., Guzman, M. A., Collier, G. H., and Stern, J. S. (1984). Self-selection and the obese Zucker rat: The effect of dietary fat dilution. *Physiol. Behav.* **33**, 119–126.

Caterson, I. D., and Taylor, K. W. (1982). Islet cell function in gold thioglucose-induced obesity in mice. *Diabetologia* **23**, 119–123.

Challis, R. A. J., Budohoski, L., Newsholme, E. A., Sennitt, M. V., and Cawthorne, M. A. (1985). Effect of a novel thermogenic beta-adrenoceptor agonist (BRL 26830) on insulin resistance in soleus muscle from obese Zucker rats. *Biochem. Biophys. Res. Commun.* **128**, 928–935.

Chan, C. B., Pederson, R. A., Buchan, A. M., Tubesing, K. B., and Brown, J. C. (1984b). Gastric inhibitory polypeptide (GIP) and insulin release in the obese Zucker rat. *Diabetes* **33**, 536–542.

Chan, C. P., and Stern, J. S. (1982). Adipose lipoprotein lipase in insulin-treated diabetic lean and obese Zucker rats. *Am. J. Physiol.* **242**, E445–E450.

Chikamori, K., Nishimura, N., Suehiro, F., Sato, K., Mori, H., and Saito, S. (1980). Alterations in glucagon secretion in obese rats with hypothalamic lesions. *Horm. Metab. Res.* **12**, 47–88.

Chlouverakis, C., and Bernardis, L. L. (1972). Ventrolateral hypothalamic lesions in obese-hyperglycaemic obese mice (ob/ob). *Diabetologia* **8**, 179–184.

Chlouverakis, C., Bernardis, L. L., and Hojnicki, D. (1973). Ventromedial hypothalamic lesions in obese-hyperglycaemic mice. *Diabetologia* **9**, 391–395.

Clark, J. T., Kalra, P. S., Crawley, W. R., and Kalra, S. P. (1984). Neuropeptide Y and human pancreatic polypeptide stimulate feeding behavior in rats. *Endocrinology (Baltimore)* **115**, 427–429.

Clark, J. T., Sahu, B., Kalra, P. S., Balasubramaniam, A., and Kalra, S. P. (1987). Neuropeptide Y (NPY)-induced feeding behavior in female rats: Comparison with human NPY ((Met[17])NPY), NPY analog ((norLeu[4])NPY) and peptide YY. *Regul. Pept.* **17**, 31–39.

Cohn, C., and Joseph, D. (1959). Changes in body composition with force feeding. *Am. J. Physiol.* **196**, 965–968.

Coleman, D. L. (1978). Obese and diabetes: Two mutant genes causing diabetes—obesity syndromes in mice. *Diabetologia* **14**, 141–148.

Collier, G. H. (1985). Satiety: An ecological perspective. *Brain Res. Bull.* **14**, 693–700.

Cook, K. S., Min, H. Y., Johnson, D., Chaplinsky, R. J., Flier, J. S., Hunt, C. R., and Spiegelman, B. M. (1987). Adipsin: A circulating serine protease homolog secreted by adipose tissue and sciatic nerve. *Science* **237**, 402–405.

Corbit, J. D., and Stellar, E. (1964). Palatability, food intake and obesity in normal and hyperphagic rats. *J. Comp. Physiol. Psychol.* **58**, 63–67.

Coscina, D. V., and Nobrega, J. N. (1982). 6-Hydroxydopamine-induced blockade of hypothalamic obesity: Critical role of brain dopamine-norepinephrine interaction. *Prog. Neuro-Psychopharmacol. Biol. Psychiatry* **6**, 369–372.

Coscina, D. V., and Nobrega, J. N. (1984). Anorectic potency of inhibiting GABA transaminase in brain: Studies of hypothalamic, dietary and genetic obesities. *Int. J. Obes.* **8**, Suppl. 1, 191–200.

Coscina, D. V., Chambers, J. W. Park, I., Hogan, S., and Himms-Hagen, J. (1985). Impaired diet-induced thermogenesis in brown adipose tissue from rats made obese with parasagittal hypothalamic knife-cuts. *Brain Res. Bull.* **14**, 585–593.

Cox, J. E., and Powley, T. L. (1981). Prior vagotomy blocks VMH obesity in pair-fed rats. *Am. J. Physiol.* **240**, E573–E583.

Crawley, J. N., and Schwaber, J. S. (1984). Abolition of the behavioral effects of cholecystokinin following bilateral radiofrequency lesions of the parvocellular subdivision of the nucleus tractus solitarius. *Brain Res.* **295**, 289–299.

Crawley, J. N., and Kiss, J. Z. (1985). Paraventricular nucleus lesions abolish the inhibition of feeding induced by systemic cholecystokinin. *Peptides (N.Y.)* **6**, 927–935.

Cruce, J. A., Thoa, N., and Jacobowitz, D. M. (1976). Catecholamines in the brains of genetically obese rats. *Brain Res.* **101**, 165–170.

Cuendot, G. S., Loten, E. G., Cameron, D. P., Renold, A. E., and Marliss, E. B. (1975). Hormone substrate responses to total fasting in lean and obese mice. *Am. J. Physiol.* **228**, 276–283.

Cunningham, J. J., Calles, J., Eisikowitz, L., Zawalich, W., and Felig, P. (1983). Increased efficiency of weight gain and altered cellularity of brown adipose tissue in rats with impaired glucose tolerance during diet-induced overfeeding. *Diabetes* **32**, 1023–1027.

Cunningham, J. J., Calles-Escandon, J., Garrido, F., Carr, D. B., and Bode, H. H. (1986). Hypercorticosteronuria and diminished pituitary responsiveness to corticotropin-releasing factor in obese Zucker rats. *Endocrinology (Baltimore)* **118**, 98–101.

Curry, D. L., and Stern, J. S. (1985). Dynamics of insulin hypersection by obese Zucker rats. *Metab. Clin. Exp.* **34**, 791–796.

Dambach, G., and Friedmann, N. (1974). Substrate-induced membrane potential changes in the perfused rat liver. *Biochim. Biophys. Acta* **367**, 366–370.

Danforth, E., Horton, E. S., Sims, E. A. H., Burger, A. G., Vagenaki's, A. G., Braverman, L. E., and Ingbar, S. H. (1979). Dietary induced alterations in thyroid hormone metabolism during over nutrition. *J. Clin. Invest.* **64**, 1336–1347.

Davis, J. D., and Campbell, C. S. (1973). Peripheral control of meal size in the rat: Effect of sham feeding on meal size and drinking rate. *J. Comp. Physiol. Psychol.* **83**, 379–387.

Davis, J. D., and Collins, B. J. (1978). Distention of the small intestines, satiety and the control of food intake. *Am. J. Clin. Nutr.* **31**, Suppl. S255–S258.

Davis, J. D., Gallagher, R. J., Ladlore, R. F., and Turavasky, A. J. (1969). Food intake controlled by blood factor. *J. Comp. Physiol. Psychol.* **167**, 1107.

Davis, J. D., Wirtshafter, D., Asin, K. E., and Brief, D. (1981). Sustained intracerebroventricular infusion of brain fuels reduces body weight and food intake in rats. *Science* **212**, 81–82.

Deb, S., Martin, R. J., and Hershberger, T. V. (1976). Maintenance requirement and energetic efficiency of lean and obese Zucker rats. *J. Nutr.* **106,** 191–197.

Debons, A. F., Siclari, E., Das, K. C., and Fuhr, B. (1982). Gold thioglucose-induced hypothalamic damage, hyperphagia, and obesity: Dependence on the adrenal gland. *Endocrinology (Baltimore)* **110,** 2014–2029.

Debons, A. F., Das, K. C., Fuhr, B., and Siclari, E. (1983). Anorexia after adrenalectormy in gold thioglucose-treated obese mice. *Endocrinology (Baltimore)* **112,** 1847–1851.

Debons, A. F., Zuerk, L. D., Tse, C. S., and Abrahamsen, S. (1986). Central nervous system control of hyperphagia in hypothalamic obesity: Dependence on adrenal glucocorticoids. *Endocrinology (Baltimore)* **118,** 1678–1681.

Deutch, A. Y., and Martin, R. J. (1983). Mesencephalic dopamine modulation of pituitary and central B-endorphin: Relation to food intake regulation. *Life Sci.* **88,** 281–287.

Deutsch, J. A. (1978). The stomach in food satiation and the regulation of appetite. *Prog. Neurobiol.* **10,** 135–153.

Deutsch, J. A., and Wang, M.-L. (1977). The stomach as a site for rapid nutrient reinforcement sensors. *Science* **195,** 89–90.

Diamond, P., Brondel, L., and LeBlanc, J. (1985). Palatability and postpandrial thermogenesis in dogs. *Am. J. Physiol.* **248,** E75–E79.

Dubuc, P. U., Cahn, P. J., and Willis, P. (1984). The effects of exercise and food restriction on obesity and diabetes in young ob/ob mice. *Int. J. Obes.* **8,** 271–278.

Duggan, J. P., and Booth, D. A. (1986). Obesity, overeating, and rapid gastric emptying in rats with ventromedial hypothalamic lesions. *Science* **231,** 609–611.

Dulloo, A. G., and Miller, D. S. (1987). Obesity: A disorder of the sympathetic nervous system. *World Rev. Nutr. Diet.* **50,** 1–56.

Dunmore, S. J., and Beloff-Chain, A. (1982). Insulin release from the perfused rat pancreas stimulated by perifusates of the pituitary neurointermediate lobes of genetically obese and lean mice. *J. Endocrinol.* **92,** 15–21.

Dunmore, S. J., Morton, J. L., and Beloff-Chain, A. (1988). Plasma levels of B-cell tropin following adrenalectomy of lean and obese (ob/ob) mice. *In* "Lessons from Experimental Diabetes II" (B. Jeanrenaud, ed.). John Libbey & Co., Ltd., London (in press).

Eisenstein, A. B., Strack, I., and Steiner, A. (1974). Increased hepatic gluconeogenesis without a rise of glucagon secretion in rats fed a high fat diet. *Diabetes* **23,** 869–875.

El-Refai, M. F., and Chan, T. M. (1986). Possible involvement of a hypothalamic dopaminergic receptor in development of genetic obesity in mice. *Biochim. Biophys. Acta* **880,** 16–25.

Enser, M., Roberts, J., and Whittington, F. (1985). Effect of gold thioglucose-induced obesity on adipose tissue weight and cellularity in male and female mice suckled in large and small litters: Investigations into sex differences and site differences. *Br. J. Nutr.* **54,** 645–654.

Fabry, P. (1973). Food intake pattern and energy balance. In "Energy Balance in Man" (M. Apfelbaum, ed.), pp. 297–303. Masson et Cie, Paris.

Faust, I. M., Johnson, P. R., and Hirsch, J. (1976). Noncompensation of adipose mass in partially lipectomized mice and rats. *Am. J. Physiol.* **231,** 538–544.

Faust, I. M., Johnson, P. R., Stern, J. S., and Hirsch, J. (1978). Diet-unduced adipocyte number increase in adult rats: A new model of obesity. *Am. J. Physiol.* **235,** E279–E286.

Faust, I. M., Johnson, P. R., and Hirsch, J. (1980). Long-term effects of early nutritional experience on the development of obesity in the rat. *J. Nutr.* **110,** 2027–2034.

Faust, I. M., Miller, W. M., Jr., Sclafani, A., Aravich, P. F., Triscari, J., and Sullivan, A.

C. (1984). Diet-dependent hyperplastic growth of adipose tissue in hypothalamic obese rats. *Am. J. Physiol.* **247**, R1038–R1046.

Fenton, P. F., and Chase, H. B. (1951). Effect of diet on obesity of yellow mice in inbred lines. *Proc. Soc. Exp. Biol. Med.* **77**, 420–422.

Ferguson-Segall, M. J., Flynn, J., Walker, J., and Margules, D. L. (1982). Increased immunoreactive dynorphin and leuenkephalin in posterior pituitary of obese (ob/ob) mice and supersensitivity to drugs that act as kappa receptors. *Life Sci.* **31**, 2233–2236.

Figlewicz, D. P., Dorsa, D. M., Stein, L. J., Baskin, D. G., Paguette, T., Greenwood, M. R. C., Woods, S. C., and Porte, D. (1985). Brain and liver insulin binding is decreased in Zucker rats carrying the fa gene. *Endocrinology (Baltimore)* **117**, 1537, 1543.

Figlewicz, D. P., Ikeda, H., Stein, L. J., *et al.* (1986). Brain insulin binding is decreased in Wistar Kyoto rats carrying the fa gene. *Peptides (N.Y.)* **7**, 61–65.

Finkelstein, J. A., and Steggles, A.-W. (1981). Levels of gastrin-cholecystokinin like immunoreactivity in brains of genetically obese and non-obese rats. *Peptides (N.Y.)* **2**, 19–21.

Finkelstein, J. A., Steggles, A.-W., Martinez, P., and Pruissman, M. (1983). Changes in cholecystokinin receptor binding in rat brain after food deprivation. *Brain Res.* **288**, 193–197.

Finkelstein, J. A., Steggles, A.-W., Martinez, P., and Pruissman, M. (1984). Cholecystokinin receptor binding levels in the genetically obese rat brain. *Peptides (N.Y.)* **5**, 11–14.

Finkelstein, J. A., Jervois, P., Menadue, M., and Willough, J. O. (1986). Growth hormone and prolactin secretion in genetically-obese Zucker rats. *Endocrinology (Baltimore)* **118**, 1233–1236.

Fisler, J. S., and Bray, G. A. (1985). Dietary obesity: Effects of drugs on food intake in S 5B/P1 and Osborne–Mendel rats. *Physiol. Behav.* **34**, 225–231.

Fisler, J. S., and Bray, G. A. (1986). Effect of fenfluramine on food intake and body weight of S 5B/P1 and Osborne–Mendel rats. (1986). *Am. J. Clin. Nutr.* **43**, 54A.

Fisler, J. S., Yoshida, T., and Bray, G. A. (1984). Catecholamine turnover in S 5B/P1 and Osborne–Mendel rats: Response to a high-fat diet. *Am. J. Physiol.* **247**, R290–R295.

Fisler, J. S., Lupien, J. R. Wood, R. D., Bray, G. A., and Schemmel, R. A. (1987). Brown fat thermogenesis in a rat model of dietary obesity. *Am. J. Physiol.* **253**, R756–R762.

Fisler, J. S., Shimizu, H, and Bray, G. A. (1989). Brain 3-hydroxybutyrate, glutamate, and GABA in a rat model of dietary obesity. *Physiol. Behav.* **45**, (in press).

Fitz, G. J., and Scharschmidt, B. F. (1987). Regulation of transmembrane electrical potential gradient in rat hepatocytes in situ. *Am. J. Physiol.* **252**, G56–G64.

Flatt, P. R., and Bailey, C. J. (1981). Development of glucose intolerance and impaired plasma insulin response to glucose in obese hyperglycemic (ob/ob) mice. *Horm. Metab. Res.* **13**, 556–560.

Flatt, P. R., Bailey, C. J., Kwasowski, P., Swanson-Flatt, S. K., and Marks, V. (1983). Abnormalities of GIP in spontaneous syndrome of obesity and diabetes in mice. *Diabetes* **32**, 433–435.

Flatt, P. R., Bailey, C. J., Kwasowski, P., Page, T., and Marks, V. (1984). Plasma immunoreactive gastric inhibitor polypeptide in obese hyperglycaemic (ob/ob) mice. *J. Endocrinol.* **101**, 249–256.

Flatt, P. R., Bailey, C. J., Kwasowski, P., Swanston-Flatt, S. K., and Marks, V. (1985). Glucoregulatory effects of cafeteria feeding and diet restriction in genetically obese hyperglycemic (ob/ob) mice. *Nutr. Rep. Int.* **32**, 847–854.

Fletcher, J. M. (1986). Effects of adrenalectomy before weaning and short or long term glucocorticoid administration on genetically obese Zucker rat. *Biochem. J.* **238**, 459–463.

Flier, J. S., Cook, K. S., Usher, P., and Spiegelman, B. M. (1987). Severely impaired adipsin expression in genetic and acquired obesity. *Science* **237**, 405–408.

Freedman, M. R., Castonguay, T. W., and Stern, J. S. (1985). Effect of adrenalectomy and corticosterone replacement on meal patterns of Zucker rats. *Am. J. Physiol.* **249**, R584–R594.

Freedman, M. R., Horwitz, B. A., and Stern, J. S. (1986a). Effect of adrenalectomy and glucocorticoid replacement on development of obesity. *Am. J. Physiol.* **250**, R595–R607.

Freedman, M. R., Stern, J. R., Reaven, G. M., and Mondon, C. E. (1986b). Effect of adrenalectomy on in vivo glucose metabolism in insulin resistant Zucker obese rats. *Horm. Metab.* **18**, 296–298.

Friedman, M. I., and Granneman, J. (1983). Food intake and peripheral factors after recovery from insulin-induced hypoglycemia. *Am. J. Physiol.* **244**, R374–R382.

Friedman, M. I., and Tordoff, M. G. (1986). Fatty acid oxidation and glucose utilization interact to control food intake in rats. *Am. J. Physiol.* **251**, R840–R845.

Friedman, M. I., Edens, N. K., and Ramirez, I. (1983). Differential effects of medium and long chanin triglycerides on food intake of normal and diabetic rats. *Physiol. Behav.* **31**, 851–855.

Friedman, M. I., Ramirez, I., Edens, N. K., and Granneman, J. (1985). Food intake in diabetic rats: Isolation of primary metabolic effects of fat feeding. *Am. J. Physiol.* **249**, R44–R51.

Frohlich, A. (1901). Ein fall von tumor der hypophysis cerebri ohne akromegalie. *Wien. Klin. Rundsch.* **15**, 883–886.

Frohman, L. A., and Bernardis, L. L. (1971). Effect of hypothalamic stimulation on plasma glucose, insulin, and glucagon levels. *Am. J. Physiol.* **221**, 1596–1603.

Frohman, L. A., Bernardis, L. L., Schnatz, J. D., and Burek, L. (1969). Plasma insulin and triglyceride levels after hypothalamus lesions in weanling rats. *Am. J. Physiol.* **216**, 1496–1501.

Fukushima, M., Tokunaga, K., Lupien, J., Kemnitz, J. W., and Bray, G. A. (1987). Dynamic and static phases of obesity following lesions in PVN and VMH. *Am. J. Physiol.* **253**, R523–529.

Gale, S. K., and Sclafani, A. (1977). Comparison of ovarian and hypothalamic obesity syndromes in the female rat: Effects of diet palatability on food intake and body weight. *J. Comp. Physiol. Psychol.* **91**, 381–392.

Garratini, S. (1986). Central mechanisms of anorectic drugs. *Recent Adv. Obes. Res.* **5**, 208–215.

Garthwaite, T. L., Martinson, D., Tseng, L. F., Hagen, T. C., and Menhal, N. A. (1980). A longitudinal hormonal profile of the genetically obese mouse. *Endocrinology (Baltimore)* **107**, 671–678.

Gates, R. J., and Lazarus, N. R. (1977). The ability of pancreatic polypeptide (APP and BPP) to return to normal the hyperglycemia, hyperinsulinaemia and weight gain of New Zealand obese mice. *Horm. Res.* **8**, 189–202.

Gates, R. J., Hunt, M., and Lazarus, N. (1974). Further studies in amelioration of characteristics of New Zealand obese (NZO) mice following implantation of islets of langerhans. *Diabetologia* **10**, 401–406.

Geary, N., and Smith, G. P. (1983). Selective hepatic vagotomy blocks pancreatic glucagon's satiety effect. *Physiol. Behav.* **31**, 391–394.

Geary, N., Smith, G. P., and Gibbs, J. (1986). Pancreatic glucagon and bombesin inhibit meal size in ventromedial hypothalamus-lesioned rats. *Regul. Pept.* **15**, 261–268.

Geiselman, P. J., Novin, D., and Kissileff, H. R. (1982). Individual differences in meal patterns as predictors of short-term and 24-hour food intake and intact and vagotomized rabbits. *In* "The Neural Basis of Feeding and Reward" (B. G. Hobel and D. Novin, eds.), pp. 175–185. Haerr Inst. Electrophys. Res., Brunswick, Maine.

Geschwind, I. I., Huseby, R. A., and Nishioka, R. (1972). The effect of melanocyte-stimulating hormone on coat color in the mouse. *Recent Prog. Horm. Res.* **28**, 91.

Gibbs, J., and Smith, G. P. (1986). Satiety: The roles of peptides from the stomach and the intestine. *Fed. Proc., Fed. Am. Soc. Exp. Biol.* **45**, 1391–1395.

Gibbs, J., Young, R. C., and Smith, G. P. (1973). Cholecystokinin decreases food intake in rats. *J. Comp. Psychol.* **84**, 488–495.

Gibbs, J., Fauser, D. J., Rowe, E. A., Rolls, B. J., Rolls, E. T., and Maddison, S. P. (1979). Bombesin suppresses feeding in rats. *Nature (London)* **282**, 208–210.

Gibson, E. L., and Booth, D. A. (1986). Feeding induced by injection of norepinephrine near the paraventricular nucleus is suppressed specifically by the early stages of strong postingestional satiety in the rat. *Physiol. Psychol.* **14**, 98–103.

Gibson, M. J., Liotta, A. S., and Krieger, D. T. (1981). The Zucker fa/fa rat: Absent circadian corticosterone periodicity and elevated B-endophin concentrations in brain and neurointermediate pituitary. *Neuropeptides* **1**, 349–362.

Gillian-Barr, H., and McCracken, K. J. (1984). High efficiency of energy utilization in 'cafeteria'- and force-fed rats kept at 29 degrees. *Br. J. Nutr.* **51**, 379–387.

Giza, B. K., and Scott, T. R. (1984). Intravenous insulin injections affect taste responses in the rat nucleus tractus soliatarius. *Soc. Neurosci. Abstr.* **10**, 534.

Glick, Z., and Modan, M. (1977). Control of food intake during continuous injection of glucose into the upper duodenum and upper ileum of rats. *Physiol. Psychol.* **5**, 7–10.

Glick, Z., and Raum, W. J. (1986). Norepinephrine turnover in brown adipose tissue is stimulated by a single meal. *Am. J. Physiol.* **251**, R13–R17.

Glick, Z., Wu, S. W., Lupien, J., Reggio, R., Bray, G. A., and Fisher, D. A. (1985). Meal induced brown fat thermogenesis and thyroid hormones in the rat. *Am. J. Physiol.* **249**, E519–E524.

Gold, R. M., Sawchenko, P. E., DeLuca, C., Alexander, J., and Eng, R. (1980). Vagal mediation of hypothalamic obesity but not of supermarket dietary obesity, *Am. J. Physiol.* **238**, R447–R453.

Goldman, C. K., Marino, L., and Leibowitz, S. F. (1985). Postsynaptic alpha-2 noradrenergic receptors mediate feeding induced by paraventricular nucleus injection of norepinephrine and clonidine. *Eur. J. Pharmacol.* **115**, 11–19.

Goldman, J. K., Schnatz, J. D., Bernardis, L. L., and Frohman, L. A. (1972). In vivo and in vitro metabolism in hypothalamic obesity. *Diabetologia* **8**, 160–164.

Goodbody, A. E., and Trayhurn, P. (1981). GDP binding to brown adipose tissue mitochondria of diabetic obese (db/db) mice. *Biochem. J.* **194**, 1019–1022.

Goodbody, A. E., and Trayhurn, P. (1982). Studies on the activity of brown adipose tissue in suckling preobese ob/ob mice. *Biochim. Biophys. Acta* **680**, 119–126.

Gosnell, B. A. (1987). Effects of dietary dehydroepiandrosterone on food intake and body weights in rats with medial hypothalamic knife cuts. *Physiol. Behav.* **39**, 687–691.

Gosnell, B. A., Romsos, D. R., Morley, J. E., and Levine, A. S. (1985). Opiates and medial hypothalamic knife-cuts cause hyperphagia through different mechanisms. *Behav. Neurosci.* **99**, 1181–1191.

Goudie, A. J., Thornton, E. W., and Wheeler, T. J. (1976). Effects of Lilly 100140, a specific inhibitor of 5-hydroxytryptamine uptake, on food intake and on 5-hydroxytryptophan-induced anorexia. Evidence for serotonergic inhibition of feeding. *J. Pharm. Pharmacol.* **28**, 318–320.

Govani, S., and Yang, H. Y. (1981). Sex differences in the content of beta-endorphin and enkephalin-like peptides in the pituitary of obese (ob/ob) mice. *J. Neurochem.* **36**, 1829–1833.

Grandison, L., and Guidotti, A. (1977). Stimulation of food intake by muscimol and beta-endorphin. *Neuropharmacology* **16**, 533–536.

Gray, T. S., and Morley, J. E. (1986). Neuropeptide Y: Anatomical distribution and possible function in mammalian nervous system. *Life Sci.* **38**, 389–401.

Gray, T. S., O'Donohue, T. L., and Magnuson, D. J. (1986). Neuropeptide Y innervation of amygdaloid and hypothalamic neurons that project to the dorsal vagal complex in rat. *Peptides (N.Y.)* **7**, 341–349.

Greenberg, J., Ellyn, F., Pullen, G., Ghrenpresin, S., Singh, S., and Cheng, J. (1985). Methionin-enkephalin and B-endorphin levels in brain, pancreas and adrenals of db/db mice. *Endocrinology (Baltimore)* **116**, 328–331.

Greenwood, M. R. C. (1985). Relationship of enzyme activity to feeding behavior in rats: Lipoprotein lipase as the metabolic gate keeper. *Int. J. Obes.* **9**, Suppl. 1, 67–70.

Greenwood, M. R. C., Quartermain, M., Johnson, P., Cruce, J., and Hirsch, J. (1974). Food motivated behavior in genetically obese and hypothalamic–hyperphagic rats and mice. *Physiol Behav.* **13**, 687–692.

Greenwood, M. R. C., Cleary, M., Steingrimsdottir, L., and Vasseli, J. (1981). Adipose tissue metabolism and genetic obesity: The LPL hypothesis. *Adv. Obes. Res.* **3**, 75–79.

Grundleger, M. L., and Thenen, S. W. (1982). Decreased insulin binding, glucose transport, and glucose metabolism in soleus muscle of rats fed a high fat diet. *Diabetes* **31**, 232–237.

Grundleger, M. L., Godbole, V. Y., and Thenen, S. W. (1980). Age-dependent development of insulin resistance of soleus muscles in genetically obese (ob/ob) mice. *Am. J. Physiol.* **239**, R363–R371.

Grunstein, H. S., James, D. E., Strolien, L. H., Smythe, G. A., and Kraegen, E. W. (1985). Hyperinsulinemia suppresses glucose utilization in specific brain regions: In vivo studies using the euglycemic clamp in the rat. *Endocrinology (Baltimore)* **116**, 604–610.

Hales, C. N., and Kennedy, G. C. (1964). Plasma glucose, non-esterified fatty acids and insulin concentrations in hypothalamic–hyperphagia rats. *Biochem. J.* **90**, 620–624.

Han, P. W. (1967). Hypothalamic obesity in rats without hyperphagia. *Trans. N.Y. Acad. Sci. [2]* **30**, 229–242.

Han, P. W., and Frohman, L. A. (1970). Hyperinsulinemia in tube-fed hypophysectomized rats bearing hypothalamic lesions. *Am. J. Physiol.* **219**, 1632–1636.

Hansen, F. M., Nilsson, P., Hustvedt, B. E., Nilsson-Ehle, P., and Lovo, A. (1983). The significance of hyperphagia and diet composition on the metabolism in ventromedial hypothalamic lesioned male rats. *Horm. Metab. Res.* **15**, 538–542.

Harris, R. B. S., Hervey, E., Hervey, G. R., and Tobin, G. (1987). Body composition of lean and obese Zucker rats in parabiosis. *Int. J. Obes.* **11**, 275–283.

Hauger, R., Hulihan-Giblin, B., Angel, A., Luu, M. D., Janowsky, A., Skolnick, P., and Paul, S. M. (1986). Glucose regulates (^{3}H)(+)-amphetamine binding and Na$^+$K$^+$ ATPase activity in the hypothalamus: A proposed mechanism for the glucostatic control of feeding and satiety. *Brain Res. Bull.* **16**, 281–288.

Havrankova, J., Roth, J., and Brownstein, M. (1979). Concentrations of insulin and of insulin receptors in the brain are independent of peripheral insulin levels: Studies of obese and streptozotocin-treated rodents. *J. Clin. Invest.* **64**, 636–642.

Havrankova, J., Roth, J., and Brownstein, M. J. (1983). Insulin receptors in brain. *Adv. Metab. Disord.* **10**, 259–268.

Hays, S. E., Goodman, F. K., and Paul, S. M. (1981). Cholecystokinin receptors in brain: Effects of obesity, drug treatment and lesions. *Peptides (N.Y.)* **2**, 1–26.

Herberg, L., Doeppen, W., Major, E., and Gries, F. A. (1974). Dietary induced hypertrophic–hyperplastic obesity in mice. *J. Lipid Res.* **6**, 580–585.

Hervey, G. R. (1959). The effects of lesions in the hypothalamus in parabiotic rats. *J. Physiol. (London)* **145**, 336–356.

Hetherington, A. W., and Ranson, S. W. (1940). Hypothalamic lesions and adiposity in the rat. *Anat. Rec.* **78**, 149–172.

Hill, J. O., Davis, J. R., Tagliaferro, A. R., and Stewart, J. (1984). Dietary obesity and exercise in young rats. *Physiol. Behav.* **33**, 31–328.

Himms-Hagen, J. (1984). Nonshivering thermogenesis. *Brain Res. Bull.* **12**, 151–160.

Himms-Hagen, J., and Desautels, M. (1978). A mitochondrial defect in brown adipose tissue of the obese (ob/ob) mouse: Reduced binding of purine nucleotides and a failure to respond to cold by an increase in binding. *Biochem. Biophys. Res. Commun.* **83**, 628–634.

Himms-Hagen, J., Hogan, S., and Zaror-Behrens, G. (1986). Increased brown adipose tissue thermogenesis in obese (ob/ob) mice fed a palatable diet. *Am. J. Physiol.* **250**, E274–E281.

Hirsch, J., and Han, P. W. (1969). Cellularity of rat adipose tissue: Effects of growth, starvation, and obesity. *J. Lipid Res.* **10**, 77–82.

Hirsch, E., Dubose, C., and Jacobs, H. L. (1982). Overeating, dietary selection patterns and sucrose intake in growing rats. *Physiol. Behav.* **28**, 819–828.

Hogan, S., and Himms-Hagen, J. (1981). Abnormal brown adipose tissue in genetically obese (ob/ob) mice effect of thyroxine. *Am. J. Physiol.* **241**, E436–E443.

Hogan, S., and Himms-Hagen, J. (1983). Brown adipose tissue of mice with gold thioglucose-induced obesity: Effect of cold and diet. *Am. J. Physiol.* **244**, E581–E588.

Hogan, S., Coscina, D. V., and Himms-Hagen, J. (1982). Brown adipose tissue of rats with obesity-inducing ventromedial hypothalamic lesions. *Am. J. Physiol.* **243**, E338–E344.

Hogan, S., Himms-Hagen, J., and Coscina, D. V. (1985). Lack of diet-induced thermogenesis in brown adipose tissue of obese medial hypothalamic-lesioned rats. *Physiol. Behav.* **35**, 287–294.

Holt, S. J., and York, D. A. (1989). Studies on the sympathetic afferent nerves of brown adipose tissue of lean and obese Zucker rats. *Brain Res.* **481**, 106–112.

Holt, S. A., York, D. A., and Fitzsimons, J. T. R. (1983). The effects of corticosterone, cold exposure and overfeeding sucrose on brown adipose tissue of obese Zucker rats (fa/fa). *Biochem. J.* **214**, 215–223.

Holt, S. J., Rothwell, N. J., Stock, M. J., and York, D. A. (1987a). Changes in energy, balance, thermogenesis and brown adipose tissue activity following hypophysectomy in obese Zucker rats. *Am. J. Physiol.* **254**, E162–E166.

Holt, S. J., Wheal, H. V., and York, D. A. (1987b). Hypothalamic control of brown adipose tissue in Zucker lean and obese rats. Effect of electrical stimulation of the ventromedial nucleus and other hypothalamic centres. *Brain Res.* **405**, 227–233.

Holtzman, S. G. (1974). Behavioral effects of separate and combined administration of naloxone and *d*-amphetamine. *J. Pharmacol. Exp. Ther.* **189**, 51–60.

Hyde, T. M., and Miselis, R. R. (1983). Effects of area postrema/caudal medial nucleus of solitary tract lesion on food intake and body weight. *Am. J. Physiol.* **244,** R577–R587.

Hyde, T. M., Eng, R., and Miselis, R. R. (1982). Brainstem mechanisms in hypothalamic and dietary obesity. *In* "The Neural Basis of Feeding and Reward" (B. G. Hoebel and D. Novin, eds.), pp. 97–114. Haerr Inst. Electrophys. Res., Brunswick, Maine.

Ikeda, H., Nishikawa, K., and Matsuo, T. (1980). Feeding responses of Zucker fatty rat to 2-deoxy-D-glucose, norepinephrine and insulin. *Am. J. Physiol.* **239,** E379–E384.

Ikeda, H., Shimakawa, K., Kito, G., Meguro, K., and Matsuo, T. (1986a). The antiobesity action of (S)-(+)-1-(4-Chlorophenyl-thiomethyl-N-methyethylaine fumarate (AD-124). *Eur. J. Pharmacol.* **125,** 201–210.

Ikeda, H., West, D. B., Pustek, J. J., Figlewicz, D. P., Greenwood, M. R. C., Porte, D., Jr., and Woods, S. C. (1986b). Intraventricular insulin reduces food intake and body weight of lean but not obese Zucker rats. *Appetite (London)* **7,** 381–386.

Inagaki, S., Kubota, Y., Kito, S., Fukuda, M., Ono, T., Yamano, M., and Tohyama, M. (1986). Ultrastructural evidence of enkephalinergic input to glucoreceptor neurons in ventromedial hypothalamic nucleus. *Brain Res.* **378,** 420–424.

Inoue, S., and Bray, G. A. (1977). The effect of subdiaphragmatic vagotomy in rats with ventromedial hypothalamic obesity. *Endocrinology (Baltimore)* **100,** 108–114.

Inoue, S., Bray, G. A., and Mullen, Y. (1977a). Effect of transplantation of pancreas on development of hypothalamic obesity. *Nature (London)* **226,** 742–744.

Inoue, S., Campfield, L. A., and Bray, G. A. (1977b). Comparison of metabolic alterations in hypothalamic and high-fat diet induced obesity. *Am. J. Physiol.* **223,** R162–R168.

Inoue, S., Bray, G. A., and Mullen, Y. S. (1978). Transplantation of pancreatic beta-cells prevents the development of hypothalamic obesity in rats. *Am. J. Physiol.* **235,** E266–E271.

Inoue, S., Mullen, Y. S., and Bray, G. A. (1983). Hyperinulinemia in rats with hypothalamic obesity: Effects of autonomic drugs and glucose. *Am. J. Physiol.* **245,** R372–R378.

Inui, Y., Nishikawa, M., Minami, Y., Kawata, S., Nozaki, S., Fujioka, S., Yamada, K., Tokunaga, K., Matsuzawa, Y., Kono, N., and Tarui, S. (1987). Morphological study of lipoprotein particles in the livers of ventromedial hypothalamus lesioned rats. *Int. J. Obes.* **11,** 527–536.

Ionescu, E., Rohner-Jeanrenaud, F., Proiotto, J., Rivest, R. A., and Jeanrenaud, B. (1988). Taste-induced changes in plasma insulin and glucose turnover in lean and genetically obese rats. *Diabetes* **37,** 773–779.

Janowitz, H. D., and Grossman, M. I. (1949). Some factors affecting the food intake of normal dogs and dogs with esophagotomy and gastric fistula. *Am. J. Physiol.* **159,** 143–148.

Jeanrenaud, B. (1985). An hypothesis on the aetiology of obesity: Dysfunction of the central nervous system as a primary cause. *Diabetologia* **28,** 502–513.

Jenkins, T. C., and Hershberger, T. V. (1978). Effect of diet, body type and sex on voluntary intake, energy balance and body composition of Zucker rats. *J. Nutr.* **108,** 124–136.

Jhanwar-Uniyal, M., Roland, C. R., and Leibowitz, S. F. (1986). Diurnal rhythm of alpha-2-noradrenergic receptors in the paraventricular nucleus and other brain areas: Relation to circulating corticosterone and feeding behavior. *Life Sci.* **38,** 473–482.

Kamatchi, G. L., Veeraragavan, K., Chandra, D., and Bapna, J. S. (1986). Antagonism of acute feeding response to 2-deoxyglucose and 5-thioglucose by GABA antagonists:

The relative role of ventromedial and lateral hypothalamus. *Pharmacol., Biochem. Behav.* **25**, 59–62.

Kanarek, R. B., and Hirsch, E. (1977). Dietary-induced overeating in experimental animals. *Fed. Proc., Fed. Am. Soc. Exp. Biol.* **36**, 154–158.

Kanarek, R. B., and Marks-Kaufman, R. (1979). Developmental aspects of sucrose-induced obesity in rats. *Physiol. Behav.* **23**, 881–885.

Kanarek, R. B., and Orthen-Gambill, N. (1982). Differential effects of sucrose, fructose and glucose on carbohydrate-induced obesity in rats. *J. Nutr.* **112**, 1546–1554.

Kanarek, R. B., Meyers, J., Meade, R. G., and Mayer, J. (1979). Juvenile-onset obesity and deficits in caloric regulation in MSG-treated rats. *Pharmacol., Biochem. Behav.* **10**, 717–721.

Kanarek, R. B., Marks-Kaufman, R., and Lipeles, B. J. (1980). Increased carbohydrate intake as a function of insulin administration in rats. *Physiol. Behav.* **25**, 779–782.

Kaneto, A., Miki, E., and Kosaka, K. (1974). Effects of vagal stimulation on glucagon and insulin secretion. *Endocrinology (Baltimore)* **95**, 1005–1010.

Kaplan, M. M., and Young, J. B. (1987). Abnormal thyroid hormone deiodination in tissue of ob/ob and db/db obese mice. *Endocrinology (Baltimore)* **120**, 886–893.

Kaplan, M. M., Young, J. B., and Shaw, E. A. (1985). Abnormal thyroid hormone binding to serum proteins in ob/ob and db/db genetically obese mice. *Endocrinology (Baltimore)* **117**, 1858–1864.

Karakash, C., Hustvedt, B. E., Lovo, A., Le Marchand, Y., and Jeanrenard, B. (1977). Consequences of ventromedial hypothalamic lesions on metabolism of perfused rat liver. *Am. J. Physiol.* **232**, E286–E293.

Kasser, T. R., Harris, R. B. S., and Martin, R. J. (1985a). Level of satiety: Fatty acid and glucose metabolism in three brain sites associated with feeding. *Am. J. Physiol.* **248**, R447–R452.

Kasser, T. R., Harris, R. B. S., and Martin, R. J. (1985b). Level of satiety: GABA and pentose shunt activities in three brain sites associated with feeding. *Am. J. Physiol.* **248**, R453–R458.

Kasser, T. R., Deutch, A., and Martin, R. J. (1986). Uptake and utilization of metabolites in specific brain sites relative to feeding status. *Physiol. Behav.* **36**, 1161–1165.

Katafuchi, T., Oomura, Y., Niijima, A., and Yoshimatsu, H. (1985a). Effects of intra-cerebroventricular 2-DG infusion and subsequent hypothalamic lesion on adrenal nerve activity in the rat. *J. Auton. Nerv. Syst.* **13**, 81–84.

Katafuchi, T., Oomura, Y., and Yoshimatsu, H. (1985b). Single neuron activity in the rat lateral hypothalamus during 2-deoxy-D-glucose induced and natural feeding behavior. *Brain Res.* **359**, 1–9.

Katafuchi, T., Yoshimatsu, H., Oomura, Y., and Sato, A. (1986). Responses of adrenal catecholamine secretion to lateral hypothalamic stimulation and lesion in rats. *Brain Res.* **363**, 141–144.

Kates, A. L., and Himms-Hagen, J. (1985). Defective cold-induced stimulation of thyroxine 5′-deiodinase in brown adipose tissue of genetically obese (ob/ob) mice. *Biochem. Biophys. Res. Commun.* **130**, 188–196.

Kaul, R., Schmidt, I., and Carlisle, H. (1985). Maturation of thermoregulation in Zucker rats. *Int. J. Obes.* **9**, 401–409.

Keesey, R. E., and Powley, T. L. (1986). The regulation of body weight. *Annu. Rev. Psychol.* **37**, 109–133.

Keesey, R. E., Boyle, P. C., Kemnitz, J. W., and Mitchell, J. S. (1976). The role of the lateral hypothalamus in determining the body weight set point. *In* "Hunger: Basic

Mechanisms and Clinical Implications" (D. Novin, W. Wyrwicka, and G. A. Bray, eds.), pp. 243–256. Raven Press, New York.

Kelly, J., Rothstein, J., and Grossman, S. P. (1979). GABA and hypothalamic feeding systems. I. Topographic analysis of the effects of microinjections of Muscimol. *Physiol. Behav.* **23,** 1123–1134.

Khan, S. G., Boyle, P. C., and Lachance, P. A. (1986). Decreased triiodothyronine binding to isolated nuclei from livers of preobese and obese ob/ob mice. *Proc. Soc. Exp. Biol. Med.* **182,** 84–87.

Kimbrough, T. D., and Weekley, L. B. (1984). The effect of a high-fat diet on brainstem and duodenal serotonin (5-HT) metabolism in Sprague–Dawley and Osborne–Mendel rats. *Int. J. Obes.* **8,** 305–310.

Kimura, H., and Kuriyama, K. (1975). Distribution of gamma-aminobutyric acid (GABA) in the rat hypothalamus: Functional correlates of GABA with activities of appetite controlling mechanisms. *J. Neurochem.* **24,** 903–907.

King, B. M., and Frohman, L. A. (1982). The role of vagally-mediated hyperinsulinemia in hypothalamic obesity. *Neurosci. Biobehav. Rev.* **6,** 205–214.

King, B. M., and Frohman, L. A. (1985). Nonirritative lesions of VMH: Effects on plasma insulin, obesity, and hyperreactivity. *Am. J. Physiol.* **248,** E669–E675.

King, B. M., and Smith, R. L. (1985). Hypothalamic obesity after hypophysectomy or adrenalectomy: Dependence on corticosterone. *Am. J. Physiol.* **249,** R522–R526.

King, B. M., Castellanos, F. X., Kastin, A. J., Berzas, M. C., Mauk, M. D., Olson, G. A., and Olson, R. D. (1979). Naloxone-induced suppression of food intake in normal and hypothalamic obese rats. *Pharmacol., Biochem. Behav.* **11,** 729–732.

King, B. M., Banta, A. R., Tharel, G. N., Bruce, B. K., and Frohman, L. A. (1983). Hypothalamic hyperinsulinemia and obesity: Role of adrenal glucocorticoids. *Am. J. Physiol.* **245,** E194–E199.

King, B. M., Calvert, C. B., Esquerre, K. R., Kaufman, J. H., and Frohman, L. A. (1984). Relationship between plasma corticosterone and insulin levels in rats with ventromedial hypothalamic lesions. *Physiol. Behav.* **32,** 991–994.

Kissileff, H. R., Pi-Sunyer, F. X., Thornton, J., and Smith, G. P. (1981). C-terminal octapeptide of cholecystokinin decreases food intake in man. *Am. J. Clin. Nutr.* **34,** 154–160.

Kissileff, H. R., Thornton, J., and Becker, E. (1982). A quadratic equation adequately describes the cumulative food intake curve in man. *Appetite (London)* **3,** 255–272.

Knehans, A. W., and Romsos, D. R. (1982). Reduced norepinephrine turnover in brown adipose tissue of ob/ob mice. *Am. J. Physiol.* **242,** E253–E261.

Knehans, A. W., and Romsos, D. R. (1983). Norepinephrine turnover in obese (ob/ob) mice: Effects of age, fasting, and acute cold. *Am. J. Physiol.* **244,** E567–E574.

Knehans, A. W., and Romsos, D. R. (1984). Effects of diet on norepinephrine turnover in obese (ob/ob) mice. *J. Nutr.* **114,** 2080–2088.

Koopmans, H. S. (1983). A stomach hormone inhibits food intake. *J. Auton. Nerv. Syst.* **9,** 157–171.

Koopmans, H. S. (1985). Internal signals cause large changes in food intake in one-way crossed intestines rats. *Brain Res. Bull.* **14,** 595–603.

Koopmans, H. S., and Heird, W. C. (1977). Hunger satiety dissociated from pancreatic enzyme flow. *Proc. Int. Conf. Food Fluid Intake, 6th.*

Koopmans, H. S., and Pi-Sunyer, F. X. (1986). Large changes in food intake in diabetic rats fed high-fat and low-fat diets. *Brain Res. Bull.* **17,** 861–871.

Koopmans, H. S., Sclafani, A., Fichtner, C., and Aravich, P. F. (1982). The effects of ileal transportation on food intake and body weight loss in VMH-obese rats. *Am. J. Clin. Nutr.* **35**, 284–293.

Koopmans, H. S., Ferri, G.-L., Sarson, D. L., Polak, J. M., and Bloom, S. R. (1984). The effects of ileal transposition and jejunoileal bypass on food intake and GI hormone levels in rats. *Physiol. Behav.* **33**(4), 601–609.

Kow, L.-M., and Pfaff, D. W. (1985). Actions of feeding-relevant agents on hypothalamic glucose-responsive neurons in vitro. *Brain Res. Bull.* **15**, 509–513.

Kraegen, E. W., James, D. W., Storlien, L. H., Burleigh, K. M., and Chisholm, D. J. (1986). In vivo insulin resistance in individual peripheral tissues of the high fat fed rat: Assessment by euglycemic clamp plus deoxyglucose administration. *Diabetologia* **29**, 192–198.

Kraly, F. S., and Smith, G. P. (1978). Combined pregastric and gastric stimulation by food is sufficient for normal meal size. *Physiol. Behav.* **21**, 405–408.

Kramer, T. H., Sclafani, A., Kindya, K., and Pezner, M. (1983). Conditioned taste aversion in lean and obese rats with ventromedial hypothalamic knife cuts. *Behav. Neurosci.* **97**, 110–119.

Krauchi, K., Wirz-Justice, A., Morimasa, T., Willener, R., and Feer, H. (1984). Hypothalamic alpha-2 and beta-adrenoceptor rhythms are correlated with circadian feeding: Evidence from chronic methamphetamine treatment and withdrawal. *Brain Res.* **321**, 83–90.

Krieger, D. T. (1979). Restoration of corticosteroid periodicity in obese rats by limited A.M. food access. *Brain Res.* **171**, 67–75.

Kulkosky, P. J., Breckenridge, C., Krinsky, R., and Woods, S. C. (1976). Satiety elicited by the C-terminal octapeptide of cholecystokinin–pancreozymin in normal and VMH-lesioned rats. *Behav. Biol.* **18**, 227–234.

Kyrokouli, S. E., Stanley, B. G., and Leibowitz, S. F. (1986). Galanin: Stimulation of feeding induced by medial hypothalamic injection of this novel peptide. *Eur. J. Pharmacol.* **122**, 159–160.

Landau, B. R., Takaoka, Y., Abrams, M. A., Genuth, S. M., Van Houten, M., Posner, B. I., White, R. J., Ohgaku, S., Horvat, A., and Hemmelgarn, E. (1983). Binding of insulin by monkey and pig hypothalamus. *Diabetes* **32**, 284–292.

Landsberg, L., Saville, M. E., and Young, J. B. (1984). Sympathoadrenal system and regulation of thermogenesis. *Am. J. Physiol.* **247**, E181–E189.

Langhans, W., and Scharrer, E. (1987a). Evidence for a vagally mediated satiety signal derived from hepatic fatty acid oxidation. *J. Auton. Nerv. Syst.* **18**, 13–18.

Langhans, W., and Scharrer, E. (1987b). Role of fatty acid oxidation in control meal pattern. *Behav. Neural Biol.* **47**, 7–16.

Langhans, W., and Scharrer, E. (1987c). Evidence for a role of the sodium-pump of hepatocytes in the control of food-intake. *J. Auton. Nerv. Syst.* **20**, 199–205.

Langhans, W., Wiesenreiter, F., and Scharrer, E. (1983). Different effects of subcutaneous D,L-3-hydroxybutyrate and acetoacetate injections on food intake in rats. *Physiol. Behav.* **31**, 483–486.

Langhans, W., Damaske, U., and Scharrer, E. (1985a). Different metabolites might reduce food intake by the mitochondrial generation of reducing equivalents. *Appetite (London)* **6**, 143–152.

Langhans, W., Egli, G., and Scharrer, E. (1985b). Selective hepatic vagotomy eliminates the hypophagic effect of different metabolites. *J. Auton. Nerv. Syst.* **13**, 255–262.

Larson, B. A., Sinha, Y. N., and Vanderlaan, W. P. (1976). Serum growth hormone and prolactin during and after development of obese hyperglycemic syndrome in mice. *Endocrinology (Baltimore)* **98**, 139–145.

Laughton, W., and Powley, T. L. (1981). Bipiperidyl mustard produced brain lesions and obesity in the rat. *Brain Res.* **221,** 415–420.

Lavau, M., and Susini, C. (1975). (U-^{14}C)Glucose metabolism in vivo in rats rendered obese by a high fat diet. *J. Lipid Res.* **16,** 134–142.

Lavau, M., Fried, S. K., Susini, C., and Freychet, P. (1979). Mechanism of insulin resistance in adipocytes of rats fed a high fat diet. *J. Lipid Res.* **20,** 8–16.

Lavau, M., Bazin, R., and Guerre-Millo, M. (1985). Increased capacity for fatty acid synthesis in white and brown adipose tissues from 7-day-old obese Zucker pups. *Int. J. Obes.* **9,** 61–66.

LeBlanc, J., and Blondel, L. (1985). Role of palatability on meal-induced thermogenesis in human subjects. *Am. J. Physiol.* **248,** E333–E336.

LeBlanc, J., Cabanac, M., and Samson, P. (1984). Reduced postprandial heat production with gavage as compared with meal feeding in human subjects. *Am. J. Physiol.* **246,** E95–E101.

Lee, T. F., Wang, C. M., and Russell, J. C. (1987). Enhancement of cold-stimulated thermogenesis in the corpulent rat (LA/N cp) by aminophylline. *Am. J. Physiol.* **252,** R737–R742.

Leibowitz, S. F. (1970). Reciprocal hunger-regulating circuits involving alpha- and beta-adrenergic receptors located, respectively, in the ventromedial and lateral hypothalamus. *Proc. Natl. Acad. Sci. U.S.A.* **67,** 1063–1070.

Leibowitz, S. F. (1980). Neurochemical system of the hypothalamus: Control of feeding and drinking behavior and water–electrolyte excretion. *In* "Handbook of the Hypothalamus" (P. J. Morgan and J. Panksepp, eds.), Vol. 3, pp. 299–437. Dekker, New York.

Leibowitz, S. F. (1986). Brain monoamines and peptides: Role in the control of eating behavior. *Fed. Proc., Fed. Am. Soc. Exp. Biol.* **45,** 1396–1403.

Leibowitz, S. F., and Hor, L. (1982). Endorphinergic and alpha-noradrenergic systems in the paraventricular nucleus: Effects on eating behavior. *Peptides (N.Y.)* **3,** 421–428.

Leibowitz, S. F., and Stanley, B. G. (1986a). Brain peptides and the control of eating behavior. *In* "Neural and Endocrine Peptides and Receptors" (T. W. Moody, ed.), pp. 333–352. Plenum, New York.

Leibowitz, S. F., and Stanley, B. G. (1986b). Neurochemical controls of appetite. *In* "Feeding Behavior: Neurol and Humoral Controls" (R. Ritter, S. Ritter, and C. D. Barnes, eds.), pp. 191–234. Academic Press, Orlando, Florida.

Leibowitz, S. F., Hammer, N. J., and Chang, K. (1981). Hypothalamic paraventricular nucleus lesions produce overeating and obesity in the rat. *Physiol. Behav.* **27,** 1031–1040.

Leibowitz, S. F., Hammer, N. J., and Chang, K. (1983). Feeding behavior induced by central norepinephrine injection is attenuated by discrete lesions in the hypothalamic paraventricular nucleus. *Pharmacol., Biochem. Behav.* **19,** 945–950.

Leibowitz, S. F., Roland, C. R., Hor, L., and Squillari, V. (1984). Noradrenergic feeding elicited via the paraventricular nucleus is dependent upon circulating corticosterone. *Physiol. Behav.* **32,** 857–864.

Leibowitz, S. F., Brown, O., Tretter, J. R., and Kirschgessner, A. (1985). Norepinephrine, clonidine and tricyclic antidepressants selectively stimulate carbohydrate ingestion through noradrenergic system of the paraventricular nucleus. *Pharmacol., Biochem. Behav.* **23,** 541–550.

Le Magnen, J. (1983). Body energy balance and food intake: A neuroendocrine regulatory mechanism. *Physiol. Rev.* **63,** 314–385.

Leveille, G. A., Pardini, R. S., and Tillotsan, J. A. (1967). Influence of medium-chain triglycerides on lipid metabolism in the rat. *Lipids* **2,** 287–294.

Levin, B. E. (1986). Neurological regulation of body weight. *CRC Crit. Rev. Clin. Neurobiol.* **2**, 1–60.

Levin, B. E., and Sullivan, A. C. (1979a). Catecholamine levels in discrete brain nuclei of 7 month old genetically obese rats. *Pharmacol., Biochem. Behav.* **11**, 77–82.

Levin, B. E., and Sullivan, A. C. (1979b). Catecholamine synthesising enzymes in various brain regions of the genetically obese Zucker rat. *Brain Res.* **171**, 560–566.

Levin, B. E., and Sullivan, A. C. (1984). Dietary obesity and neonatal sympathectomy II. Thermoregulation and brown adipose tissue metabolism. *Am. J. Physiol.* **247**, R988–R994.

Levin, B. E., and Sullivan, A. C. (1987). Glucose-induced norepinephrine levels and obesity resistance. *Am. J. Physiol.* **253**, R475–R481.

Levin, B. E., Triscari, J., and Sullivan, A. C. (1981). Defective catecholamine metabolism in peripheral organs of genetically obese Zucker rats. *Brain Res.* **224**, 353–366.

Levin, B. E., Triscari, J., and Sullivan, A. C. (1982). Sympathetic activity in thyroid treated Zucker rats. *Am. J. Physiol.* **243**, R170–R178.

Levin, B. E., Triscari, J., and Sullivan, A. C. (1983a). Studies of origins of abnormal sympathetic function in obese Zucker rats. *Am. J. Physiol.* **245**, E87–E93.

Levin, B. E., Triscari, J., and Sullivan, A. C. (1983b). Altered sympathetic activity during development of diet-induced obesity in rat. *Am. J. Physiol.* **244**, R347–R355.

Levin, B. E., Triscari, J., and Sullivan, A. C. (1983c). Relationship between sympathetic activity and diet-induced obesity in two rat strains. *Am. J. Physiol.* **245**, R367–R371.

Levin, B. E., Stoddard-Apter, S., and Sullivan, A. C. (1984a). Central activation and peripheral function of sympatho-adrenal and cardiovascular systems in the Zucker rat. *Physiol. Behav.* **32**, 295–299.

Levin, B. E., Finnegan, M. B., Marquet, E., Triscari, J. Comai, K., and Sullivan, A. C. (1984b). Effects of diet and obesity on brown adipose tissue metabolism. *Am. J. Physiol.* **246**, E418–E425.

Levin, B. E., Triscari, J., Marquet, E., and Sullivan, A. C. (1984c). Dietary obesity and neonatal sympathectomy. I. Effects on body composition and brown adipose. *Am. J. Physiol.* **247**, R979–R987.

Levin, B. E., Finnegan, M. B., Triscari, J., and Sullivan, A. C. (1985). Brown adipose and metabolic features of chronic diet-induced obesity. *Am. J. Physiol.* **248**, R717–R723.

Levin, B. E., Triscari, J., and Sullivan, A. C. (1986a). The effect of diet and chronic obesity on brain catecholamine turnover in the rat. *Pharmacol., Biochem. Behav.* **24**, 299–304.

Levin, B. E., Triscari, J., and Sullivan, A. C. (1986b). Metabolic features of diet-induced obesity without hyperphagia in young rats. *Am. J. Physiol.* **251**, R433–R440.

Levin, B. E., Triscari, J., Hogan, S., and Sullivan, A. C. (1987). Resistance to diet-induced obesity: Food intake, pancreatic sympathetic tone, and insulin. *Am. J. Physiol.* **252**, R471–R478.

Levine, A. S., and Morley, J. E. (1984). Neuropeptide Y: A potent inducer of consummatory behavior in rats. *Peptides (N.Y.)* **5**, 1025–1030.

Levine, A. S., Rogers, B., Kneip, J., Grace, M., and Morley, J. E. (1983). Effect of centrally administered corticotropin-releasing factor (CRF) on multiple feeding paradigms. *Neuropharmacology* **22**, 337–339.

Lorden, J. F., and Caudle, A. (1986). Behavioral and endocrinological effects of single injections of monosodium glutamate in the mouse. *Neurobehav. Toxicol. Teratol.* **8**, 509–519.

Lorenz, D. N., and Goldman, S. A. (1982). Vagal mediation of the cholecystokinin satiety effect in rats. *Physiol. Behav.* **29**, 599–604.

Louis-Sylvestre, J., Servant, J.-M., Molimard, R., and Le Magnen, J. (1980). Effect of liver denervation on feeding pattern of rats. *Am. J. Physiol.* **239,** R66–R70.

Louis-Sylvestre, J., Giachetti, I., and Le Magnen, J. (1984). Sensory versus dietary factors in cafeteria-induced overweight. *Physiol. Behav.* **32**(6), 901–905.

Luiten, P. G. M., ter Horst, J. G., and Steffens, A. B. (1987). The hypothalamus, intrinsic connections and outflow pathways to the endocrine system in relation to the control of feeding and metabolism. *Prog. Neurobiol.* **28,** 1–54.

Lupien, J. R., and Bray, G. A. (1985). Influence of fenfluramine on GDP-binding to brown adipose tissue mitochondria. *Pharmacol., Biochem. Behav.* **23,** 509–513.

Lupien, J. R., Glick, Z., Saito, M., and Bray, G. A. (1985). Guanosine diphosphate binding to brown adipose tissue mitochondria is increased after single meal. *Am. J. Physiol.* **249,** R694–R698.

Maggio, C. A., Greenwood, M. R. C., and Vasselli, J. R. (1983). The satiety effects of intragastric macronutrient infusions in fatty and lean Zucker rats. *Physiol. Behav.* **31,** 367–372.

Maggio, C. A., Yang, M. U., and Vasselli, J. R. (1984). Developmental aspects of macronutrient selection in genetically obese and lean rats. *Nutr. Behav.* **2,** 95–110.

Malaisse, W. J., Lemonnier, D., Malaisse-Legae, F., and Mendel Brum, I. M. (1975). Secretion of and high sensitivity to insulin in obese rats fed a high fat diet. *Horm. Metab. Res.* **1,** 9–13.

Maller, O. (1964). The effect of hypothalamic and dietary obesity on taste preferences in rats. *Life Sci.* **3,** 1281–1291.

Mandenoff, A., Lenoir, T., and Apfelbaum, M. (1982). Tardy occurrence of adipocyte hyperplasia in cafeteria-fed rats. *Am. J. Physiol.* **242,** R349–R351.

Marchington, D., Rothwell, N. J., Stock, M. J., and York, D. A. (1983). Energy balance, diet-induced thermogenesis and brown adipose tissue in lean and obese (fa/fa) Zucker rats after adrenalectomy. *J. Nutr.* **113,** 1395–1402.

Margules, D. L., Moisset, B., Lewis, M., Shibuya, H., and Pert, C. (1978). B-Endorphin is associated with overeating in genetically obese mice (ob/ob) and rats (fa/fa). *Science* **202,** 988–993.

Martin, J. M., Konijnendijk, W., and Bouman, P. R. (1974). Insulin and growth hormone secretion in rats with ventromedial hypothalamic lesions maintained on restricted food intake. *Diabetes* **23,** 203–208.

Martin, R. J., and Jeanrenaud, B. (1985). Growth hormone in obesity and diabetes: Inappropriate hypothalamic control of secretion. *Int. J. Obes.* **9,** Suppl. 1, 99–104.

Martin, R. J., Wangsness, P. J., and Gahagan, J. H. (1978). Diurnal changes in serum metabolites and hormones in lean and obese Zucker rats. *Horm. Metab. Res.* **10,** 187–192.

Matsumura, M., Yamanoi, A., Sato, K., Tsuda, M., Chikamori, K., Mori, H., and Saito, S. (1984). Alterations in the levels of beta-endorphin-like immunoreactivity in plasma and tissues of obese rats with hypothalamic lesions. *Horm. Metab. Res.* **16,** 105–106.

Mayer, J. (1960). The obese hyperglycemic syndrome of mice as an example of metabolic obesity. *Am. J. Clin. Nutr.* **8,** 712–718.

McCabe, J. J., Bitran, D., and Leibowitz, S. F. (1986). Amphetamine-induced anorexia: Analysis with hypothalamic lesions and knife cuts. *Pharmacol., Biochem. Behav.* **24,** 1047.

McCaleb, M. L., and Myers, R. D. (1982). 2-Deoxy-D-glucose and insulin modify release of norepinephrine from rat hypothalamus. *Am. J. Physiol.* **242,** R596–R601.

McCaleb, M. L., Myers, R. D., Singer, G., and Willis, G. (1979). Hypothalamic norepinephrine in the rat during feeding and push-pull perfusion with glucose, 2-D-G, or insulin. *Am. J. Physiol.* **236,** R312–R321.

McGinty, D., Epstein, A. N., and Teitelbaum, P. (1965). The contribution of oropharyngeal sensations to hypothalamic hyperphagia. *Anim. Behav.* **13**, 413–418.

McHugh, P. R., and Moran, T. H. (1978). The accuracy of regulation of caloric ingestion in the rhesus monkey. *Am. J. Physiol.* **235**, R29–R34.

McKay, L. D., Kenney, N. J., Edens, N. K., Williams, R. H., and Woods, S. C. (1981). Intracerebroventricular beta-endorphin increases food intake of rats. *Life Sci.* **29**, 1429–1434.

McLaughlin, C. L., and Baile, C. A. (1978). Cholecystokinin, amphetamine and diazepam and feeding in lean and obese Zucker rats. *Pharmacol., Biochem. Behav.* **10**, 87–93.

McLaughlin, C. L., and Baile, C. A. (1980a). Feeding responses of weanling Zucker obese rats to cholecystokinin and bombesin. *Physiol. Behav.* **25**, 341–346.

McLaughlin, C. L., and Baile, C. A. (1980b). Decreased sensitivity of Zucker obese rats to the putative satiety agent cholecystokinin. *Physiol. Behav.* **25**, 543–548.

McLaughlin, C. L., and Baile, C. A. (1981). Obese mice and the satiety effects of cholecystokinin, bombesin and pancreatic polypeptide. *Physiol. Behav.* **26**, 433–437.

McLaughlin, C. L., and Baile, C. A. (1983). Nalmefene decreases meal size and food and water intake and weight gain in Zucker rats. *Physiol. Behav.* **19**, 235–240.

McLaughlin, C. L., and Baile, C. A. (1984a). Feeding behavior responses of Zucker rats to naloxone. *Physiol. Behav.* **32**, 755–761.

McLaughlin, C. L., and Baile, C. A. (1984b). Increased sensitivity of Zucker obese rats to Naloxone is present at weaning. *Physiol. Behav.* **32**, 929–933.

McLaughlin, C. L., and Baile, C. A. (1985). Autoimmunization against beta-endorphin increases food intakes and body weights of obese rats. *Physiol. Behav.* **35**, 365–370.

McLaughlin, C. L., Peikin, S. R., and Baile, C. A. (1983a). Food intake response to modulation of secretion of cholecystokinin in Zucker rats. *Am. J. Physiol.* **244**, R676–R685.

McLaughlin, C. L., Peikin, S. R., and Baile, C. A. (1983b). Trypsin inhibitor effects on food intake and weight gain in Zucker rats. *Physiol. Behav.* **31**, 487–491.

McLaughlin, C. L., Peikin, S. R., and Baile, C. A. (1984). Decreased pancreatic CCK receptor binding and CCK stimulated amylase release in Zucker obese rats. *Physiol. Behav.* **32**, 961–965.

McLaughlin, C. L., Baile, C. A., Dellaferra, M. A., and Kasser, T. G. (1985). Meal-stimulated increased concentration of CCK in the hypothalami of Zucker obese and lean rats. *Physiol. Behav.* **35**, 215–220.

McLaughlin, C. L., Baile, C. A., and Dellaferra, M. A. (1986). Changes in brain CCK concentrations with peripheral CCK injections in Zucker rats. *Physiol. Behav.* **36**, 477–482.

Melnyk, R. B. (1987). Decreased binding to hypothalamic insulin receptors in young genetically obese rats. *Physiol. Behav.* **40**, 237–241.

Mercer, S. W., and Trayhurn, P. (1987). Effect of high fat diets on energy balance and thermogenesis in brown adipose tissue of lean and genetically obese ob/ob mice. *J. Nutr.* **117**, 2147–2153.

Meyer, J. (1985). Biochemical effects of corticosteroids on neural tissues. *Annu. Rev. Physiol.* **65**, 946–1020.

Micevych, P., Yaksh, T. L., Go, V. L. W., and Finkelstein, J. A. (1985). Effect of opiates on the release of cholecystokinin from in vitro hypothalamus and frontal cortex of Zucker lean (FA/−) and obese (fa/fa) rats. *Brain Res.* **337**, 382–385.

Mickelsen, O., Takahashi, S., and Craig, C. (1955). Experimental obesity I. Production of obesity in rats by feeding high-fat diets. *J. Nutr.* **57**, 541–554.

Milam, K. M., Stern, J. S., Storlien, L. M., and Keesey, R. E. (1980). Effect of lateral hypothalamic lesions on regulation of body weight and adiposity in rats. *Am. J. Physiol.* **239**, R337–R343.

Milam, K. M., Keesey, R. E., and Stern, J. S. (1982a). Body composition and adiposity in LH-lesioned and pair fed Zucker rats. *Am. J. Physiol.* **242**, E437–E444.

Milam, K. M., Keesey, R. E., Storlien, L. H., and Stern, J. S. (1982b). Development study of adipose cellularity in lateral hypothalamic-lesioned Zucker obese rats. *Am. J. Physiol.* **242**, R311–R317.

Mohr, B. (1840). Hypertrophie der Hypophysis cerebri und dadurch bedingter Druck auf die Hirngrundflache, insebesondere auf die Sehnerven, das Chiasm derselben und den linkseitigen Hirnschenkel. *Wochenschr. Gesamte Heilkd.* **6**, 565–571.

Montiel, F., Ortiz-Caro, J., Villa, A., Pascual, A., and Aranda, A. (1987). Glucocorticoids regulate insulin binding in a rat glial cell line. *Endocrinology (Baltimore)* **121**, 258–265.

Morley, J. E. (1987). Neuropeptide regulation of appetite and weight. *Endocr. Rev.* **8**, 256–287.

Morley, J. E., and Levine, A. S. (1981). Dynorphin-(1-13) induces spontaneous feeding in rats. *Life Sci.* **29**, 1901–1903.

Morley, J. E., and Levine, A. S. (1982). Corticotropin-releasing factor, grooming and ingestive behavior. *Life Sci.* **31**, 1459–1464.

Morley, J. E., Levine, A. S., Kneip, J., and Grace, M. (1982). The effect of vagotomy on the satiety effects of neuropeptides and naloxone. *Life Sci.* **30**, 1943–1947.

Morley, J. E., Levine, A. S., Gosnell, B. A., Kneip, J., and Grace, M. (1983). The kappa opioid receptor, ingestive behaviors and the obese (ob/ob) mouse. *Physiol. Behav.* **31**, 603–606.

Mrosovsky, N. (1975). The amplitude and period of circannual cycles of body weight in golden-mantled ground squirrels with medial hypothalamic lesions. *Brain Res.* **99**, 97–116.

Murase, T., and Inoue, S. (1985). Hepatic triglycerides lipase is not an insulin-dependent enzyme in rats. *Metab., Clin. Exp.* **34**, 531–534.

Nagai, K., Nishio, T., Nakagawa, H., Nakamura, S., and Fukuda, Y. (1978). Effect of bilateral lesions of the suprachiasmatic nuclei on the circadian rhythm of food-intake. *Brain Res.* **142**, 384–389.

Naim, M., Brand, J. G., Kare, M. R., and Carpenter, R. G. (1985). Energy intake, weight gain and fat deposition in rats fed flavored, nutritionally controlled diets in a multichoice ("cafeteria") design. *J. Nutr.* **115**, 1447–1458.

Nakai, T., Tamai, T., Takai, H., Hayashi, S., Fujiwara, R., and Miyabo, S. (1986). Decreased ketonaemia in the monosodium glutamate-induced obese rats. *Life Sci.* **38**, 2009–2013.

Niijima, A. (1981). Visceral afferents and metabolic function. *Diabetologia* **20**, 325–330.

Niijima, A. (1983a). Electrophysiological study on nervous pathway from splanchnic nerve to vagus nerve in rat. *Am. J. Physiol.* **244**, R888–R890.

Niijima, A. (1983b). Glucose-sensitive afferent nerve fibers in the liver and their role in food intake and blood glucose regulation. *J. Auton. Nerv. Syst.* **9**, 207–220.

Niijima, A. (1984a). The effect of D-glucose on the firing rate of glucose-sensitive vagal afferents in the liver in comparison with the effect of 2-deoxy-D-glucose. *J. Auton. Nerv. Syst.* **10**, 255–260.

Niijima, A. (1984b). Reflex control of the autonomic nervous system activity from the glucose sensors in the liver in normal and midpontine-transected animals. *J. Auton. Nerv. Syst.* **10**, 279–285.

Niijima, A. (1986). Effect of glucose and other hexoses on efferent discharges of brown adipose tissue nerves. *Am. J. Physiol.* **251**, R240–R242.

Niijima, A., Rohner-Jeanrenaud, F., and Jeanrenaud, B. (1984). Role of ventromedial hypothalamus on sympathetic efferents of brown adipose tissue. *Am. J. Physiol.* **247**, R650–R654.

Nishio, T., Shiosaka, S., and Nakagawa, H. (1979). Circadian feeding rhythm after hypothalamic knife-cut isolating suprachiasmatic nucleus. *Physiol. Behav.* **23**, 763–769.

Nishizawa, Y., and Bray, G. A. (1978). Ventromedial hypothalamic lesions and the mobilization of fatty acids. *J. Clin. Invest.* **61**, 714–721.

Nishizawa, Y., and Bray, G. A. (1980). Evidence of a circulating ergostatic factor: Studies on parabiotic rats. *Ann. J. Physiol.* **239**, R344–R351.

Nordby, G., Hustvedt, B. E., and Norum, K. R. (1979). The hepatic secretion of lecithin: Cholesterol acyl transferase in rats with increased secretion of triglycerides due to ventromedial hypothalamic lesions. *Scand. J. Clin. Lab. Invest.* **39**, 235–240.

Novin, D., Sanderson, J. D., and Vanderweele, D. A. (1974). The effect of isotonic glucose on eating as a function of feeding condition and infusion. *Physiol. Behav.* **13**, 3–7.

Novin, D., Sanderson, J., and Gonzalez, M. (1979). Feeding after nutrient infusions: Effects of hypothalamic lesions and vagotomy. *Physiol. Behav.* **22**, 107–113.

Novin, D., Rogers, R. C., and Hermann, G. (1981). Visceral afferent and efferent connections in the brain. *Diabetologia* **20**, 331–336.

Obst, B. E., Schemmel, R. A., Czajka-Narins, D., and Merkel, R. (1981). Adipocyte size and number in dietary obesity resistant and susceptible rats. *Am. J. Physiol.* **240**, E47–E53.

Ogundipe, O. O., and Bray, G. A. (1974). The influence of diet and fat cell size on glucose, metabolism, lipogenesis and lipolysis in the rat. *Horm. Metab. Res.* **6**, 351–356.

Ohshima, K., Shargill, N. S., Chan, T. M., and Bray, G. A. (1984). Adrenalectomy reverses insulin resistance in muscle from obese (ob/ob) mice. *Am. J. Physiol.* **246**, E193–E197.

Ohshima, K., Okada, S., Onai, T., Shimizu, H., Satoh, N., Maruta, S., Mori, M., Shimomura, Y., Kobayashi, I., and Kobayashi, S. (1985). The characteristics of obese rats induced by medial basal hypothalamic deafferentation. *Proc. Congr. Jpn. Soc. Study Obes., 5th* pp. 114–115.

Ohtake, M., Bray, G. A., and Azukizawa, M. (1977). Studies on hypothermic and thyroid function in the obese (ob/ob) mouse. *Am. J. Physiol.* **233**, R110–R115.

Oku, J., Bray, G. A., and Fisler, J. S. (1984a). Effects of oral and parenteral quinine on rats with ventromedial hypothalamic knife-cut obesity. *Metab., Clin. Exp.* **33**, 538–544.

Oku, J., Bray, G. A., Fisler, J. S., and Schemmel, R. (1984b). Ventromedial hypothalamic knife-cut lesions in rats resistant to dietary obesity. *Am. J. Physiol.* **246**, R943–R948.

Oku, J., Inoue, S., Glick, Z., Bray, G. A., and Walsh, J. M. (1984c). Cholecystokinin, bombesin and neurotensin in brain tissue from obese animals. *Int. J. Obes.* **8**, 171–182.

Olney, J. W. (1969). Brain lesions, obesity, and other disturbances in mice treated with monosodium glutamate. *Science* **164**, 719.

Ono, T., Sasaki, K., Nishino, H., Fukuda, M., and Shibata, R. (1986). Feeding and diurnal related activity of lateral hypothalamic neurons in freely behaving rats. *Brain Res.* **373**, 92–102.

Oomura, Y. (1976). Significance of glucose, insulin and free fatty acid on the hypothalamic feeding and satiety neurons. *In* "Hunger: Basic Mechanisms and Clinical Implications," (D. N. Novin, W. Wyrwicka, and G. A. Bray, eds.), pp. 145–157. Raven Press, New York.

Oomura, Y. (1983). Glucose as a regulator of neuronal activity. *Adv. Metab. Disord.* **10**, 31–65.

Oomura, Y., and Yoshimatsu, H. (1984). Neural network of glucose monitoring system. *J. Auton. Nerv. Syst.* **10**, 359–372.

Oomura, Y., Ono, T., Ooyama, H., and Wayner, M. J. (1969). Glucose and osmosensitive neurones of the rat hypothalamus. *Nature (London)* **222**, 282–284.

Opsahl, C. A., and Powley, T. L. (1974). Failure of vagotomy to reverse obesity in genetically obese Zucker rat. *Am. J. Physiol.* **226**, 34–38.

Orosco, M., Jacquot, C., and Cohen, Y. (1981). Brain catecholamine levels and turnover in various models of obese animals. *Gen. Pharmacol.* **12**, 267–271.

Orosco, M., Trouvin, J. H., Cohen, Y., and Jacquot, C. (1986). Ontogeny of brain monoamines in lean and obese female Zucker rats. *Physiol. Behav.* **36**, 907–911.

Parameswaran, S. V., Steffens, A. B., Hervey, G. R., and de Ruiter, L. (1977). Involvement of a humoral factor in regulation of body weight in parabiotic rats. *Am. J. Physiol.* **232**, R150–R157.

Penicaud, L., Rohner-Jeanrenaud, F., and Jeanrenaud, B. (1986). In vivo metabolic changes as studied longitudinally after ventromedial hypothalamic lesions. *Am. J. Physiol.* **250**, E662–E668.

Penicaud, L., Terretaz, F. J., Kinebanyat, M. F., Leturque, A., Dore, E., Girard, J., Jeanrenaud, B., and Picou, L. (1987). Development of obesity in Zucker rats. Early insulin resistance in muscles but normal sensitivity in white adipose tissue. *Diabetes* **36**, 626–631.

Peters, R. H., Blythe, B. L., and Sensenig, L. D. (1985). Electrolytic current parameters in the dorsolateral tegmental obesity syndrome in rats. *Physiol. Behav.* **34**, 57–60.

Planche, E., Joliff, M., DeGasquet, P., and LeLiepvre, X. (1983). Evidence of a defect in energy expenditure in the 7-day-old Zucker rat (fa/fa). *Am. J. Physiol.* **245**, E107–E113.

Plata-Salaman, C. R., Oomura, Y., and Shimizu, N. (1986a). Dependence of food intake on acute and chronic ventricular administration of insulin. *Physiol. Behav.* **37**, 717–734.

Plata-Salaman, C. R., Oomura, Y., and Shimizu, N. (1986b). Endogenous sugar acid derivative acting as a feeding suppressant. *Physiol. Behav.* **38**, 1–15.

Porte, D., and Woods, S. C. (1981). Regulation of food intake and body weight by insulin. *Diabetologia* **20**, 274–278.

Powley, T. L. (1977). The ventromedial hypothalamic syndrome, satiety, and a cephalic phase hypothesis. *Psychol. Rev.* **84**, 89–126.

Powley, T. L., and Morton, S. (1976). Hypophysectomy and regulation of body weight in genetically obese Zucker rats. *Am. J. Physiol.* **230**, 982–987.

Powley, T. L., and Opsahl, C. A. (1974). Ventromedial hypothalamic obesity abolished by subdiaphragatic vagotomy. *Am. J. Physiol.* **226**, 25–33.

Powley, T. L., Walgren, M. D., and Laughton, W. B. (1983). Effects of guanethidine sympathectomy on ventromedial hypothalamic obesity. *Am. J. Physiol.* **245**, R408–R420.

Praissman, M., and Izzo, R. S. (1986). A reduced pancreatic protein secretion in response to cholecystokinin in the obese rat correlates with a reduced receptor capacity for CCK. *Endocrinology (Baltimore)* **119**, 546–553.

Puthuraya, K. P., Oomura, Y., and Shimizu, N. (1985). Effect of endogenous sugar acids on the ventromedial hypothalamic nucleus of the rat. *Brain Res.* **332**, 165–168.

Raasmaja, A., and York, D. A. (1987). Alpha[1] and B-adrenergic receptors in brown adipose tissue of lean and obese Zucker rats: The effect of sucrose feeding, cold acclimation and adrenalectomy. *Biochem. J.* **249,** 831–838.

Radcliffe, J. D., and Webster, A. F. (1976). Regulation of food intake during growth in fatty and lean female Zucker rats given diets of different protein content. *Br. J. Nutr.* **36,** 457–469.

Radcliffe, J. D., and Webster, A. F. (1978). Sex, body, composition and regulation of food intake during growth in the Zucker rat. *Br. J. Nutr.* **39,** 483–492.

Radcliffe, J. D., and Webster, A. F. (1979). The effect of varying the quality of dietary protein and energy on food intake and growth in the Zucker rat. *Br. J. Nutr.* **41,** 111–124.

Ramirez, I. (1986). Hypophagia following dietary obesity. *Physiol. Behav.* **38,** 95–98.

Ramirez, I. (1987a). Diet texture, moisture and starch type in dietary obesity. *Physiol. Behav.* **41,** 149–154.

Ramirez, I. (1987b). Feeding a liquid diet increases energy intake, weight gain and body fat in rats. *J. Nutr.* **117,** 2127–2134.

Ramirez, I., and Friedman, M. I. (1983). Food intake and blood fuels after oil consumption: Differential effects in normal and diabetic rats. *Physiol. Behav.* **31,** 847–850.

Rattigan, S., Howe, P. R. C., and Clark, M. G. (1986). The effect of a high-fat diet and sucrose drinking option on the development of obesity in spontaneously hypertensive rats. *Br. J. Nutr.* **56,** 73–80.

Rayer, P. F. O. (1823). Observations sur les maladies de l'appendice sus-sphenoïdal (glande pituitaire) du cerveau. *Arch. Gen. Med.* **3,** 350–367.

Recant, L., Voyles, N. R., Luciano, M., and Pert, C. B. (1980). Naloxone reduces weight gain, alters B-endorphin and reduces insulin output from pancreatic islets of genetically obese mice. *Peptides (N.Y.)* **1,** 309–313.

Recant, L., Voyles, N., Wade, A., Awoke, S., and Bhathena, S. J. (1983). Studies on the role of opiate peptides in two forms of genetic obesity: ob/ob mouse and fa/fa rat. *Horm. Metab. Res.* **15,** 589–593.

Reisin, E., Suarez, D. H., and Frohlich, E. D. (1980). Haemodynamic changes associated with obesity and high blood pressure in rats with ventromedial hypothalamic lesions. *Clin. Sci.* **59,** 397s–399s.

Ricquier, D., Bouillard, F., Tomelin, P., Mory, G., Bazin, R., Arch, J., and Penicaud, L. (1986). Expression of uncoupling protein mRNA in thermogenic brown adipose tissue. *J. Biol. Chem.* **261,** 13905–13910.

Ritter, S. (1986). Glucoprivation and the glucoprivic control of food intake. *In* "Feeding Behavior: Neural and Humoral Controls" (R. Ritter, S. Ritter, and C. D. Barnes, eds.), pp. 271–313. Academic Press, Orlando, Florida.

Robeson, B. L., Eisen, E. J., and Leatherwood, M. J. (1981). Adipose cellularity, serum glucose, insulin and cholesterol in polygenic obese mice fed high-fat or high-carbohydrate diets. *Growth* **45,** 198–215.

Rohner-Jeanrenaud, F., and Jeanrenaud, B. (1980). Consequences of ventromedial hypothalamic lesions upon insulin and glucagon secretion by subsequently isolated perfused pancreases in the rat. *J. Clin. Invest.* **65,** 902–910.

Rohner-Jeanrenaud, F., and Jeanrenaud, B. (1985). Involvement of the cholinergic system in insulin and glucagon oversecretion in preobesity. *Endocrinology (Baltimore)* **116,** 830–834.

Rohner-Jeanrenaud, F., Seydoux, J., Chinet, A., Bas, S., Giacobino, J.-P., Assimacopoulos-Jeannet, F., Jeanrenaud, B., and Girardier, L. (1983a). Defective diet-induced but normal cold-induced brown adipose tissue adaptation in hypothalamic obesity in rats. *J. Physiol. (Paris)* **78,** 833–837.

Rohner-Jeanrenaud, F., Hochstrasser, A.-C., and Jeanrenaud, B. (1983b). Hyperinsulinemia of preobese and obese fa/fa rats is partly vagus nerve mediated. *Am. J. Physiol.* **244,** E317–E322.

Rohner-Jeanrenaud, F., Proietto, J., Ionesco, E., and Jeanrenaud, B. (1986). Mechanism and abnormal oral glucose tolerance of genetically obese fa/fa rat. *Diabetes* **35,** 1350–1355.

Roland, C. R., Bhakthavatsalam, P., and Leibowitz, S. F. (1986). Interaction between corticosterone and alpha-2-noradrenergic system of the paraventricular nucleus in relation to feeding behavior. *Neuroendocrinology* **42,** 296–305.

Rolls, B. J., Rowe, E. A., and Turner, R. C. (1980). Persistent obesity in rats following a period of consumption of a mixed, high energy diet. *J. Physiol. (London)* **298,** 415–427.

Rolls, B. J., Van Duijenvoorde, P. M., and Rowe, E. A. (1983). Variety in the diet enhances intake in a meal and contributes to the development of obesity in the rat. *Physiol. Behav.* **31,** 21–17.

Romsos, D. R. (1985). Norepinephrine turnover in obese mice and rats. *Int. J. Obes.* **9,** 55–62.

Romsos, D. R., and Ferguson, D. (1982). Self-selected intake of carbohydrate, fat, and protein by obese (ob/ob) and lean mice. *Physiol. Behav.* **28,** 301–305.

Rossier, J., Rogers, J., Shibasaki, R., Guilleman, R, and Bloom, F. E. (1979). Opioid peptides and a-melanocyte stimulating hormone in genetically obese (ob/ob) mice during development. *Proc. Natl. Acad. Sci. U.S.A.* **76,** 2077–2080.

Rostene, W. H., Bazin, R, Morgat, J. L., Dussaillant, M., and Broer, Y. (1985). Quantitative autoradiographic localization of neurotensin binding sites in lean and obese Zucker rats. *Horm. Metab. Res.* **17,** 692–693.

Rothwell, N. J., and Stock, M. J. (1978a). A paradox in the control of energy intake in the rat. *Nature (London)* **273,** 146–147.

Rothwell, N. J., and Stock, M. J., (1978b). Mechanism of weight gain and loss in reversible obesity in the rat. *J. Physiol. (London)* **276,** 60–61.

Rothwell, N. J., and Stock, M. J. (1979). A role for brown adipose tissue in diet-induced thermogenesis. *Nature (London)* **281,** 31–35.

Rothwell, N. J., and Stock, M. J. (1981a). Acute effects of food, 2-deoxyglucose and noradrenaline on metabolic rate and brown adipose tissue in normal and atropinized lean and obese Zucker rats. *Pfluegers Arch.* **392,** 172–177.

Rothwell, N. J., and Stock, M. J. (1981b). A role for insulin in the diet-induced thermogenesis of cafeteria-fed rats. *Metab., Clin. Exp.* **30,** 673–678.

Rothwell, N. J., and Stock, M. J. (1982). Energy expenditure of "cafeteria"-fed rats determined from measurements of energy balance and indirect calorimetry. *J. Physiol. (London)* **328,** 371–377.

Rothwell, N. J., and Stock, M. J. (1983). Acute effects of fat and carbohydrate on metabolic rate in normal, cold-acclimated and lean and obese (fa/fa) Zucker rats. *Metab., Clin. Exp.* **32,** 371–376.

Rothwell, N. J., and Stock, M. J. (1984a). Brown adipose tissue. *Recent Adv. Physiol.* **10,** 349–384.

Rothwell, N. J., and Stock, M. J. (1984b). Energy balance, thermogenesis and brown adipose tissue activity in tube-fed rats. *J. Nutr.* **114,** 1965–1970.

Rothwell, N. J., and Stock, M. J. (1986). Energy balance and brown fat activity in adrenalectomized male, female and castrated male rats. *Metab., Clin. Exp.* **35,** 657–660.

Rothwell, N. J., and Stock, M. J. (1987a). Stimulation of thermogenesis and brown fat activity in rats fed medium chain triglyceride. *Metab., Clin. Exp.* **36,** 128–130.

Rothwell, N. J., and Stock, M. J. (1987b). Effect of diet and fenfluramine on thermogenesis in the rat: Possible involvement of serotonergic mechanisms. *Int. J. Obes.* **11**, 319–324.

Rothwell, N. J., Stock, M. J., and Wyllie, M. G. (1981). Na$^+$,K$^+$-ATPase activity and noradrenaline turnover in brown adipose tissue of rats exhibiting diet-induced thermogenesis. *Biochem. Pharmacol.* **30**, 1709–1712.

Rothwell, N. J., Saville, M. E., and Stock, M. J. (1982a). Sympathetic and thyroid influences on metabolic rate in fed, fasted and refed rats. *Am. J. Physiol.* **243**, R339–346.

Rothwell, N. J., Stock, M. J., and Tzybir, R. S. (1982b). Energy balance and mitochondrial function in liver and brown fat of rats fed "cafeteria" diets of varying protein. *J. Nutr.* **112**, 1663–1672.

Rothwell, N. J., Saville, M. E., and Stock, M. J. (1983a). Metabolic responses to fasting and refeeding in lean and genetically obese rats. *Am. J. Physiol.* **244**, R615–R620.

Rothwell, N. J., Stock, M. J., and Trayhurn, P. (1983b). Reduced lipogenesis in cafeteria-fed rats exhibiting diet-induced thermogenesis. *Biosci. Rep.* **3**, 217–224.

Rothwell, N. J., Saville, M. E., and Stock, M. J. (1983c). Role of insulin in thermogenic responses to refeeding in 3-day-fasted rats. *Am. J. Physiol.* **245**, E160–E165.

Rothwell, N. J., Stock, M. J., and Tyzbir, R. S. (1983d). Mechanisms of thermogenesis induced by low protein diets. *Metab., Clin. Exp.* **32**, 257–261.

Rothwell, N., Stock, M. J., and York, D. A. (1984). Effects of adrenalectomy on energy balance, diet-induced thermogenesis and brown adipose tissue in adult cafeteria-fed rats. *Comp. Biochem. Physiol. A* **78**, 565–569.

Rothwell, N. J., Stock, M. J., and Warwick, B. P. (1985a). Involvement of insulin in the acute thermogenic responses to food and nonmetabolizable substances. *Metab., Clin. Exp.* **34**, 43–47.

Rothwell, N. J., Stock, M. J., and Warwick, B. P. (1985b). Energy balance and brown fat activity in rats fed cafeteria diets or high-fat, semisynthetic diets at several levels of intake. *Metab., Clin. Exp.* **34**, 474–480.

Rowland, N. E., Bellush, L. L., and Carlton, J. (1985). Metabolic and neurochemical correlates of glucoprivic feeding. *Brain Res. Bull.* **14**, 617–624.

Russek, M. (1970). Demonstration of the influence of an hepatic glucosensitive mechanism on food intake. *Physiol. Behav.* **5**, 1207–1209.

Rutman, R. J., Lewis, F. S., and Bloomer, W. D. (1966). Bipiperidyl mustard, a new obesifying agent in the mouse. *Science* **153**, 1000–1002.

Saito, M., and Bray, G. A. (1984). Adrenalectomy and food restriction in the genetically obese (ob/ob) mouse. *Am. J. Physiol.* **248**, E20–E25.

Saito, A., Williams, J., and Goldfine, I. (1981). Alterations in brain cholecystokinin receptors and fasting. *Nature (London)* **289**, 599–600.

Saito, M., Minokoshi, Y., and Shimazu, T. (1985). Brown adipose tissue after ventromedial hypothalamic lesions in rats. *Am. J. Physiol.* **246**, R20–R25.

Sakaguchi, T., and Bray, G. A. (1987a). Intrahypothalamic injection of insulin decreases firing rate of sympathetic nerves. *Proc. Natl. Acad. Sci. U.S.A.* **84**, 2021–2014.

Sakaguchi, T., and Bray, G. A. (1987b). The effect of intrahypothalamic injections of glucose on sympathetic efferent firing rate. *Brain Res. Bull.* **18**, 591–595.

Sakaguchi, T., and Bray, G. A. (1989). Effect of norepinephrine, serotonin and tryptophan on the firing rate of sympathetic nerves. *Brain Res.* (in press).

Sakaguchi, T., Arase, K., and Bray, G. A. (1988a). Effect of intrahypothalamic hydroxybutyrate on sympathetic firing rate. *Met., Clin. Exp.* **37**, 731–735.

Sakaguchi, T., Takahashi, M., and Bray, G. A. (1988b). The lateral hypothalamus and sympathetic firing rate. *Am. J. Physiol.* **255**, R507–R512.

Sakata, T., Oomura, Y., Fukushima, M., Tsutsui, K., Hashimoto, K., Kuhara, T, and

Matsumoto, I. (1980). Circadian and long-term variation of certain metabolites in fasted rat: Implications. *Brain Res. Bull.* **5**, 23–28.

Sakata, T., Ookuma, K., Fukagawa, K., Fujimoto, K., Yoshimatsu, H., Shiraishi, T., and Wada, H. (1988). Blockade of the histamine H_1-receptor in the rat ventromedial hypothalamus and feeding elicitation. *Brain Res.* **441**, 403–407.

Salmon, D. M. W., and Flatt, J. P. (1985). Effect of dietary fat content on the incidence of obesity among ad libitum fed mice. *Int. J. Obes.* **9**, 443–449.

Sauter, A., Goldstein, M., Engel, J., and Ueta, K. (1983). Effect of insulin on central catecholamines. *Brain Res.* **260**, 330–333.

Sawchenko, P. E., Gold, R. M., and Alexander, J. (1981). Effects of selective vagotomies on knife-cut induced hypothalamic obesity: Differential results on lab chow vs high-fat diets. *Physiol. Behav.* **26**, 293–300.

Sawchenko, P. E., Swanson, L. W., and Vale, W. W. (1984). Co-expression of corticotropin-releasing factor and vasopressin immunoreactivity in parvocellular neuro-secretory neurons of the adrenalectomized rat. *Proc. Natl. Acad. Sci. U.S.A.* **81**, 1883–1887.

Scallett, A. C., and Olney, J. W. (1986). Components of hypothalamic obesity: Bipiperidyl-mustard lesions add hyperphagia to monosodium glutamate-induced hyperinsulinemia. *Brain Res.* **374**, 380–384.

Scharrer, E., and Langhans, W. (1986). Control of food intake by fatty acid oxidation. *Am. J. Physiol.* **250**, R1003–R1006.

Schechter, M. D. (1986). Fenfluramine discrimination in obese and lean Zucker rats: Serotonergic mediation of effect. *Eur. J. Pharmacol.* **125**, 135–141.

Schechter, M. D., and Finkelstein, J. A. (1985). Effect of dopamine agonists and fenfluramine on discriminative behavior in obese and lean Zucker rats. *Pharmacol., Biochem. Behav.* **23**, 7–11.

Schemmel, R. (1976). Physiological considerations of lipid storage and utilization. *Am. Zool.* **16**, 661–670.

Schemmel, R., Mickelson, O., and Gill, J. L. (1970). Dietary obesity in rats: Body weight and body fat accretion in seven strains of rats. *J. Nutr.* **100**, 1041–1048.

Schemmel, R., Hu, D., Mickelson, O., and Romsos, D. R. (1982a). Dietary obesity in rats: Influence on carbohydrate metabolism. *J. Nutr.* **112**, 223–230.

Schemmel, R. A., Teague, R. J., and Bray, G. A. (1982b). Obesity in Osborne–Mendel and S 5B/P1 rats: Effects of sucrose solutions, castration, and treatment with estradiol or insulin. *Am. J. Physiol.* **243**, R347–R353.

Schick, R. R., Yaksh, T. L., and Go, V. L. W. (1986). An intragastric meal releases the putative satiety factor cholecystokinin from hypothalamic neurons in cats. *Brain Res.* **370**, 349–353.

Schneider, B., Monahan, J., and Hirsch, J. (1979). Brain cholecystokinin and nutritional status in rats and mice. *J. Clin. Invest.* **64**, 1348–1356.

Schulz, R., Wilhelm, A., and Dirlich, G. (1984). Intracerebral injection of different antibodies against endogenous opioids suggested alpha-neo-endorphin participation in control of feeding behavior. *Naunyn. Schmiedeberg's Arch. Pharmacol.* **326**, 222–226.

Schwartz, J. H., Young, J. B., and Landsberg, L. (1983). Effect of dietary fat on sympathetic nervous system activity in the rat. *J. Clin. Invest.* **72**, 361–370.

Sclafani, A. (1978). Food motivation in hypothalamic hyperphagic rats reexamined. *Neurosci. Biobehav. Rev.* **2**, 339–355.

Sclafani, A. (1981). The role of hyperinsulinema and the vagus nerve in hypothalamic hyperphagia reexamined. *Diabetologia* **20**, 402–410.

Sclafani, A. (1984). Animal models of obesity: Classification and characterization. *Int. J. Obes.* **8**, 491–508.

Sclafani, A. (1987a). Carbohydrate taste, appetite, and obesity: An overview. *Neurosci. Biobehav. Rev.* **11**, 131–153.

Sclafani, A. (1987b). Carbohydrate-induced hyperphagia and obesity in the rat: Effects of saccharide type, form, and taste. *Neurosci. Biobehav. Rev.* **11**, 155–162.

Sclafani, A., and Aravich, P. F. (1983). Macronutrient self-selection in three forms of hypothalamic obesity. *Am. J. Physiol.* **244**, R686–R694.

Sclafani, A., and Gorman, A. N. (1977). Effects of age, sex, and prior body weight on the development of dietary obesity in adult rats. *Physiol. Behav.* **18**, 1021–1026.

Sclafani, A., and Grossman, S. P. (1969). Hyperphagia produced by knife cuts between the medial and lateral hypothalamus in the rat. *Physiol. Behav.* **4**, 533–537.

Sclafani, A., and Kirchgessner, A. L. (1986a). The role of the medial hypothalamus in the control of food intake; an update. *In* "Feeding Behavior: Neural and Humoral Controls" (R. Ritter, S. Ritter, and C. D. Barnes, eds.), pp. 27–66. Academic Press, Orlando, Florida.

Sclafani, A., and Kirchgessner, A. L. (1986b). Influence of taste and nutrition on the sugar appetite of rats. *Nutr. Behav.* **3**, 57–74.

Sclafani, A., and Krammer, T. H. (1985). Dietary selection in vagotomized rats. *J. Auton. Nerv. Syst.* **9**, 247–258.

Sclafani, A., and Springer, D. (1976). Dietary obesity in adult rats: Similarities to hypothalamic and human obesity syndromes. *Physiol. Behav.* **17**, 461–471.

Sclafani, A., Koopmans, H. S., Vasselli, J. R., and Reichman, M. (1978). Effects of intestinal bypass surgery on appetite, food intake, and body weight in obese and lean rats. *Am. J. Physiol.* **234**, E389–E398.

Sclafani, A., Aravich, P., and Schwartz, J. (1979). Hypothalamic hyperphagic rats overeat bitter sucrose octa acetate diets but not quinine diets. *Physiol. Behav.* **22**, 759–766.

Sclafani, A., Aravich, P. F., and Landman, M. (1981). Vagotomy blocks hypothalamic hyperphagia in rats on a chow diet and sucrose solution, not on a mixed palatable diet. *J. Comp. Physiol. Psychol.* **95**, 720–734.

Seydoux, J., Rohner-Jeanrenaud, F., Assimacopoulos-Jeannet, F., Jeanrenaud, B., and Girardier, L. (1981). Functional disconnection of brown adipose tissue in hypothalamic obesity in rats. *Pfluegers Arch.* **390**, 1–4.

Seydoux, J., Assimacopoulos-Jeannet, F., Jeanrenaud, B., and Girardier, L. (1982a). Alterations of brown adipose tissue in genetically obese (ob/ob) mice. I. Demonstration of loss of metabolic response to nerve stimulation and catecholamines and its partial recovery after fasting or cold adaptation. *Endocrinology (Baltimore)* **110**, 432–438.

Seydoux, J., Ricquier, D., Rohner-Jeanrenaud, F., Assimacopoulos-Jeannet, F., Giacobino, J. P., Jeanrenaud, B., and Girardier, L. (1982b). Decreased guanine nucleotide binding and reduced equivalent production by brown adipose tissue in hypothalamic obesity. *FEBS Lett.* **146**, 161–164.

Shargill, N. S., York, D. A., and Marchington, D. R. (1983). Regulation of hepatic tyrosine aminotransferase in genetically obese rats. *Biochim. Biophys. Acta* **156**, 297–307.

Shargill, N. S., Al-Baker, I., and York, D. A. (1987). Normal levels of serum corticosterone and hepatic glucocorticoid receptors in obese fa/fa rats. *Biosci. Rep.* **7**, 843–851.

Sheppard, M. C., Bailey, C. J., Flatt, P. R., Swanston-Flatt, S. K., and Shennan, K. I. J. (1985). Immunoreactive neurotensin in spontaneous syndromes of obesity and diabetes in mice. *Acta Endocrinol. (Copenhagen)* **108**, 532–536.

Shimazu, T., Noma, M., and Saito, M. (1986). Chronic infusion of norepinephrine into the ventromedial hypothalamus induces obesity in rats. *Brain Res.* **369**, 215–223.

Shimizu, N., Oomura, Y., and Sakata, T. (1984). Modulation of feeding by endogenous sugar acids acting as hunger or satiety factors. *Am. J. Physiol.* **246**, R542–R550.

Shimizu, H., Shargill, N. S., Bray, G. A., Yen, T. T., and Geselchen, P. D. (1989). Effects of MSH on food intake, body weight and coat color of the yellow obese mouse. *Life Sci.* (in press).

Shimomura, Y., Bray, G. A., and York, D. A. (1981). Effects of thyroid hormone and adrenalectomy on (Na$^+$ + K$^+$) ATPase in the ob/ob mouse. *Horm. Metab. Res.* **13**, 579–582.

Shimomura, Y., Oku, J., Glick, Z., and Bray, G. A. (1982). Opiate receptors, food intake and obesity. *Physiol. Behav.* **28**, 441–445.

Shimomura, Y., Bray, G. A., and Lee, M. (1987). Adrenalectomy and steroid treatment in obese (ob/ob) and diabetic (db/db) mice. *Horm. Metab. Res.* **19**, 295–299.

Shor-Posner, G., Azar, P., Insinga, S., and Leibowitz, S. F. (1985). Deficits in the control of food intake after hypothalamic paraventricular nucleus lesions. *Physiol. Behav.* **35**, 883–890.

Shor-Posner, G., Azar, A. P., Filart, R., Tempel, D., and Leibowitz, S. F. (1986a). Morphine-stimulated feeding: Analysis of macronutrient selection and paraventricular nucleus lesions. *Pharmacol., Biochem. Behav.* **24**, 931–939.

Shor-Posner, G., Grinker, J. A., Marinescu, C., Brown, O., and Leibowitz, S. F. (1986b). Hypothalamic serotonin in the control of meal patterns and macronutrient selection. *Brain Res. Bull.* **17**, 663–671.

Silva, J. E., and Larsen, P. R. (1986). Hormonal regulation of iodothyronine 5'deiodinase in rat brown adipose tissue. *Am. J. Physiol.* **251**, E639–E643.

Sims, E. A. H., (1986). Energy balance in human beings: The problems of plenitude. *Vitam. Horm. (N.Y.)* **43**, 1–101.

Sinha, Y. N., Salocks, C. B., and Vanderlaan, W. P. (1976). Control of prolactin and growth hormone secretion in mice by obesity. *Endocrinology (Baltimore)* **99**, 881–886.

Sinha, Y. N., Thomas, J. W., Salocks, C. B., Wickes, M. A., and Vanderlaan, W. P. (1977). Prolactin and growth hormone secretion in diet-induced obesity in mice. *Horm. Metab. Res.* **9**, 277–282.

Smith, C. K., and Romsos, D. R. (1985). Effects of adrenalectomy on energy balance obese mice are diet dependent. *Am. J. Physiol.* **249**, R13–R22.

Smith, F. J., and Campfield, L. A. (1986). Pancreatic adaptation in VMH obesity: In vivo compensatory response to altered neural input. *Am. J. Physiol.* **251**, R70–R76.

Smith, G. P., and Gibbs, J. (1984). Gut peptides and postprandial satiety. *Fed. Proc., Fed. Am. Soc. Exp. Biol.* **43**, 2889–2892.

Smith, G. P., Jerome, C., Cushin, B. J., Eterno, R., and Simansky, K. J. (1981a). Abdominal vagotomy blocks the satiety effect of cholecystokinin in the rat. *Science* **213**, 1036–1037.

Smith, G. P., Jerome, C., and Gibbs, J. (1981b). Abdominal vagotomy does not block the satiety effect of bombesin in the rat. *Peptides (N.Y.)* **2**, 409–411.

Smith, M. H., Salisbury, R., and Weinberg, H. (1961). The reaction of hypothalamic-hyperphagic rats to stomach preloads. *J. Comp. Physiol. Psychol.* **54**, 660–664.

Smith, U., Kral, J., and Bjorntorp, P. (1974). Influence of dietary fat and carbohydrate on the metabolism of adipocytes of different size in the rat. *Biochim. Biophys. Acta* **337**, 278–285.

Smutz, E. R., Hirsch, E., and Jacobs, H. L. (1975). Caloric compensation in hypothalamic obese rats. *Physiol. Behav.* **14**, 305–309.

Spear, G. S., Ohshima, K., Bray, G. A., and Couple, M. V. (1987). Effect of adrenalectomy on the pancreas of db/db mice. *Horm. Metab. Res.* **18**, 743–746.

Stanley, B. G., and Leibowitz, S. F. (1984). Neuropeptide Y: Stimulation of feeding and drinking by injection into the paraventricular nucleus. *Life Sci.* **33**, 2635–2642.

Stanley, B. G., and Leibowitz, S. F. (1985). Neuropeptide Y injected in the paraventricular hypothalamus: A powerful stimulant of feeding behavior. *Proc. Natl. Acad. Sci. U.S.A.* **82**, 3940–3943.

Stanley, B. G., Kyrkouli, S. E., Lampert, S., and Leibowitz, S. F. (1986). Neuropeptide Y chronically injected into the hypothalamus: A powerful neurochemical inducer of hyperphagia and obesity. *Peptides (N.Y.)* **7**, 1189–1192.

Steffens, A. B., and Strubbe, J. H. (1987). Regulation of body weight and food intake. *Sci. Prog.* **71**, 545–562.

Steffens, A. B., Flik, G., Kuipers, F., Lotter, E. C., and Luiten, P. G. M. (1984). Hypothalamically-induced insulin release and its potentiation during oral and intravenous glucose loads. *Brain Res.* **301**, 351–361.

Stein, L. J., Dorsa, D. M., Baskin, D. G., Figlewicz, D. P., Ikeda, H., Frankmann, S. P., Greenwood, M. R. C., Porte, D., Jr., and Woods, W. C. (1983). Immunoreactive insulin levels are elevated in the cerebrospinal fluid of genetically obese Zucker rats. *Endocrinology (Baltimore)* **113**, 2299–2301.

Stein, L. J., Figlewicz, D. P., Dorsa, D. M., Baskin, D. G., Reed, D., Braget, D., Midkiff, M., Porte, D., Jr., and Woods, S. C. (1985). Effect of insulin infusion on cerebrospinal fluid concentrations in heterozygous lean and obese Zucker rats. *Int. J. Obes.* **9**, A145.

Stern, J. S., and Keesey, R. E. (1981). The effect of ventromedial hypothalamic lesions on adipose cell number in the rat. *Nutr. Rep. Int.* **23**, 295–301.

Stolz, D. J., and Martin, R. J. (1982). Role of insulin in food intake, weight gain and lipid deposition in the Zucker obese rat. *J. Nutr.* **112**, 997–1002.

Stone, M., Schemmel, R., and Czajka-Narins, D. M. (1980). Growth and development of kidneys, heart and liver in S 5B/P1 and Osborne–Mendel rats fed high or low-fat diets. *Int. J. Obes.* **4**, 65–78.

Storlien, L. H., James, D. E., Burleigh, K. M., Chisholm, D. J., and Kraegen, E. W. (1986). Fat feeding causes widespread in vivo insulin resistance, decreased energy expenditure, and obesity in rats. *Am. J. Physiol.* **251**, E576–E583.

Storlien, L. H., Kraegen, E. W., Chisholm, D. J., Ford, G. L., Bruce, D. G., and Pascoe, W. S. (1987). Fish oil prevents insulin resistance induced by high-fat feeding in rats. *Science* **237**, 885–888.

Strauss, E., and Yallow, R. S. (1979). Cholecystokinin in the brain of obese and nonobese mice. *Science* **203**, 68–69.

Stricker, E. M., Rowland, N., and Saller, C. F. (1977). Homeostasis during hypoglycemia: Central control of adrenal secretion and peripheral control of feeding. *Science* **196**, 79–81.

Strubbe, J. H., and Mein, C. G. (1977). Increased feeding in response to bilateral injections of insulin antibodies in the VMH. *Physiol. Behav.* **17**, 309–314.

Stuckey, J. A., Gibbs, J., and Smith, G. P. (1985). Neural disconnection of gut from brain blocks bombesin-induced satiety. *Peptides (N.Y.)* **6**, 1249–1252.

Sundin, U., and Nachad, M. (1983). Tropic response of rat brown fat by glucose feeding: Involvement of sympathetic nervous system. *Am. J. Physiol.* **244**, C142–C149.

Susini, C., and Lavau, M. (1978). In-vitro and in-vivo responsiveness of muscle and adipose tissue to insulin in rats rendered obese by a high-fat diet. *Diabetes* **27**, 114–120.

Tache, Y., and Gunion, M. (1985). Corticotropin releasing factor: Central action to influence gastric secretion. *Fed. Proc., Fed. Am. Soc. Exp. Biol.* **44**, 255–258.

Takasaki, Y. (1978). Studies on brain lesion by administration of monosodium L-glutamate to mice. I. Brain lesions in intact mice caused by administration of monosodium-L-glutamate. *Toxicology* **9**, 293–305.

Tanaka, K., Shimada, M., Nakao, K., and Kusonoki, T. (1978). Hypothalamic lesion induced by injection of monosodium glutamate in suckling period and subsequent development of obesity. *Exp. Neurol.* **62**, 191–199.

Teague, R. J., Kanarek, R., Bray, G. A., Glick, Z., and Orthen-Gambill, N. (1981). Effect of diet on the weight of brown adipose tissue in rodents. *Life Sci.* **29**, 1531–1536.

Terrettaz, J., Assimacopoulos-Jeannet, F., and Jeanrenaud, B. (1986). Severe hepatic and peripheral insulin resistance as evidence by euglycemic clamps in genetically obese fa/fa rats. *Endocrinology (Baltimore)* **118**, 674–678.

Tews, J. K. (1981). Dietary GABA decreases body weight of genetically obese mice. *Life Sci.* **29**, 2535–2542.

Thurlby, P., and Trayhurn, T. (1980). Regional blood flow in genetically obese (ob/ob) mice. *Pfluegers Arch.* **385**, 193–201.

Tokunaga, K., Fukushima, M., Kemnitz, J. W., and Bray, G. A. (1986a). Effect of vagotomy on serum insulin in rats with paraventricular or ventromedial hypothalamic lesions. *Endocrinology (Baltimore)* **119**, 1708–1711.

Tokunaga, K., Fukushima, M., Kemnitz, J. W., and Bray, G. A. (1986b). Comparison of ventromedial and paraventricular lesions in rats that become obese. *Am. J. Physiol.* **251**, R1221–R1227.

Tokunaga, K., Fujioka, S., Matsuzawa, Y., Tarui, S., Fukushima, M., and Bray, G. A. (1987). Differences in glucose metabolism between PVN and VMH lesioned rats. *Int. J. Obes.* **11**, Suppl. 2, 36.

Tokunaga, K., Fukushima, M., Lupien, J. R., Bray, G. A., Kemnitz, J. W., and Schemmel, R. (1989). Effects of food restriction and adrenalectomy in rats with VMH or PVN lesions. *Physiol. Behav.* **45**, (in press).

Tordoff, M. G., Hopfenbeck, J., and Novin, D. (1982). Hepatic vagotomy (partial hepatic denervation) does not alter ingestive responses to metabolic challenges. *Physiol. Behav.* **28**, 417–424.

Tordoff, M. G., Glick, Z., Butcher, L. L., and Novin, D. (1984). Guanethidine sympathectomy does not prevent meal-induced increases in the weight or oxygen consumption of brown fat. *Physiol. Behav.* **33**, 975–979.

Trayhurn, P. (1977). Thermogenic defect in pre-obese ob/ob mice. *Nature (London)* **266**, 60–62.

Trayhurn, P., and James W. P. T. (1978). Thermoregulation and non-shivering thermogenesis in the genetically obese (ob/ob) mouse. *Pfluegers Arch.* **373**, 189–193.

Triandafillou, J., and Himms-Hagen, J. (1983). Brown adipose tissue in genetically obese (fa/fa) rats: Response to cold and diet. *Am. J. Physiol.* **244**, E145–E150.

Triscari, J., Nauss-Karol, C., Levin, B. E., and Sullivan, A. C. (1985). Changes in lipid metabolism in diet-induced obesity. *Metab., Clin. Exp.* **34**, 580–587.

Turkenkopf, I. J., Johnson, P. R., and Greenwood, M. R. C. (1983). Development of pancreatic and plasma insulin in prenatal and suckling Zucker rats. *Am. J. Physiol.* **24**, E220–E225.

Underberger, S. J., Fisler, J. S., York, D. A., and Bray, G. A. (1987). Fenfluramine prevents dietary obesity in Osborne–Mendel rats. *Clin. Res.* **35**, 166A.

Ungerstedt, U. (1971). Adipsia and agphagia after 6-hydroxydopamine induced degeneration of the nigro-striatal dopamine system. *Acta Physiol. Scand., Suppl.* **367**, 95–112.

van der Kroon, P. H. W., Wittgen-Struik, G., and Vermeulen, L. (1981). The role of hyperphagia and hypothyroidism in the development of the obese-hyperglycemic syndrome in mice (ob/ob). *Int. J. Obes.* **5**, 353–358.

van der Kroon, P. H. W., Boldewijn, H., and Langeveld-Soeter, N. (1982). Congenital hypothyroidism in latent obese (ob/ob) mice. *Int. J. Obes.* **6**, 83–90.

Vander Tuig, J. G., Trostler, N., Romsos, D., and Leveille, G. (1979). Heat production of lean and obese (ob/ob) mice in response to fasting, food restriction and thyroxine. *Proc. Soc. Exp. Biol. Med.* **160**, 266–271.

Vander Tuig, J. G., Knehans, A. W., and Romsos, D. R. (1982). Reduced sympathetic nervous activity in rats with ventromedial hypothalamic lesions. *Life Sci.* **30**, 913–920.

Vander Tuig, J. G., Ohshima, K., Yoshida, T., Romsos, D. R., and Bray, G. A. (1984). Adrenalectomy increases norepinephrine turnover in brown adipose tissue of obese (ob/ob) mice. *Life Sci.* **34**, 1423–1432.

Vander Tuig, J. G., Kerner, J., and Romsos, D. R. (1985). Hypothalamic obesity, brown adipose tissue, and sympathoadrenal activity in rats. *Am. J. Physiol.* **248**, E607–E617.

Vander Tuig, J. G., Kerner, J., Crist, K. A., and Romsos, D. A. (1986). Impaired thermoregulation in cold-exposed rats with hypothalamic obesity. *Metab., Clin. Exp.* **35**, 960–966.

Vanderweele, D. A., and Van Itallie, T. B. (1983). Sham feeding is inhibited by dietary-induced obesity in rats. *Physiol. Behav.* **31**, 533–537.

Vanderweele, D. A., Novin, D., Rezek, M., and Sanderson, J. D. (1974). Duodenal versus hepatic-portal glucose perfusion: Evidence for a duodenal satiety mechanism. *Physiol. Behav.* **12**, 467–473.

Van Itallie, T. B., and Kissileff, H. R. (1985). Physiology of energy intake: An inventory control model. *Am. J. Clin. Nutr.* **42**, 914–923.

Walgren, M. C., and Powley, T. L. (1985). Effects of intragastric hyperalimentation on pair-fed rats with ventromedial hypothalamic lesions. *Am. J. Physiol.* **248**, R172–R180.

Wangness, P. J., Dilettuso, B. A., and Martin, R. J. (1978). Dietary effects on body weight, feed intake and diurnal feeding behavior of genetically obese rats. *J. Nutr.* **108**, 256–264.

Weekley, L. B., Maher, R. W., and Kimbrough, T. D. (1982). Alterations of tryptophan metabolism in a rat strain (Osborne–Mendel) predisposed to obesity. *Comp. Biochem. Physiol. A* **72A**, 747–752.

Weingarten, H. P., and Powley, T. L. (1980). Ventromedial hypothalamic lesions elevate basal and cephalic phase gastric acid output. *Am. J. Physiol.* **239**, G221–G229.

Weingarten, H. P., and Watson, S. D. (1982). Sham feeding as a procedure for assessing the influence of diet palatability on food intake. *Physiol. Behav.* **28**, 401–407.

Weingarten, H. P., Chang, P. K., and McDonald, T. J. (1985). Comparison of the metabolic and behavioral disturbances following paraventricular and ventromedial hypothalamic lesions. *Brain Res. Bull.* **14**(6), 551–559.

Weiss, G. F., Papadakos, P., Knudson, K., and Leibowitz, S. F. (1986). Medial hypothalamic serotonin: Effects on deprivation and norepinephrine-induced eating. *Pharmacol., Biochem. Behav.* **25**, 1223–1230.

Wellman, P. J., Elissalde, M., Watkins, P. A., and Pinto, A. (1984). Hyperinsulinemia and obesity in the dorsolateral tegmental rat. *Physiol. Behav.* **32**, 1–4.

West, D. B., Williams, R. H., Braget, D. J., and Woods, S. C. (1982). Bombesin reduces food intake of normal and hypothalamically obese rats and lowers body weight when given chronically. *Peptides (N.Y.)* **3**, 61–67.

West, D. B., Fey, D., and Woods, S. C. (1984). Cholecystokinin persistently suppresses meal size but not food intake in free-feeding rats. *Am. J. Physiol.* **246**, R776–R787.

West, D. B., Prinz, W. A., Francendese, A. A., and Greenwood, M. R. C. (1987). Adipocyte blood flow is decreased in obese Zucker rats. *Am. J. Physiol.* **253**, R228–R233.

Wexler, B. C., and McMurtry, J. P. (1985). Anti-opiate (naloxone) suppression of cushingoid degenerative changes in obese/SHR rats. *Int. J. Obes.* **9**, 77–91.

Wickler, S. J., Horwitz, B. A., and Stern, J. S. (1986). Blood flow to brown fat in lean and obese adrenalectomized Zucker rats. *Am. J. Physiol.* **251**, R851–R856.

Wiley, J. H., and Leveille, F. A. (1973). Metabolic consequences of dietary medium-chain triglycerides in the rat. *J. Nutr.* **103**, 829–835.

Wirtshafter, D., and Davis, J. D. (1977). Body weight reduction by long-term glycerol treatment. *Science* **198**, 1271–1274.

Wong, B. T., and Fuller, R. W. (1987). Serotonergic mechanisms in feeding. *Int. J. Obes.* **11**, Suppl. 3, 125–133.

Woods, S. C., Lotter, E. C., McKay, L. D., and Porte, D., Jr. (1979). Chronic intracerebroventricular infusions of insulin reduce food intake and body weight of baboons. *Nature (London)* **282**, 503–505.

Woods, S. C., McKay, L. D., Stein, L. J., West, D. B., Lotter, E. C., and Porte, D., Jr. (1980). Neuroendocrine regulation of food intake and body weight. *Brain Res. Bull.* **5**, 1–5.

Woods, S. C., West, D. B., Stein, L. J., McKay, L. D., Lotter, E. C., Porte, S. G., Kenney, N. J., and Porte, D. (1981). Peptides and the control of meal size. *Diabetologia* **20**, 305–313.

Yamashita, J., Hirata, Y., and Hayashi, S.-I. (1986). Changes in histological features and nerve growth factor content of submandibular gland in the genetically obese mouse (ob/ob). *Int. J. Obes.* **10**, 461–465.

Yeh, Y.-Y., and Zee, P. (1976). Relation of ketosis to metabolic changes induced by acute medium-chain triglyceride feeding in rats. *J. Nutr.* **106**, 58–67.

York, D. A. (1987). Neural activity in hypothalamic and genetic obesity. *Proc. Nutr. Soc.* **46**, 105–117.

York, D. A., and Al-Baker, I. (1984). Effect of corticotropin on brown adipose tissue mitochondrial GDP binding in obese rats. *Biochem. J.* **223**, 263–266.

York, D. A., and Bray, G. A. (1972). Dependence of hypothalamic obesity on insulin, the pituitary and the adrenal gland. *Endocrinology (Baltimore)* **90**, 885–894.

York, D. A., Hershman, J. H., Utiger, R., and Bray, G. A. (1972). Thyrotropin secretion in genetically obese rats. *Endocrinology (Baltimore)* **90**, 67–72.

York, D. A., Bray, G. A., and Yukimura, Y. (1978a). An enzymatic defect in the obese mouse: Loss of thyroid induced sodium potassium dependent ATPase. *Proc. Natl. Acad. Sci. U.S.A.* **75**, 477–481.

York, D. A., Otto, W., and Taylor, T. F. (1978b). Thyroid status of obese (ob/ob) mice and its relationship to adipose tissue metabolism. *Comp. Biochem. Physiol. B* **59B**, 59–65.

York, D. A., Shargill, N. S., and Godbole, V. (1981). Serum insulin and lipogenesis in the suckling fatty fa/fa rat. *Diabetologia* **21**, 143–148.

York, D. A., Holt, S. J., and Marchington, D. (1985a). Regulation of sympathetic activity by corticosterone in obese fa/fa rats. *Int. J. Obes.* **9**, Suppl. 2, 89–96.

York, D. A., Marchington, D., Holt, S. J., and Allars, J. (1985b). Regulation of sympathetic activity in lean and obese Zucker (fa/fa) rats. *Am. J. Physiol.* **249,** E299–E305.

Yoshida, T., and Bray, G. A. (1984). Catecholamine turnover in rats with ventromedial hypothalamic lesions. *Am. J. Physiol.* **246,** R558–R565.

Yoshida, T., Kemnitz, J. W., and Bray, G. A. (1983). Lateral hypothalamic lesions and norepinephrine turnover in rats. *J. Clin. Invest.* **72,** 919–927.

Yoshida, T., Nishioka, H., Nakamura, Y., and Kondo, M. (1984). Reduced norepinephrine turnover in mice with monosodium glutamate-induced obesity. *Metab., Clin. Exp.* **33,** 1060–1063.

Yoshida, T., Nishioka, H., Nakamura, Y., Kanatsuna, T., and Kondo, M. (1985b). Reduced norepinephrine turnover in brown adipose tissue of pre-obese mice treated with monosodium-L-glutamate. *Life Sci.* **36,** 931–938.

Yoshida, T., Fisler, J. S., Fukushima, M., Bray, G. A., and Schemmel, R. A. (1987). Effects on diet, lighting, and food intake on norepinephrine turnover in dietary obesity. *Am. J. Physiol.* **252,** R402–R408.

Yoshimatsu, H., Niijima, A., Oomura, Y., Yamabe, K., and Katafuchi, T. (1984). Effects of hypothalamic lesion on pancreatic autonomic nerve activity in the rat. *Brain Res.* **303,** 147–152.

Yoshimatsu, H., Oomura, Y., Katafuchi, T., Niijhima, A., and Sato, A. (1985). Lesions of the ventromedial hypothalamic nucleus enhance sympatho-adrenal function. *Brain Res.* **339,** 390–392.

Young, J. B., and Landsberg, L. (1977). Suppression of sympathetic nervous system during fasting. *Science* **196,** 1473–1475.

Young, J. B., and Landsberg, L. (1980). Impaired suppression of sympathetic activity during fasting in the gold thioglucose treated mouse. *J. Clin. Invest.* **65,** 1086–1094.

Young, J. B., and Landsberg, L. (1983). Diminished sympathetic nervous system activity in genetically obese (ob/ob) mice. *Am. J. Physiol.* **245,** E148–E154.

Young, J. K., and Grizard, J. (1985). Sensitivity to satiating and taste qualities of glucose in obese Zucker rats. *Physiol. Behav.* **34,** 415–421.

Young, P. T., and Green, J. T. (1953). Quantity of food ingested as a measure of relative acceptability. *J. Comp. Physiol. Psychol.* **46,** 288–294.

Young, R. A., Fang, S.-L., Prosky, J., and Braverman, L. E. (1984). Hepatic conversion of thyroxine to triiodothyronine in obese and lean Zucker rats. *Life Sci.* **34,** 1783–1789.

Young, R. C., Gibbs, J., Antin, J., Holt, J., and Smith, G. P. (1974). Absence of satiety during sham feeding in the rat. *J. Comp. Physiol. Psychol.* **87,** 795–800.

Yukimura, Y., and Bray, G. A. (1978). Effects of adrenalectomy on body weight and the size and number of fat cells in the Zucker rat. *Endocr. Res. Commun.* **5,** 189–198.

Yukimura, Y., Bray, G. A., and Wolfsen, A. R. (1978). Some effects of adrenalectomy in the fatty rat. *Endocrinology (Baltimore)* **103,** 1924–1928.

Zaragoza-Hermans, N., and Felber, J. P. (1970). Studies on the metabolic effects induced in the rat by a high fat diet. I. Carbohydrate metabolism in vivo. *Horm. Metab. Res.* **2,** 323–329.

Zaragoza-Hermans, N., and Felber, J.-P. (1972). Studies of the metabolic effects induced in the rat by a high fat diet. II. Disposal of orally administered (^{14}C)-glucose. *Horm. Metab. Res.* **4,** 25–30.

Zaror-Behrens, G., and Himms-Hagen, J. (1983). Cold stimulated sympathetic activity in brown adipose tissue of obese ob/ob mice. *Am. J. Physiol.* **244,** E361–E366.

Estrogen Regulation of Protein Synthesis and Cell Growth in Human Breast Cancer*

KEVIN J. CULLEN AND MARC E. LIPPMAN

Georgetown University Medical Center
Vincent T. Lombardi Cancer Research Center
Washington, D.C. 20007

I. INTRODUCTION

It has long been recognized that estrogens are an important factor in the regulation of growth in human breast cancer. Over 90 years ago Beatson reported that oophorectomy could induce tumor regression in premenopausal women with metastatic breast carcinoma (1).

Abundant epidemiological evidence supports the notion that estrogens are important in the genesis of breast cancer. Breast cancer occurs in women 100 times more frequently than it does in men, despite the fact that the male breast contains glandular epithelium just as the female breast does, and the male breast epithelium demonstrates the same proliferative response to estrogen seen in the female.

---

*We dedicate this chapter to Helen B. O'Bannon, who died recently of breast cancer in her forty-ninth year. Vice President of the University of Pennsylvania, former Secretary of Welfare for the State of Pennsylvania, economist, mother of four, and a member of the 1985 National Institutes of Health Consensus Development Committee on the Adjuvant Treatment of Breast Cancer, Helen worked tirelessly for educational, civic, and women's issues. Her loss is deeply felt by family and colleagues alike.

In addition, the length of a woman's menstrual life, the time during which she is exposed to significant levels of estrogen, is positively correlated with the risk of breast cancer. Early menarche and late natural menopause increase overall breast cancer risk (2). In fact, geographic differences in breast cancer incidence (severalfold greater in the United States and in western Europe compared with Japan, for example) appear to be due to differences in environmental factors, such as diet, which alter age of menarche and menopause, rather than genetic differences in geographically distinct areas (3).

Surgical menopause decreases breast cancer risk in proportion to the reduction in menstrual life. If estrogen replacement is given following oophorectomy, however, the protective effects in terms of breast cancer risk are lost (4).

Estrogen levels themselves, however, do not appear to correlate with the risk for breast cancer development. Plasma estrogen concentrations in a group of patients with breast cancer were not significantly different from those of matched controls (5).

The hormonal modulations involved in breast cancer risk are clearly not limited to estrogen alone. Full-term pregnancy, in general, reduces breast cancer risk. Women with a full-term pregnancy before the age of 20 have half the breast cancer risk of nulliparous women (6), while women who undergo early abortion (less than 3 months of gestation) had a doubled breast cancer risk in one study (7). A possible explanation for this observation is that the hormonal changes associated with full-term pregnancy, such as exposure to high levels of progesterone and prolactin, exert a differentiating effect on mammary epithelium which reduces the subsequent risk of cancer. However, this theory does not fully explain the finding that women undergoing a late first pregnancy actually have a higher breast cancer risk than do nulliparous women (3,6), so the timing of the hormonal changes associated with full-term pregnancy is important in the determination of risk as well. The promotional effects of hormones on prior carcinogenic events may predominate in the setting of late pregnancy.

Despite the strong association between estrogens and the risk of breast cancer, the exact mechanism linking estradiol with breast tumor development is not clear. Several mechanisms for estradiol-associated tumor development are conceivable, and one or more could be important.

First, estrogens could be acting as true carcinogens—that is, inducing a genomic mutation or mutations leading to malignant transformation. Diethylstilbestrol (DES), for example, is a synthetic estrogen which has been associated with cervical cancer in the daughters of women who took the drug during pregnancy as a progestational agent. In cellular studies, DES can interrupt the mitotic apparatus, leading to cellular aneuploidy (8). Alternatively, estradiol has been postulated to be toxic to DNA directly through semiquinone compounds formed during estrogen metabolism (9,10). In a Syrian hamster model of estrogen-mediated tumor development, animals treated with estradiol develop renal tumors. However, animals treated with 2-fluoroestradiol do not develop tumors, despite the fact that both compounds have identical physiological effects *in vivo* and *in vitro*. The fluorinated compound differs from native estradiol in that it is not metabolized to a reactive 2-OH intermediate (11), suggesting that the carcinogenic effects of estrogens can be separated from physiological hormonal effects.

Second, estrogens could be acting as tumor-promoting agents by stimulating the growth of malignant cells transformed by another mechanism. An example of this is the model in which rats treated with the carcinogen 7,12-dimethylbenz(*a*)anthracene (DMBA) develop breast cancers which are estrogen dependent and grow only if the animal has functioning ovaries or a pharmacological source of estrogen (12).

Third, estrogens may be acting as permissive agents in tumor development, functioning as a facilitator necessary for some other cellular process of malignant transformation to take place. In survivors of the atomic bombings of Hiroshima and Nagasaki, the incidence of breast cancer was highest among those women who were between 10 and 19 years of age at the time of exposure to the bomb's radiation. This age group corresponds to the time around puberty, when estrogen-induced breast epithelial proliferation is at its greatest, possibly explaining why women in this age group were more sensitive to the carcinogenic effects of ionizing radiation than were older or younger women (13).

Abundant clinical evidence has shown that after the development of a malignant breast tumor, estrogens can continue to function in the control of tumor growth. Jensen in 1967 demonstrated that radiolabeled estradiol could specifically bind to some breast tumor specimens and that this binding correlated with the clinical response to endocrine therapies (14). Early studies showed that in patients with tumors having detectable estrogen receptor, 73% responded to endocrine therapy, whereas less than 10% of patients with estrogen receptors-negative tumors responded to similar treatment (15). More recent data have shown that the presence of both estrogen and progesterone receptors is a better predictor for response to endocrine therapy than is the presence of estrogen receptor alone. In patients with tumors that are both estrogen receptor and progesterone receptor positive, there is an approximately 80% objective response rate to endocrine therapy (16).

In the remainder of this chapter we will attempt to outline the important cellular processes which are under estrogenic control and which can influence cellular growth. Central to these are the production of (1) secreted growth factors that can act in an autocrine or paracrine fashion to stimulate breast tumor growth and (2) cellular products that are important in the replication of DNA and other cellular components.

II. ESTROGEN REGULATION OF NORMAL BREAST DEVELOPMENT

Estradiol is required for mammary ductal growth during adolescence as well as lobuloalveolar proliferation during pregnancy (17). The pubertal breast, however, is under a large number of interacting hormonal influences, and the precise role of estradiol itself is difficult to quantify. As breast development begins at the time of puberty, there are marked increases in estradiol, androgens, and gonadotropins (18,19). Increases in circulating estradiol, however, appear to be most closely correlated with breast development (20). While estradiol is necessary for breast development, some of the estrogen-induced breast growth appears to take place through several indirect mechanisms. Estradiol, for example, induces the production of other hormones, such as thyroid-stimulating hormone and prolactin, in *in vitro* pituitary cell culture systems (21,22). *In vivo,* these hormones may exert secondary stimulatory effects on the proliferating breast epithelium and stroma. In addition, estrogen alters the end-organ effects of other hormones. Rats treated with estrogen show enhanced sensitivity to the effects of prolactin in the stimulation of protein synthesis (23).

Gonadotropins as well are important in the modulation of estrogen-induced breast development. In patients with gonadal dysgenesis, estradiol treatment causes normal breast development in the presence of an intact hypothalamic–pituitary axis, while normal breast development is not restored by estradiol treatment if there is concomitant gonadotropin deficiency (24). Similarly, estrogen treatment of ovariectomized mice will result in breast glandular proliferation (25), but if the animal has undergone pituitary ablation as well, estrogen will not induce breast development (26).

Other hormones may have a direct stimulatory effect on breast development independent of estrogen, or may serve to antagonize the effects of estrogen. Plasma insulin-like growth factor I (IGF-I; somatomedin C) concentrations, for example, correlate positively with breast size (27). Androgens suppress the breast response to estrogens, and the relative excess of androgens appears to explain why boys do not undergo breast enlargement at puberty (18). Transient gynecomastia is common in boys at this age, and may be due to a temporary relative dominance of estrogen effect over androgen effect (28).

In a mouse model of mammary development, androgen treatment causes condensation of mesenchymal cells around the mammary gland bud and is accompanied by death of the glandular epithelial cells. However, mesenchymal cells are necessary for this reaction, because androgens will not cause this effect directly on epithelium in the absence of surrounding mesenchyme. Further, there is no androgen effect on breast epithelium if the epithelial cells are grown with mesenchymal cells from androgen-insensitive mice bearing a testicular feminization mutation. Experimental combination of breast mesenchyme with epithelium from other organs shows that mesenchyme-mediated inhibition of epithelial growth is specific for breast epithelium and is not seen in epithelial cells from other organs (29).

Interactions between breast epithelium and surrounding stroma are important in the response to estradiol as well. In mouse cell culture experiments, estrogen-induced proliferation of mammary epithelial cells is detected in epithelial cells only when cultured with mammary stromal cells (30). Furthermore, there appears to be more than one mechanism by which stromal cells participate in the mammary epithelial response to estrogen. Mammary epithelial cells treated with estradiol in the presence of killed fibroblasts or fibroblast-conditioned media show induction of progesterone receptor, but not increased DNA synthesis or epithelial cell proliferation. Estradiol-induced cell proliferation in epithelial cells requires direct contact with live fibroblasts. Under these conditions, epithelial cells in turn promote estrogen-induced stimulation of fibroblast cell proliferation (31), suggesting that the stromal–epithelial interactions involved in mammary growth regulation are bidirectional.

These and similar studies have suggested that estrogen induction of normal mammary gland growth is at least in part indirect, and not through direct mitogenic effects of estrogen on epithelial cells themselves. This notion is supported by immunocytochemical studies of breast biopsy specimens from normal, nonlactating women which detected estrogen receptor in less than 10% of epithelial cells and not at all in stromal cells (32,33).

Other studies suggest that overall regulation of breast growth may reflect a careful balance of both stimulatory and inhibitory growth factors. Mouse mammary bud development is inhibited by transforming growth factor-β (TGF-β) released from pellets implanted in the immediate proximity of the developing breast. The inhibited cells are histologically normal and proliferate normally upon withdrawal of TGF-β (34). TGF-β will be discussed in greater detail later in this review, but its production in breast cells is influenced by estrogen as well, further interlacing the mechanisms that regulate overall breast development.

Therefore, while estrogen is critically necessary in breast development, it is not sufficient to produce breast development by itself. Many other hormonal and cellular interactions are involved in the overall regulation of mammary gland growth and development.

In contrast, estrogens do not appear to have as significant a role in the regulation of lactation. *In vitro* mouse mammary models have shown that estrogen is not sufficient to induce the synthesis of milk proteins but does enhance the effect of other lactogenic factors such as thyroid hormone, insulin, glucocorticoids, and prolactin (35). Laboratory data from a primate system have shown that estrogens may, in fact, have an inhibitory effect on milk secretion (36).

III. Estrogen Regulation of Protein Synthesis via the Estrogen Receptor

It has been known for over 30 years that radiolabeled estrogen is bound specifically to estrogen target tissues (37). This estrogen-binding component was subsequently recognized as a specific soluble receptor protein which was first isolated by centrifugation of homogenized uterine tissues (38). The estrogen receptor protein was initially found in both cytosolic and nuclear cell fractions.

Jensen and others interpreted the early labeled estradiol experiments as inferring a two-step mechanism by which estradiol was bound by a cytosolic estrogen receptor and then transported to the nucleus (39). Following ligand binding and transfer to the nucleus, the estrogen–receptor complex was assumed to bind to specific acceptor sites on the genome. In so doing, it activated transcription of specific genes which produced mRNA encoding the effector proteins of estrogen action (40). Subsequent work utilizing monoclonal antibodies to the estrogen receptor in intact cells demonstrated that unoccupied receptor sites in the intact cell were located in the nucleus and not in the cytoplasm (41). Similarly, when rat pituitary cells were enucleated by centrifugation, the majority of the estrogen receptor was found in the nuclear fraction, not in the cytoplasmic fraction (42). The apparent cytosolic steroid binding which formed the basis of the nuclear translocation hypothesis of estrogen receptor action represented an artifact of cell homogenization, and it appears that both ligand binding and subsequent interaction of the ligand–receptor complex with the genome take place in the nucleus.

Several nuclear proteins have been described which bind the estrogen receptor, including a 90-kDa heat-shock protein (43), a 29-kDa phosphoprotein (44), and others (45,46). These binding proteins may serve an intermediary function in the interaction between the ligand-bound receptor and nuclear DNA, but the precise function of these proteins is still speculative at present.

Chambon and colleagues have reported the cDNA sequence for the human estrogen receptor (47). Interestingly, the sequence of the estrogen receptor revealed extensive homology with the erbA protein of the oncogenic avian erythroblastosis virus, as do sequences previously described for the glucocorticoid, thyroid, mineralocorticoid, and several other receptors (48).

Site-directed mutagenesis studies with estrogen receptor deletion mutants have shown a central 83-amino acid DNA-binding site separated by a hinge region from a carboxy-terminal estrogen-binding domain of approximately 250 residues in length. Both the DNA-binding and ligand-binding regions of the estrogen receptor show a high degree of homology between chicken and human sequences, indicating marked conservation of receptor structure between widely divergent species (49).

It is now generally felt that, following the binding of estrogen, the DNA-binding region of the estrogen receptor develops an increased affinity for specific sequences in estrogen-regulated genes (50).

A proposed model for the DNA-binding site of the estrogen receptor as well as other steroid receptors consists of a cysteine-rich region coordinated around two zinc ions in a double-"finger" structure (51). Point mutations in the finger regions can abolish estrogen effect (52). After binding of the steroid, the receptor undergoes a conformational change which facilitates binding of the estrogen–receptor complex finger region contained in amino acids 185–250 to specific gene enhancer elements (52). In the rat prolactin gene, the finger structure in the DNA-binding region of the estrogen receptor binds to a 13-bp estrogen-regulatory element (ERE) in the distal upstream enhancer located approximately 1.5 kb from the transcription start site (53). Very similar sequences are seen in the ERE of the estrogen-regulated vitellogenin gene of both the chicken and *Xenopus,* which has permitted the definition of at least one consensus sequence for an ERE (54, 55).

Binding of the estrogen–receptor complex to the ERE in the distal enhancer segment has been postulated to be a necessary step in the initiation of transcription of the estrogen-regulated gene, since mutation of either the DNA-binding site of the estrogen receptor or the ERE can prevent transcription (52). However, the mechanisms by which the transcription start site is activated following binding of the estrogen receptor to the ERE are not yet understood. Likewise, the mechanism for turning off gene transcription following estrogen-mediated activation is not known.

The sequence homology seen in a wide range of species for both ligand- and DNA-binding sites of the estrogen receptor as well as estrogen-regulated enhancer elements in the activated genes is an indication of the tremendous conservation of the fundamental mechanism of the estrogen response over evolutionary time.

While the estrogen receptor appears to be a ligand-regulated, positive transcription factor for numerous genes, as will be discussed later in this paper, there is evidence that in certain circumstances the estrogen receptor may have an inhibitory function, and this inhibition is conferred by areas of the receptor distinct from the DNA-binding and steroid-binding domains (52). The significance of this inhibitory function is not known.

IV. Estrogen-Mediated Control of Cell Growth

A tremendous body of research has developed over the last 15 years regarding estrogen regulation of cellular growth and replication. In humans, the bulk of available data comes from experiments performed in breast tumor cell culture. A large number of estrogen-sensitive and -insensitive breast tumor cell lines have been established and characterized in this way. Several hormone-sensitive rodent mammary tumor models have been described which have been useful in the study of growth regulation by estrogen (56). More recently, the study of human tumor cells grown in nude mice has provided some new insights into the hormonal regulation of tumor growth, but this model system, like the others, has significant limitations (57).

While the studies of estrogen-dependent and -independent tumors in each of these model systems have led to significant new insights in cell physiology and molecular biology, they all suffer from a substantial common flaw. The regulation of growth of breast cancer *in vivo* is the product of complex interactions among stromal, vascular, and epithelial tumor elements. Since these interactions are as yet very poorly understood, no model system currently available can hope to reproduce them accurately. Even those experimental results produced from a single model system must be viewed with some caution since, for example, considerable differences in the characteristics and behavior of the same breast tumor cell line carried in different laboratories have been reported (58).

Before discussing in detail the mechanisms of estrogen action, it is important to examine the net effects of estrogen on cell growth which have been analyzed both *in vivo* and *in vitro*. Castrated female rodents show breast epithelial proliferation as well hyperplasia and hypertrophy of estrogen target tissues, such as uterus and vagina, upon estradiol replacement (59,60). MCF-7 cells implanted in nude mice show a proliferative response to estradiol and, in fact, require estrogen for tumor take and subsequent growth (61,62). Early analysis of estradiol effects in estrogen receptor-positive MCF-7 breast carcinoma cells grown in defined medium free of estrogen showed a 3-fold increase in nucleoside uptake in cells treated with 10^{-8} M estradiol, compared with controls. A 2-fold increase in cell number was noted with estrogen treatment. Higher concentrations of estrogen (10^{-5} M) resulted in cell death. Tamoxifen-treated cells were growth inhibited below control levels, but this effect was reversible with the addition of estradiol (63,64). Additional studies have demonstrated cell proliferation *in vitro* in estrogen receptor-positive breast tumor cell lines treated with physiological concentrations of estradiol (65–70).

Other groups, however, failed to demonstrate the mitogenic effects of estradiol in cell culture (71,72). However, these studies did show that the growth-inhibitory effects of antiestrogens could be reversed with estrogen. Part of the difficulty in interpreting these conflicting studies was explained by the finding of the Katzenellenbogen group that phenol red, the pH indicator universally present in tissue culture media prior to that point, is a weak estrogen, binding to estrogen receptor at approximately 0.001% the affinity of estradiol. At the concentrations in which it is found in most media preparations (15–45 μM), phenol red is a significant mitogen for MCF-7 cells (73). The presence of phenol red in the media used in the previous studies could significantly mask estradiol effects, in that control sera free of estrogen contained significant quantities of this estrogenlike compound.

Subsequent studies analyzing growth of estrogen receptor-positive cells in media free of serum and phenol red have confirmed that physiological concentrations of estradiol are significantly mitogenic (74,75).

Given these overall estrogen effects, it is useful to look at estrogen regulation of cell growth by dividing the subject into several broad areas. First, there are a number of intracellular growth regulators which are under estrogen control and which can influence cell replication directly through control of DNA synthesis, or which can act as secondary messengers for estrogen action. Second, there is an enlarging group of estrogen-regulated, secreted growth factors which has been of considerable recent interest. These factors can influence the growth not only of the cells which produce them, but there is evidence that they can play a role in the regulation of the growth of surrounding cells and tissues as well. We will examine these factors in some detail. Third, there are several proteolytic factors whose production is influenced by estrogen and which may be important in the modulation of tumor invasiveness and metastatic potential. Finally, there are numerous additional proteins which may be important in growth regulation, but which have been less well characterized or whose function is not yet fully understood.

A. INTRACELLULAR GROWTH REGULATORS

1. *DNA-Replicative Enzymes*

Net cellular DNA synthesis as determined by ^{32}P inorganic orthophosphate labeling shows a 2-fold increase in estrogen-treated MCF-7 cells, compared with control cells grown in the absence of estrogen (76). This effect is maximal at an estradiol concentration of 10^{-9} M. There is a steady reduction in the stimulatory effect on DNA synthesis at higher concentrations of estradiol, and at a concentration of 10^{-5} M, E_2 is actually inhibitory, with lower net DNA synthesis than in estrogen-free controls. Increased DNA synthesis is most apparent at optimal estradiol concentrations after 36–48 hours of steroid treatment in these studies, and is preceded by increases in the activity of several cellular enzymes that control DNA synthesis.

McGuire and colleagues examined DNA polymerase activity in estrogen-sensitive MCF-7 human breast cancer cells (77). Antiestrogens were able to significantly reduce DNA polymerase activity in a dose-dependent fashion. This effect was reversible with the addition of estrogen to tamoxifen-inhibited cells. Thymidine kinase, an enzyme involved in the salvage pathway biosynthesis of deoxynucleotides, was shown to undergo a 4-fold increase in activity under estrogen stimulation of MCF-7 cells (78). Enzyme kinetic studies suggest that estrogen stimulation of thymidine kinase activity is due to an increase in synthesis rather than a change in the molar activity of the enzyme, or changes in enzyme degradation. Tamoxifen treatment decreased thymidine kinase activity to approximately half of control levels (78).

Estrogen-induced increases in thymidine kinase activity are accompanied by an increase in steady-state levels of thymidine kinase mRNA. Conversely, antiestrogen treatment of sensitive cells resulted in reduced steady-state mRNA levels. Using isolated cell nuclei analyzed in a transcriptional run-off technique, levels of thymidine kinase transcription were elevated 2-fold in estrogen-treated cells, compared with controls. This result shows that the increase in the thymidine kinase mRNA level is due, at least in part, to transcriptional activation as a result of estrogen treatment (79). Posttranscriptional events may also influence steady-state thymidine kinase mRNA levels, as has been suggested in other experiments (80).

Several enzymes involved in *de novo* pyrimidine synthesis have been shown to increase up to 2-fold after 48 hours of estrogen treatment. These include carbamoyl-phosphate synthetase, aspartate transcarbamylase, orotate pyrophosphorylase, and orotidine decarboxylase (81). All can contribute to increased net DNA synthesis as a result of estrogen stimulation, but the mechanism of estrogen effect on the activity of these enzymes has not been clearly defined.

Dihydrofolate reductase (DHFR), an enzyme which produces reduced folates for the formation of thymidine, purines, and amino acids, increases following estradiol treatment in estrogen receptor-positive cells (82). A subclone of MCF-7 cells was selected for study because of its resistance to methotrexate, a chemotherapy agent which specifically inhibits DHFR. This cell line was found to contain amplified DHFR gene sequences and a 50-fold increase in DHFR levels, but retained functional estrogen receptor, as well as the estrogen-induced increase in DHFR synthesis and activity seen in the parent cell line. Tamoxifen treatment of these methotrexate-resistant cells resulted in a decrease in the rate of DHFR synthesis and in the net DHFR levels (83).

2. Cyclic Adenosine Monophosphate

Cyclic adenosine monophosphate (cAMP) is recognized as an important intracellular regulator of numerous cellular processes. cAMP induces gene transcription in a variety of tissues responsive to hormones or other regulatory factors (84). In estrogen-sensitive tissues, an in-

verse correlation exists between estrogen stimulation and intracellular cAMP levels (85).

Studies of human tumor cells grown in culture have shown that
cAMP or its derivatives can inhibit the tumor cell growth rate without
affecting cell viability (86). Growth of human MCF-7 breast cancer
cells is arrested by treatment with cAMP itself (87) or by cholera toxin,
which increases intracellular cAMP levels (88).

Similar results are seen in rat mammary tumor models, using cancers induced by the anthracycline DMBA. cAMP treatment of these
hormone-responsive tumors results in growth arrest (89). Hormone-
independent tumors showed a less consistent response to cAMP in this
model, but no direct toxic effects of cAMP treatment were observed
(89). In estrogen-sensitive uterine tissues estrogen induces a decrease
in cAMP levels in ovariectomized animals. In intact animals cAMP
levels fall during the portion of the menstrual cycle when plasma
estrogen levels are maximal (85). In rats with hormone-dependent
DMBA tumors cAMP levels rise following ovariectomy and are accompanied by tumor regression (90). Identical results are seen after treatment with high doses of either estrogen or tamoxifen (91).

Analyses of human breast biopsies and mastectomy specimens show
an inverse correlation between both estrogen and progesterone receptor levels and the quantity of cAMP-binding proteins, confirming in
humans similar observations made in the DMBA rat mammary tumor
system (92).

cAMP levels themselves, however, do not appear to correlate well
with the biological behavior of the tumors. Neoplastic tissues have
shown very wide ranges of cAMP levels (93).

cAMP also appears to influence expression of certain cellular oncogenes in a negative way. p21 is the protein product of the *ras* proto-
oncogene, which in mutated form is responsible for cellular transformation. In the DMBA tumor model, p21 levels fall after estrogen
withdrawal or treatment with cAMP. These effects are reversed by
subsequent estrogen supplementation (94). These results suggest that
cAMP may act to suppress the expression of this cellular oncogene.

cAMP and estradiol appear, then, to have antagonistic net effects in
the regulation of breast cancer cell growth. Since cAMP is felt to
induce expression of specific genes by phosphorylation of proteins at
upstream enhancer elements (84), it conceivably could be acting to
induce the expression of growth-inhibitory factors. Because it is part
of a ubiquitous messenger system in eukaryotic cells, it may represent
another site for the perturbation of normal growth-regulatory mechanisms in neoplastic cells.

Although the majority of laboratory evidence has shown that increased levels of intracellular cAMP are accompanied by growth inhibition in mammary tumor models, some investigators have reported that treatment of cultured breast cancer cells with either cAMP or cholera toxin produces a substantial mitogenic stimulus. This has been reported in both estrogen-sensitive stimulus. This has been reported in both estrogen-sensitive MCF-7 cells and estrogen receptor-negative HS578-T cells (95). One group has hypothesized that the growth inhibition seen with cAMP treatment is an artifact of the use of dibutyryl cAMP, the nonpolar cAMP analog used in these experiments because it can traverse the cell membrane, and that the inhibition of growth seen is secondary to the butyrl moiety of the molecule and not the cAMP itself (96). The greater body of evidence, particularly the findings in the well-characterized DMBA-induced rat tumor model, favors the general growth-inhibitory effect of cAMP.

B. Secreted Growth Factors

In addition to the enzymes discussed in the previous section, which influence cellular replication and DNA synthesis, estrogens are able to induce the production of numerous polypeptide growth factors in breast cancer cell lines. These factors in turn stimulate the growth of normal and tumor cells *in vitro*. *In vivo,* these factors may potentially act in either an autocrine or a paracrine fashion to promote tumor growth. Recent evidence suggests these growth factors are among the key determinants of tumor growth in human breast cancer. In estrogen-dependent tumors the production of these growth factors is regulated by estrogen, while in estrogen-independent tumors some of these factors may be produced in a constitutive or nonregulated manner, bypassing the need for estrogen stimulation.

While most of the growth factors described to date stimulate cancer cell growth, at least one protein, TFG-β, is inhibitory. Taken together, one can propose a model in which the net regulation of tumor growth, at least in part, represents the cumulative effect of these stimulatory and inhibitory growth factors on the tumor epithelium and stroma.

The discussion that follows will concentrate on the growth factors which have been better characterized in human breast cancer, particularly with regard to estrogen regulation. This does not imply that other factors are not important, only that sufficient information on their growth-controlling activity and hormonal regulation awaits further experimentation. It is likely that the list of estrogen-regulated and estrogen-independent growth factors important in breast cancer will continue to expand rapidly with time.

1. *Transforming Growth Factor-α*

Transforming growth factor-α (TGF-α) is a polypeptide with a molecular weight of 5600, composed of 50 amino acid residues. It has been described in a variety of malignant and nonmalignant cell types. Fibroblasts produce a 17- to 19-kDa TGF-α precursor which appears to be membrane bound and is subsequently cleaved to the lower-molecular-weight form (97–99). Mature TGF-α shows significant homology to epidermal growth factor (EGF) (100,101). TGF-α was initially characterized by its ability to induce anchorage-independent growth of normal rat kidney (NRK) fibroblasts in soft agar, and acquired the name of a transforming growth factor for that reason. The transformed phenotype induced by TGF-α in NRK cells is reversible, however, and the cells are unable to sustain anchorage-independent growth when TGF-α is withdrawn (102).

The biological activity of TGF-α is mediated by binding to the EGF receptor, whose protein structure is homologous to the product of the v-*erbB* oncogene (103). TGF-α and EGF can compete with each other on an equimolar basis in EGF receptor-binding studies (104,105). TGF-α and EGF share many biological functions in addition to their structural similarities, and both are able to stimulate epidermal cell growth (106–108). Purified EGF is a potent mitogen for breast cancer cells, including MCF-7 cells (109).

To date, TGF-α has been described in a sizable number of neoplastic and proliferating tissues (110). In contrast, production of EGF in these tissues has not been documented until recently. A single report has appeared showing EGF mRNA production determined by Northern blot analysis in T47-D breast carcinoma cells (111).

Experiments with conditioned media from MCF-7 cells show production of a 30,000-molecular-weight activity which is mitogenic for MCF-7 cells and which reacts in a TGF-α radioimmunoassay. The activity also competes with authentic EGF for binding to the EGF receptor and demonstrates transforming activity for NRK fibroblasts (112). In estrogen-sensitive MCF-7 cells, TGF-α levels increase significantly following treatment with estradiol (113). Further experiments showed that fractionation of MCF-7-conditioned media by column chromatography in acid conditions yielded two principal peaks of TGF-α activity, one at a molecular weight of 30,000 and the second at a molecular weight of approximately 7000. Each of these peaks retained immunological and biological activity (114).

Using a 1.3-kb cDNA probe for the TGF-α precursor, the predicted 4.8-kb mRNA transcript was found in multiple breast cancer cell lines at variable levels of expression. Interestingly, the estrogen-insensitive cell line MDA MB-231 showed the highest level of message. In addition, TGF-α mRNA was detected in 70% of 40 primary breast tumors tested. Estrogen treatment of MCF-7 cells caused a greater than 2-fold induction of TGF-α message.

Biologically active TGF-α can be identified in conditioned media from primary culture of human mammary epithelial cells as well as cultures of benzo[a]pyrene-immortalized normal mammary epithelial cells. In situ hybridization of frozen sections has demonstrated TGF-α expression in a normal lactating mammary gland as well (115).

While these studies demonstrate the presence of TGF-α in normal as well as malignant mammary cells, it is not yet known whether estrogen can induce TGF-α in normal breast cells, as has been demonstrated in malignant cell lines.

Experiments in nude mice provide in vivo evidence of estrogen regulation of TGF-α mRNA transcription. In ovariectomized nude mice estrogen-sensitive MCF-7 cells will form tumors only when injected in the presence of a supplemental source of estrogen (116). When tumors from such animals are examined following withdrawal of estrogen, there is a steady decrease in the level of detectable TGF-α message over time (112).

Since the biological effects of TGF-α protein are mediated via the EGF receptor, it is not surprising that these effects can be blocked experimentally by interference with ligand/receptor binding. Antibody to human TGF-α inhibits NRK colony formation in media containing low concentrations of TGF-α. MCF-7 colony formation in soft agar in the presence of fetal calf serum is also significantly inhibited by an anti-TGF-α antibody. Similarly, anchorage-dependent, estrogen-stimulated growth of MCF-7 cells is inhibited by antibody to the EGF receptor (114). However, other groups have reported that an anti-EGF receptor antibody will block TGF-α-stimulated growth, but not estrogen-induced growth of MCF-7 cells (117). This implies that, in this model system, TGF-α alone is not the primary determinant of the overall mitogenic effects of estrogen treatment.

A recent study in breast cancer tumor specimens has demonstrated that there may be an inverse correlation between the level of EGF receptor and the levels of estrogen and progesterone receptors. EGF binding was elevated in cells negative for estrogen and progesterone receptors, as compared to estrogen receptor-positive cells (118). Since the EGF receptor is the protein product of the protooncogene c-erbB, the overexpression of this receptor seen in estrogen-insensitive tumors could be related to the aggressive behavior and poor prognosis associated with estrogen insensitivity. While c-*erbB* overexpression in estrogen receptor-negative tumors seems to take place at the level of gene transcription (119), amplification of this gene in a breast cancer cell line has also been reported (120). It is unclear whether c-*erbB* expression by itself is sufficient to promote tumor growth, but in the presence of TGF-α or EGF, c-*erbB* expression can induce tumor mitogenesis (121).

Likewise, despite the fact that TGF-α is called a transforming growth factor because it promotes anchorage-independent cell growth in fibroblasts, it is controversial whether TGF-α expression is sufficient to cause cellular transformation. Several groups have reported transformation of fibroblasts in TGF-α transfection experiments (122,123). Other experiments, however, in which TGF-α was overexpressed in fibroblasts did not lead to malignant transformation (124).

Based on this combined body of experimental evidence, TGF-α serves as the model of an autocrine growth factor. It is produced after estrogen stimulation in estrogen-dependent cancer cells, it is produced constitutively in estrogen-independent cells, and it can serve as a mitogen for the cells that produce it. The autostimulatory effects of TGF-α can be modified by antibodies that block access of the growth factor to its specific receptor. The role of TGF-α in cellular transformation is less clear.

2. *Platelet-Derived Growth Factor*

Platelet-derived growth factor (PDGF) was originally identified as a component of the α granules of human platelets (125,126). It is an important mitogen for mesenchymal cells, and in its active form is a 32-kDa protein heterodimer consisting of an A and B chain linked by disulfide bonds (127). Although the usual active form is considered to be the AB heterodimer, AA and BB homodimers have been identified and are biologically active (128). The B chain of PDGF is the protein product of the c-*sis* protooncogene located on chromosome 22 (129). The A chain, in contrast, is encoded by a gene located on chromosome 7 (130). Cells transformed by simian sarcoma virus, as well as human tumor cells with active *sis* genes, secrete biologically active PDGF B chain (131). This suggests that the inappropriate expression of PDGF-related oncogenes may play a role in the malignant transformation of some cells.

The PDGF receptor is a 172- to 180-kDa glycoprotein with an internal tyrosine kinase domain (132,133). The human PDGF receptor has been cloned and, when transfected into fibroblasts the expressed receptor, is able to bind all three isoforms (i.e., AA, BB, AB) of PDGF. All three forms initiated tyrosine kinase activity and mitogenesis (134). A second population of PDGF receptor may exist which shows preferential binding for the BB dimer. Human dermal fibroblasts appear to express this receptor form in significant excess of the better-characterized AB receptor isoform (135).

Conditioned media from each of ten breast cancer cell lines contained activity that competed with authentic PDGF for PDGF receptor binding (136). The activity also was mitogenic for fibroblasts, and this effect could be blocked by anti-PDGF antibodies. There was no significant difference in the amount of receptor-active PDGF produced by estrogen-sensitive or -insensitive cells. mRNA for PDGF A chain of three transcript sizes, previously reported in other tumors, was found in eight of ten cell lines, while a 4.2-kb B chain transcript was found in nine of ten cell lines (136,137).

PDGF mRNA expression increases severalfold in MCF-7 cells exposed to 10 nM estradiol. In addition, PDGF activity in conditioned media increased approximately 3-fold with estradiol treatment. However, estrogen-independent MDA MB-231 cells grown in serum-free medium produce 50% more PDGF activity than estrogen-stimulated MCF-7 cells (137).

Immunoprecipitation with anti-PDGF antibodies reveals a 30-kDa protein in the conditioned media of MCF-7 cells which is converted to a 15- and 16-kDa bands under reducing conditions, suggesting that the larger-molecular-weight protein is the AB dimer, which was reduced to its component monomers (136,137).

Normal human mammary epithelial cells derived from reduction mammoplasties produce a factor that can compete with authentic PDGF for binding to the PDGF receptor. Using riboprobes for both the A and B chains of PDGF in an RNase protection assay, the normal mammary cells produce easily detectable amounts of mRNA for the A chain, but little message for the B chain. This finding contrasts with the results in breast cancer cell lines, where easily detectable message for both the A and B chains was found (138). Since the B chain is the product of the protooncogene c-*sis,* it is possible that the overexpression of this gene product may be related to the development of the malignant phenotype in these cells.

Although secretion of PDGF by breast cancer cells is regulatable, the receptor for PDGF is not expressed. Other epithelial tumors have also been found to express PDGF, but they lack the PDGF receptor as well (139). Several studies have demonstrated that PDGF is, in fact, not mitogenic for human breast cancer epithelial cell lines when added to serum-free defined media (108,140).

Since PDGF is a potent mitogen for fibroblasts and other mesenchymal cells, but epithelial cells lack the receptor for PDGF and do not respond to it despite the fact that they produce it in biologically important quantities, it appears that PDGF may be acting as an estrogen-regulated paracrine growth factor in human breast cancer. Malignant mammary epithelial cells may be able to export PDGF locally to stimulate the proliferation of surrounding tumor stromal elements, and so influence a particular aspect of overall tumor growth.

PDGF can induce fibroblasts to secrete immunoreactive insulin-like growth factor I (IGF-I), which, as discussed below, is a potent mitogen for breast cancer epithelial cells (141). This raises the interesting possibility of a positive paracrine loop, whereby breast epithelial cells produce PDGF, which stimulates surrounding fibroblasts to produce IGF-I, which in turn is stimulatory for the epithelial cells for the fibroblasts.

3. 52K Protein/Cathepsin D

Rochefort and Westley noted in 1979 that MCF-7 cells treated with estradiol secreted a 46,000-Da peptide into conditioned media which was detectable by gel electrophoresis (142). Subsequent studies have shown that, under estrogen influence, the protein is secreted in abundance, accounting for up to 40% of the secreted proteins of estrogen-stimulated MCF-7 cells. Studies of neuraminidase digestion and fucose incorporation suggested that the secreted product was a glycoprotein with a molecular weight of 52,000 (143). Electron-microscopic studies of estrogen-treated cells show the glycoprotein is accumulated in cytoplasmic secretory granules and subsequently released into conditioned media (144).

The protein is found in primary cultures derived from malignant effusions of breast cancer patients in the majority of specimens tested. The protein is inducible in primary culture by the addition of estrogen, but interestingly, the amount of 52K protein was lowest and was not inducible by estrogen in a patient who was estrogen receptor negative (145).

Other peptides with potential mitogenic activity, including insulin, EGF, and prolactin, do not induce increased production of the 52K protein, indicating that the production of the glycoprotein is not a universal response to mitogens in general, but is specific for estrogen.

More recently, 52K protein purified by immunoaffinity chromatography has been shown to be mitogenic for MCF-7 cells. At a concentration of 1 ng/ml, DNA content as assayed by tritiated thymidine increases roughly 2-fold over control MCF-7 cells (146). Scanning electron microscopy shows that the addition of a 52K protein induces microvilli on the cell surface similar to those seen during estrogen treatment (146).

While estrogens stimulate 52K protein production and antiestrogens are inhibitory, progestins also inhibit the 52K protein (147). Interestingly, the inhibitory effects of progestins are seen even in cells resistant to antiestrogens such as tamoxifen, suggesting that this progestin-mediated growth inhibition is not dependent on functional estrogen receptors, but is acting through some other mechanism.

The 52K protein has been found in numerous estrogen-sensitive and -insensitive breast cancer cell lines. Unlike other secreted growth factors discussed in this section, however, the estrogen-sensitive cell lines, such as MCF-7 and ZR-75-1, produce substantially more of the factor than do estrogen receptor-negative lines such as BT-20 and MDA MB-231 (148).

A model for the production and processing of the 52K protein has been proposed in which a polypeptide chain of 48K is cotranslationally N-glycosylated with at least two mannose chains to yield a 52K cellular glycoprotein. The protein is also phosphorylated primarily on the mannose side chains. In MCF-7 cells this protein is either secreted into the medium as the 52K mature glycoprotein or is processed internally to 48K and 34K forms. It appears that the mature 52K glycoprotein is able to bind to the surface of other cells through the cation-independent mannose 6-phosphate receptor (148). The cation-independent mannose 6-phosphate receptor is felt to be important in the internalization and packaging of lysosomal enzymes into cellular lysosomes. It is also a putative receptor for IGF-II (149), which will be discussed in a later section. Virtually all breast cancer cell lines express mRNA for this receptor (150). ^{35}S-labeling studies and electron-microscopic immunocytochemistry have shown that the 52K protein is taken up by MCF-7 cells and is processed into a 48K protein (151). Competition studies show that the uptake of the 52K protein into MCF-7 cells is inhibited by excess exogenous mannose 6-phosphate (152). The majority of the internalized processed protein appears to be contained in lysosomelike intracellular vesicles (153). Biochemical studies have shown that the 52K protein is secreted as an inactive proenzyme which, at acidic pH, functions as an acidic proteinase. Its enzymatic activity is inhibited by pepstatin. It is inactive at neutral pH (152).

The molecular weight, enzymatic activity, and immunoreactivity of the 52K protein were found to be very similar to the acidic protease cathepsin D. Sequencing of the 52K cDNA of MCF-7 cells showed virtual identity for the sequence of procathepsin D isolated from human kidney. The gene maps to chromosome 11 in the P-15 band, close to the H-*ras* gene (154).

Northern blot analysis shows that the mRNA for this protein is inducible by estradiol in MCF-7 cells. It is also produced at constitutively high levels in the estrogen receptor-negative cell line BT-20. Despite the higher level of mRNA expression in this estrogen receptor-negative cell line, as previously noted, less 52K activity was found in the conditioned media of BT-20 cells than in those from estrogen-sensitive cells such as MCF-7 and ZR-75-1 (148).

The 52K protein/cathepsin D may play multiple roles in the regulation of breast cancer growth. Since it has been shown to be mitogenic for cells that produce it and have the appropriate receptor, cathepsin D could be functioning as an autocrine growth factor. However, the acid proteolytic activity of the enzyme suggests that it may be functionally important in facilitating tumor invasion into normal tissues, tumor migration, and metastatic potential, as Rochefort and others have hypothesized (153).

4. *IGFs—General Characteristics*

IGF-I and IGF-II are a closely related pair of polypeptides with molecular weights of approximately 7500. As their names imply, they show considerable homology to insulin, or more precisely proinsulin (155–157).

IGF-I is also known as somatomedin C, the mediator of the effects of human growth hormone. IGF-I secretion in the normal human is stimulated directly by growth hormone. In acromegaly, for example, elevated growth hormone levels are accompanied by elevated IGF-I levels, and blood tests for serum IGF levels are useful in establishing the diagnosis of acromegaly in these patients. In contrast, the function of IGF-II is less clear. IGF-II is found in considerable quantity in fetal tissues and has been postulated to play a role in the regulation of fetal development (157). In animal models, IGF-II levels drop at the time of birth. However, considerable quantities of IGF-II are detectable in the adult, and the role of this hormone in adult life is not understood at present (158). IGF-I and IGF-II bind distinct, specific cell surface receptors, each of which have been characterized and cloned. The biological roles of the IGF-I and IGF-II receptors (also called the type 1 and type 2 IGF receptors, respectively) appear to be quite distinct as well.

The IGF-I receptor is very similar in structure to the insulin receptor, with two α chains and two β chains. The α chains comprise the extracellular ligand-binding site, while the β chains include the transmembrane and intracellular domains of the receptor, the latter possessing tyrosine kinase activity (159,160).

The IGF-II receptor, in contrast, exists as a single transmembrane chain, and does not possess intracellular tyrosine kinase activity (161). It has also been identified as the cation-independent mannose 6-phosphate receptor, which is important in the transport and packaging of lysosomal enzymes, as well as the 52K/cathepsin D protein discussed earlier (148,162). Recently, competitive binding studies have indicated that the binding sites for mannose 6-phosphate and IGF-II represent separate domains of the receptor (163).

IGF-I binds to both the IGF-I (type I) and insulin receptors. In a recent human study, IGF-I infused as an intravenous bolus caused a drop in serum glucose similar to that of insulin (164). Neither IGF-I nor insulin appears to bind significantly to the IGF-II receptor (165,166). In contrast, IGF-II can bind to both the insulin and IGF-I receptors, although the relative affinity of binding has been variously reported in several studies (167,168). This may be of significance, because evidence discussed in the following section suggests some of the biological function of IGF-II is mediated via the IGF-I receptor.

Both IGF-I and IGF-II are potent mitogens for the human breast cancer cell lines MCF-7 and T47-D. When added to serum-free medium, 5 nM IGF-I or 10 nM IGF-II show greater mitogenic potency than 1 nM estradiol (74).

Determination of production of both IGF-I and IGF-II protein by radioimmunoassay and other methods is complicated by the presence of numerous IGF-binding proteins. Binding proteins of several molecular weights are produced by a variety of breast cancer cell lines (169). These binding proteins make interpretations of IGF protein data much more difficult (170). Additionally, evidence from other systems suggests that the IGF-binding proteins discussed earlier may significantly influence the interaction of IGFs with their specific cellular receptors, and so alter growth factor bioavailability and action (171).

Assessment of the physiological roles of IGF-I and IGF-II is further complicated by the fact that, like insulin, the IGFs are produced as larger precursor hormones which are proteolytically cleaved to a smaller active peptide. Larger-molecular-weight species of IGFs have been isolated which may have significant biological activity. Processing of the precursor hormones may not be uniform in all circumstances and could significantly influence the biology of the secreted factors (172,173).

a. *IGF-I/IGF-I-Related Peptide.* A few years ago in our laboratory, we examined the production of IGF-I by breast cancer cell lines. Radioimmunoassay of conditioned media indicated that all breast cell lines examined produced an IGF-I-like material which was immunoreactive and mitogenic when given to cells grown in serum-free media (74). Addition of estrogen to estrogen receptor-positive cells incubated in serum-free media enhanced secretion of this factor substantially. It was noted, however, that of all breast cancer cell lines examined it was the estrogen receptor-negative cell lines, particularly MDA MB-231, which produced the largest quantities of this factor in a constitutive fashion that was not influenced by estrogen.

Northern blot analysis of breast cancer cell lines with IGF-I cDNA shows multiple and sometimes inconsistent hybridizing bands, the strongest of which corresponds to ribosomal RNA (74). In addition to this inconsistency on Northern blot analysis, the IGF-immunoreactive material from conditioned media displays a molecular weight of approximately 40,000 on sizing columns. There is, however, a peak detected by IGF-I radioimmunoassay very close to the size of authentic IGF-I after acid ethanol extraction of conditioned medium (74).

Because of the difficulties in interpreting the RNA and protein data for IGF-I, subsequent studies utilized the RNase protection assay as another means of examining these tumor cell lines. Previously, this assay was reported to be ten to 100 times more sensitive than Northern blot analysis in detecting specific mRNA. The assay is also significantly more specific than Northern blotting because virtual sequence identity is required between probe and cellular mRNA to obtain a positive signal (174).

Using this RNase protection assay, there was no detectable IGF-I message in any of the breast cancer cell lines studied. Examination of RNA extracted from patient breast tumor specimens, however, showed that the authentic IGF-I message was easily detectable in most of the samples (175). These data raise the possibility that the authentic IGF-I message does not arise from tumor epithelial cells but rather from stromal elements or other parts of the tumor. *In situ* hybridization of breast tumor specimens with an IGF-I riboprobe showed that this appears to be the case. In a tumor biopsy specimen, the area of histologically malignant tumor is without IGF-I mRNA signal, but the IGF-I message is easily seen in surrounding nonmalignant tissue. Examination at higher magnification shows that the expression is predominantly stromal in origin (175).

Others have reported that a truncated form of IGF-I which lacks three or four amino-terminal peptide residues is produced by MCF-7 cells. This form of the polypeptide appears to have considerably higher biological activity than the full 70-amino acid residue compound, but is produced in only picogram quantities by these cells. No RNA data were reported in this study (176).

The regulation of expression and production of these binding proteins and their physiological role in human breast cancer is under active investigation in numerous laboratories at the present time.

αIR-3, a monoclonal antibody to the type I IGF receptor, inhibits the growth of MCF-7 cells grown in serum-containing media, with or without estrogen (177). More recently, experiments in nude mice have shown that this antibody can prevent the formation of tumors by estrogen-independent MDA MB-231 cells (178). These cells produce large amounts of an IGF-I-like protein constitutively (74), but they do not have mRNA for authentic IGF-I (175).

From the data available at present, it appears that authentic IGF-I is produced primarily in fibroblast and stromal tissue rather than in breast cancer epithelial cells themselves. Thus, it is likely to be acting primarily as a paracrine growth factor. In addition, the breast cancer epithelial cell lines appear to be producing an IGF-I-like species which is immunologically and biologically similar to authentic IGF-I, but which presumably represents a different gene product. Attempts are being made to characterize this factor further.

In addition to stimulation of IGF-I-like factor by estrogen, insulin, EGF, and TGF-α all increase immunoreactive IGF-I-like secretion in MCF-7 cells. TGF-β and glucocorticoids as well as antiestrogens produce the opposite effect. Growth hormone, basic fibroblast growth factor, PDGF, and prolactin do not affect either growth rate or secretion of the IGF-I-related protein in these cells (179,180).

b. IFG-II. The function of IGF-II in the adult, as we stated earlier, is not known. The role of this growth factor in human cancer is likewise unclear, but several studies indicate that IGF-II is mitogenic for a number of cancer cell lines (108,181,182).

Of ten breast cancer cell lines examined, only T47-D consistently expressed authentic IGF-II message, as determined by both Northern blot analysis and the more sensitive RNase protection assay (75). Other studies, however, have reported IGF-II mRNA transcripts determined by Northern blot analysis in both MCF-7 and MDA MB-231 cells (182).

IGF-II mRNA expression is estrogen inducible in T47-D cells. After 8 hours of treatment with 1 nM estradiol, T47-D cells grown in serum-free media show an increase of approximately 5-fold in IGF-II mRNA levels. The weak estrogen phenol red also increases IGF-II mRNA expression, and this effect can be blocked by pretreatment with tamoxifen (75).

With the exception of T47-D cells, no breast cancer epithelial cell lines examined showed authentic IGF-II message (75). This was similar to the picture seen with RNase protection probes for authentic IGF-I message, where no cancer cell lines were found to produce IGF-I mRNA despite their almost universal production of an IGF-I-related immunoreactive protein.

With breast tumor biopsies, however, the RNase protection assay easily detected IGF-II mRNA in 24 of 26 cancer specimens. Additionally, four of five human skin fibroblast lines also expressed IGF-II message (75). Specimens of histologically normal breast taken from areas surrounding either fibroadenoma or tumor showed considerable IGF-II message, as was the case in fibroadenoma specimens themselves.

Preliminary IGF-II *in situ* hybridization data with normal breast and fibroadenoma specimens show that the message is found predominantly in stromal cells and not in epithelial cells. In breast tumor specimens, however, *in situ* hybridization shows some IGF-II expression in malignant epithelium as well (183,184). Again, this parallels the result found with IGF-I expression in breast tumor *in situ* specimens (75).

It appears then that IGF-II, like IGF-I, is produced predominantly in tumor stromal elements and probably plays a paracrine role in the regulation of breast tumor growth. The finding that at least one breast epithelial tumor cell line makes IGF-II in an estrogen-regulated fashion suggests that in some cases IGF-II may be able to act as an autocrine factor as well.

5. TGF-β

The estrogen-regulated growth factors discussed until this point have all been stimulatory. TGF-β on the other hand, appears to play an opposite role, serving as a potent inhibitor of breast tumor cell growth.

Laboratory evidence suggesting the existence of growth-inhibitory factors such as TGF-β can be derived from an experiment in which conditioned media from MCF-7 cells which were growth-arrested by treatment with antiestrogens inhibited the growth of other estrogen-dependent cells. This suggested that, just as estrogen could induce the production of growth-stimulatory factors such as TGF-α and the IGFs, antiestrogens could promote the production of growth inhibitors (185). This inhibitory effect, due to TGF-β, may represent a balancing arm in the estrogen-mediated effects on growth control of human breast cancer.

TGF-β is a 25-kDa protein comprised of two identical 12.5-kDa poly-peptides which are linked by disulfide bridges. It was initially purified from platelets and various normal tissues. Like TGF-α, TGF-β can stimulate the anchorage-dependent growth of fibroblasts in soft agar (186). However, quite unlike TGF-α, TGF-β is a potent growth inhib-itor for many epithelial cell lines (187,188). TGF-β inhibits mammary ductal development in animal models and may act coordinately with numerous other factors such as estrogen and EGF in the control of normal mammary development (34,189). TGF-β acts through a specif-ic high-molecular-weight cell surface receptor that does not appear to have tyrosine kinase activity (190,191).

Breast cancer cell lines express a 2.5-kb mRNA for TGF-β which matches the expected message based on studies with other cell types (185,192).

Radioimmunoassay of TGF-β in conditioned media from MCF-7 cells shows marked induction of TGF-β secretion by treatment with antiestrogens. Conversely, stimulation of cell growth with either in-sulin or estradiol causes a decrease in TGF-β secretion below control levels (185).

LY-II, a mutant cell line derived from MCF-7 cells, differs from the parent line in that it has lost the ability to respond to antiestrogen treatment, despite retaining a functional estrogen receptor and es-trogen responsiveness. In this line TGF-β production is no longer in-duced by antiestrogen treatment, but the cells retain the TGF-β recep-tor and the ability to be inhibited by exogenous TGF-β (185). In this laboratory model then, one possible explanation for the loss of the ability to respond to antiestrogen treatment is the loss of the ability to produce an inhibitory factor such as TGF-β. Clearly, an intact es-trogen receptor is not necessary for the effects of TGF-β, since es-trogen-independent lines such as MDA MB-231 are fully sensitive to the inhibitory effects of this polypeptide (185).

The regulation of TGF-β secretion by estrogens and antiestrogens in MCF-7 cells does not appear to take place at the level of steady-state mRNA. The fall in assayable TGF-β with estrogen treatment and the rise in TGF-β with antiestrogen treatment were not accompanied by detectable differences in mRNA levels by Northern blot analysis. This suggests that posttranscriptional events as yet undefined are responsi-ble for the noted changes in TGF-β activity (185).

A 62-kDa TGF-β precursor can be activated by proteolytic cleavage to a 25,000 molecular-weight active TGF-β (193,194). Moreover, other serum proteins may bind to TGF-β and influence its biological ac-tivity. Specifically, α_2-macroglobulin has been shown to covalently bind and inactivate TGF-β (195).

An MCF-7 variant resistant to the effects of TGF-β has been isolated. Interestingly, the cell line is growth-inhibited by estradiol, while the parental MCF-7 cells show the typical mitogenic response to estradiol. In addition, this estrogen-inhibited mutant showed a markedly different pattern of polypeptide secretion when compared with the parental MCF-7 cells (196). Other cell lines have been identified as well which are resistant to the effects of TGF-β (197).

The finding that TGF-β secretion is diminished by estrogen treatment in cell lines suggests the possibility that some of the mitogenic effects of estradiol may be mediated through the release of static inhibitory effects of factors such as TGF-β. Conversely, growth inhibition by antiestrogens may, in part, be mediated through TGF-β secretion, but some have argued that this alone is not sufficient to explain the growth-inhibitory effects mediated by tamoxifen-like drugs (198). At the present time, it is impossible to make a conclusive statement based on the available studies regarding the relative contribution of TGF-β secretion in mediating the response to estrogens and antiestrogens.

V. Other Estrogen-Regulated Proteins

In addition to effects on secreted growth factors and other proteins discussed above, estrogens induce production of numerous other proteins in breast cancer cell lines. The biology and function of these other proteins are, in general, less clearly defined, and in a number of instances, completely unknown.

A. Proteolytic Enzymes

Several estrogen-inducible proteins have proteolytic activity and may be important in the process of tumor invasion and metastasis.

1. *Plasminogen Activator*

Plasminogen activator has been described as a component of many human tumors. The enzyme converts plasminogen to the active protease plasmin, which has significant proteolytic and thrombolytic activities. In some systems it appears that tumorigenicity is enhanced by plasminogen activator production (199). MCF-7 cells increase production of plasminogen activator more than two times over control upon treatment with estradiol. Increases in plasminogen activator activity are produced as early as 8 hours after adding estrogen in concentrations as low as 10^{-10} M (200). Significantly higher concentrations of the androgen testosterone (10^{-6} M) showed a similar effect, while antiestrogens were able to inhibit plasminogen activator production by MCF-7 cells (201).

Analysis of human breast tumor explants showed that plasminogen activator activity was significantly increased in approximately 50% of the tumors that were both estrogen and progesterone receptor positive. No estradiol-mediated increase in plasminogen activator activity was seen in any of the tumors that were not positive for both estrogen and progesterone receptor (202). Of the two principal types of plasminogen activator, the tissue type and the urokinase type, only the tissue-type plasminogen activator appears to be related to estrogen receptor and estradiol sensitivity (203).

2. Collagenase

Collagenase activity has been examined in a number of cell culture and tumor biopsy experiments. MCF-7 cells secrete collagenases which are able to lyse type I and type IV collagen. Type I collagen is found in tissue stroma and in bone, while type IV is the principal form in cellular basement membranes. Estradiol treatment caused a 2- to 3-fold increase in collagenase activity in MCF-7 cells (204). Collagenase produced by another estrogen-sensitive line, ZR-75-1, displayed a molecular weight of 60,000 and required activation to exert its proteolytic effect. The estrogen-sensitive plasminogen activator may be important in the activation of collagenase (205,206). Therefore, estrogen may cause an increase in both collagenase precursors as well as the enzyme which activates them.

Immunohistochemical analysis of breast tumor specimens with an antibody against a type IV collagenase showed intense epithelial staining in each of 25 cases of invasive carcinoma studied. Interestingly, no fibroadenomas, fibrocystic disease biopsies, or normal breast specimens were positive in this study (207). Another study of type I collagenase activity in breast tumor specimens showed uniformly high secretion by fibroadenomas compared with benign fibrocystic lesions, while carcinoma specimens showed a wide range of collagenolytic activity which did not correlate with histological type (208). Electron-microscopic examination of infiltrating breast carcinomas shows a characteristic collagen fibrillar degeneration, which is reproduced *in vitro* by treatment of reconstituted fibrils with human collagenase, but not other proteolytic enzymes (209). When breast tumor samples were tested in an *in vitro* bone culture system, the ability to induce osteolysis, presumably due to type I collagenase activity, was positively correlated with the subsequent development of bone metastasis and hypercalcemia (210).

These studies are somewhat difficult to compare, since, in general, they rely on digestion of nonstandardized substrate preparations to infer enzyme activity, rather than immunological or other assay methods which would be more specific. However, they do demonstrate in both tumors and cell culture significant proteolytic activity, suggesting that the ability to digest basement membrane collagen and other collagen substrates is important in breast tumor invasion and metastasis. The MCF-7 cell culture model suggests further that estrogen may be important in the regulation of collagenase production in these tumors.

3. 52K Protein/Cathepsin D

Finally, as discussed in a previous section, the 52K protein described by Rochefort, which is one of the major secreted proteins in MCF-7 cells, is an acid protease which is significantly inducible by estradiol treatment (143).

B. PROGESTERONE RECEPTOR

In addition to the nuclear estrogen receptor, hormonally sensitive human breast tumors and cell lines generally express a specific receptor for progesterone (211). Cyclic changes in human endometrial progesterone receptor levels have been known for some time (212). This led to the investigation of progesterone receptor synthesis in estrogen-responsive MCF-7 cells by McGuire and colleagues. Progesterone receptor levels were found to increase 3- to 6-fold after 4 days of treatment with 10^{-10} M estradiol. Progesterone receptor induction was suppressed by tamoxifen, but the inhibitory effects of tamoxifen could be overcome by supraphysiological doses of estrogen (213). This observation has been confirmed by numerous other investigators (214). More recently, Northern blot analysis has shown that progesterone receptor mRNA levels increase up to 7-fold after exposure of MCF-7 cells to estradiol (215).

Using density shift techniques which involve growing cells in media containing heavy isotopes of amino acids, it has been possible to demonstrate that the increase in progesterone receptor content after estradiol stimulation is due to an increase in progesterone receptor synthesis and not decreased degradation (215).

Many studies have shown that the existence of progesterone receptors is closely correlated with that of estrogen receptors (216). Combined detection of estrogen and progesterone receptors provides the strongest indicator of hormone responsiveness in clinical breast cancer (16). Although stimulation of the progesterone receptor can induce synthesis of specific proteins (217), it does not play a direct role in the control of breast cancer cell growth.

C. LAMININ RECEPTOR

Laminin, a complex glycoprotein, is a major structural component of cellular basement membranes. It binds extracellular matrix components such as type IV collagen and proteoglycans (218). Many normal and malignant cells contain high-affinity cell surface receptors for laminin, and breast cancer cells express significantly more of the receptor than do cells from benign lesions (219). This relative overexpression of laminin receptor may enhance adherence of tumor cells to basement membranes and may ultimately foster metastasis (218).

MCF-7 cells treated with estradiol show increases in the cell surface receptor protein for laminin. E_2 treatment increases binding of radiolabeled laminin as well as attachment to laminin-coated membranes (220). The laminin receptor, it is postulated, contributes to the invasiveness of tumor cells by mediating attachment of tumor to basement membrane laminin (218).

D. ESTROGEN-REGULATED PROTEINS OF UNKNOWN FUNCTION

A number of other protein products under estrogen regulation have been described whose significance has yet to be defined.

McGuire et al. described a 24K estrogen-inducible protein in conditioned media from MCF-7 cells (221). The protein has been subsequently purified and sequenced, and is identical to the 27-kDa heat-shock protein first described in HeLa cells. Its function, nevertheless, is still unclear (222). McGuire has also found that lactate dehydrogenase (LDH) is estrogen-inducible in MCF-7 cells (223). The increased LDH activity was observed only in cell lysates and not in conditioned media.

Chambon's group found an estradiol-induced increase in mRNA coding for a 7000-molecular-weight protein designated pS2. Estrogen added to MCF-7 cells grown in estrogen-free conditions caused an increase in the content of pS2 mRNA within 30 minutes and a continued increase toward a plateau approximately 24 hours later. The protein coded by this message is of unknown function, and the regulated mRNA was found accidently while attempting to clone the cDNA coding for the 52K protein/cathepsin D (224). While the function of pS2 is not known, these experiments demonstrate that alteration of gene expression by estradiol is a very rapid event, taking place on the order of minutes to hours.

Finally, in their studies of their 52K glycoprotein, Westley and Rochefort also found estrogen-induced synthesis of a larger 160K glycoprotein. This has been less well characterized than its 52K counterpart, and its identity and function remain obscure (143).

VI. Mechanisms of Estrogen Resistance

Since the discovery of estrogen binding by breast tumors and the elaboration of the role of the estrogen receptor, it has been observed that a substantial percentage of breast tumors are estrogen receptor negative at the time of diagnosis and are very unlikely to respond to endocrine therapies. These tumors tend to be more aggressive clinically and carry a poorer prognosis than do their estrogen receptor-positive counterparts.

Moreover, tumors initially estrogen-sensitive often lose estrogen responsiveness with the passage of time, or under the selective pressure of antiestrogen therapy.

Although tumors *in vivo* and *in vitro* can clearly lose estrogen receptors, that event alone cannot completely explain the change in the biology of tumors that have become estrogen insensitive. Other intracellular events distinct from the simple loss of the estrogen receptor are necessary for the phenotypic conversion to a hormone-independent tumor. These tumors not only fail to respond to endocrine treatment, but grow more rapidly clinically, are less well-differentiated histologically, have greater metastatic potential, and are frequently more resistant to other nonendocrine therapies as well.

While these additional cellular events have not been fully defined, it is possible that conversion to estrogen insensitivity is accompanied by the constitutive or unregulated production of cellular growth factors such as those discussed in the previous sections. These growth factors are able to stimulate cell proliferation totally outside of estrogenic control; this may explain the ability of some hormone-independent tumors such as MDA MB-231 to grow in culture in the complete absence of serum or hormonal supplementation.

Data presented in earlier sections showed that hormone-independent MDA MB-231 tumors constitutively secrete higher levels of IGF-I-like growth factor (74) than do hormone-dependent MCF-7 cells. The same holds true for TGF-α determined by radioimmunoassay and for TGF-α mRNA determined by Northern blot analysis (114). Some estrogen-independent human breast tumors produce high levels of IGF-II mRNA (75). At least one growth factor, basic fibroblast growth factor (bFGF) is not under estrogen regulation per se, in that it does not appear to be produced by any known estrogen-sensitive breast tumor cell lines. However, mRNA for bFGF is detected in a number of estrogen-independent cell lines (225), so one can hypothesize that the conversion to estrogen independence could be accompanied by the production of growth factors not seen in the estrogen-sensitive phenotype.

It is not clear, however, how the loss of the estrogen receptor is linked to the activation of constitutive growth factor secretion. In an effort to establish a laboratory model for this phenomenon, estrogen-dependent MCF-7 cells were transfected with the v-ras^H oncogene. The transfected cells express both the oncogene mRNA and its protein product, p21. Upon transfection, the cells become estrogen independent in culture and fully tumorigenic without estrogen in nude mice (226); the wild-type cells remain dependent on estrogen for tumorigenicity in nude mice (116). Interestingly, the v-ras^H transfected cells retain estrogen receptors and show induction of progesterone receptor in response to estrogen treatment, confirming that the estrogen receptor is functional despite the loss of estrogen sensitivity. The transfectants show a blunted mitogenic response to estradiol and are virtually insensitive to antiestrogen treatment, unlike the wild-type MCF-7 line (226).

Further experiments with the ras-transfected MCF-7 cell line show that these cells secrete three to five times more TGF-α, TGF-β, and IGF-I-like protein than does the parent cell line. The overexpression of TGF-β would be expected to exert an inhibitory effect; this suggests that mitogenic effects of stimulatory factors, also overexpressed, outweigh any TGF-β mediated inhibition.

The ras-transfected cells are also less sensitive to the mitogenic effects of exogenous estrogen, IGF-I, or TGF-α. Conditioned media from these cells can replace estrogen in stimulating MCF-7 soft agar colony formation in vitro (227).

A different model of estrogen resistance was produced by Katzenellenbogen and colleagues, who developed an estrogen-independent MCF-7 cell line by prolonged carriage in media completely devoid of estradiol or the weak estrogen phenol red. The proliferation rate of the cells initially slowed, but after several months under these conditions, there was a marked increase in the basal rate of proliferation. This was accompanied by a 3-fold increase in cellular estrogen receptor compared with the wild type. These estrogen-deprived cells showed no mitogenic response to estradiol, but were sensitive to antiestrogens, and did show a typical increase in progesterone receptor in response to estrogen (228). Like the v-ras^H transfection model, these estrogen-insensitive cells have retained functional estrogen receptor, but no longer show a mitogenic response to estrogen treatment.

Both the v-ras^H transfection and estrogen deprivation experiments suggest possible mechanisms for the acquisition of the hormone-independent phenotype, but neither model reproduces the common clinical observation that estrogen independence is usually accompanied by loss of the estrogen receptor. This suggests that several steps may be involved in the development of hormone independence *in vivo,* or that there may be multiple pathways of estrogen resistance.

VII. CONCLUSIONS

Estrogen regulation of protein synthesis and cell growth represents a balance among complex molecular and cellular interactions. Through the estrogen receptor, estrogen binds to nuclear DNA and modulates the transcription of specific genes. These gene products can influence intracellular events in the estrogen-sensitive cell directly, as is the case with enzymes that support DNA synthesis.

Estrogen effects in the estrogen-sensitive cell can be indirect, mediated by autocrine growth stimulators such as TGF-α which are produced in response to estrogen, or autocrine growth inhibitors such as TGF-β, whose production is inhibited by estrogen. These factors subsequently bind to cell surface receptors and influence a secondary wave of cellular events.

Through paracrine-acting growth factors such as PDGF, estrogen can influence the growth of breast cells in a different, indirect manner. Epithelial cells which produce PDGF in response to estrogen can stimulate the growth of surrounding stromal cells which do not possess estrogen receptor and are not sensitive to estrogen in and of themselves. Likewise, estrogen-regulated proteins such as plasminogen activator and collagenase act on the tissues surrounding the breast epithelium but may importantly influence biological behavior important to growth, such as tumor invasion and metastasis.

The loss of estrogen responsiveness in a previously sensitive tumor cell is incompletely understood, but appears to involve both the loss of the estrogen receptor and the constitutive production of growth factors and perhaps other gene products in an unregulated fashion. At the present time, the intracellular mechanisms linking these two events are unknown.

REFERENCES

1. Beatson, G. T. (1896). On the treatment of inoperable cases of carcinoma of the mamma. Suggestions for a new method of treatment with illustrative cases. *Lancet* **2,** 104–107.
2. Yuasa, S., and McMahon, B. (1971). Lactation in reproductive histories of breast cancer patients in Tokyo, Japan. *Bull. W.H.O.* **42,** 195–204.
3. Pike, M. C., Henderson, B. E., and Casagrande, J. T. (1981). The epidemiology of breast cancer as it relates to menarche, pregnancy and menopause. *Banbury Rep.* **8,** 3–19.
4. Hoover, R., Gray, L. A., Cole, P., and MacMahon, B. (1976). Menopausal estrogens in breast cancer. *N. Engl. J. Med.* **295,** 401–405.
5. Bird, C. E., Cook, S., Owen, S., Sterns, E. E., and Clark, A. F. (1980). Plasma concentrations of C-19 steroids, estrogens, FSH, LH and prolactin in post menopausal women with and without breast cancer. *Oncology* **38,** 365–368.
6. MacMahon, B., Cole, P., Lin, T. M., Lowe, C. R., Mirra, A. P., Ravnihar, B., Salber, E. J., Valaoras, V. G., and Yuasa, S. (1970). Age at first birth and breast cancer risk. *Bull. W.H.O.* **43,** 209–215.
7. Pike, M. C., Henderson, B. E., Casagrande, J. T., Rosario, I., and Gray, G. E. (1981). Oral contraceptive use and early abortion as risk factors for breast cancer in young women. *Br. J. Cancer* **43,** 72–76.
8. Tsutsui, T., Maizumi, H., McLachlan, J. A., and Barrett, J. C. (1983). Aneuploidy induction and cell transformation by diethylstilbestrol: A possible chromosomal mechanism in carcinogenesis. *Cancer Res.* **43,** 3814–3821.
9. Degan, G. H., and Metzler, M. (1987). Sex hormone and neoplasia: Genotoxic effects in short term assays. *Arch. Toxicol., Suppl.* **10,** 264–278.
10. Metzler, M. (1987). Metabolic activation of xenobiotic stilbene estrogens. *Fed. Proc., Fed. Am. Soc. Exp. Biol.* **46,** 1855–1857.
11. Liehr, J. G., Stancel, G. M., Chorich, L. P., Bousfield, G. R., and Ulubelen, A. A. (1986). Hormonal carcinogenesis: Separation of estrogenicity from carcinogenicity. *Chem.-Biol. Interact.* **59,** 173–184.
12. Huggins, C., Grand, L. C., and Brilliantes, F. P. (1961). Mammary cancer induced by a single feeding of polynuclear hydrocarbons, and its suppression. *Nature (London)* **189,** 204–207.
13. McGregor, D. H., Land, C. E., Choi, K., Tokuoka, S., Liu, P. I., Wakabayashi, I., and Bebe, G. W. (1977). Breast cancer incidence in atomic bomb survivors. Hiroshima and Nagasaki 1945–1960. *J. Natl. Cancer Inst. (U.S.)* **59,** 799–807.
14. Jensen, E. V., DeSombre, E. R., Youngblood, A. N., and Jungblut, P. W. (1967). Estrogen receptors in hormone responsive tissues and tumors. *In* "Endogeneous Factors Influencing Host Tumor Balance" (R. W. Wissler et al., eds.), pp. 15–30. Univ. of Chicago Press, Chicago, Illinois.
15. Jensen, E. V. (1980). Historical perspective. *Cancer (Philadelphia)* **46,** 2759–2764.
16. Lippman, M. E. (1985). Endocrine response of cancers of man. *In* "Textbook of Endocrinology, 7th. ed." (R. H. Williams, ed.), pp. 1309–1326. Saunders, Philadelphia, Pennsylvania.
17. Topper, Y. J., and Freeman, C. S. (1980). Multiple hormone interactions in the developmental biology of the mammary gland. *Physiol. Rev.* **60,** 1049–1106.

18. Drife, J. O. (1986). Breast development in puberty. *Ann. N.Y. Acad. Sci.* **464,** 58–65.
19. Illig, R., Torresani, T., Bucher, H., and Prader, A. (1982). Transient rise in luteinizing hormone and follicle-stimulating hormone secretion during puberty studied in 113 healthy girls with tall stature. *J. Clin. Endocrinol. Metab.* **54,** 192–195.
20. Apter, D. (1980). Serum steroids and pituitary hormones in female puberty: A partly longitudinal study. *Clin. Endocrinol. (Oxford)* **12,** 107–120.
21. Lieberman, M. E., Maurer, R. A., and Gorski, J. (1978). Estrogen control of prolactin synthesis in vitro. *Proc. Natl. Acad. Sci. U.S.A.* **75,** 5946–5949.
22. Miller, W. L., Knight, M. M., and Gorski, J. (1977). Estrogen action in vitro: Regulation of thyroid stimulating and other pituitary hormones in cell culture. *Endocrinology (Baltimore)* **101,** 1455–1460.
23. Ip, C., and Dao, T. L. (1978). Effect of estradiol and prolactin on galactosyltransferase and alpha-lactalbumin activities in rat mammary gland and mammary tumor. *Cancer Res.* **38,** 2077–2083.
24. Pertzelan, A. L., Yalon, L., Kauli, R., and Laron, Z. (1982). A comparative study of the effect of oestrogen substitution therapy on breast development in girls with hypo- and hypergonadotrophic hypogonadism. *Clin. Endocrinol. (Oxford)* **16,** 359–368.
25. Bresciani, F. (1968). Topography of DNA synthesis in the mammary gland of the CH3 mouse and its control by ovarian hormones: An autoradiographic study. *Cell Tissue Kinet.* **1,** 51–63.
26. Lyons, W. R. (1958). Hormonal synergism in mammary growth. *Proc. R. Soc. Med.* **149,** 303–325.
27. Rosenfield, R. I., Furlanetto, R., and Bock, D. (1983). Relationship of somatomedin-C concentrations to pubertal changes. *J. Pediatr.* **103,** 723–728.
28. Large, D. M., and Anderson, D. C. (1980). Twenty-four hour profiles of serum prolactin during male puberty with and without gynecomastia. *Clin. Endocrinol. (Oxford)* **12,** 293–302.
29. Durnberger, H., Heuberger, B., Schwartz, P., Wasner, G., and Kratochwill, K. (1978). Mesenchyme-mediated effect of testosterone on embryonic mammary epithelium. *Cancer Res.* **38,** 4066–4070.
30. Haslam, S. Z., and Lively, M. L. (1985). Estradiol responsiveness of normal mouse epithelial cells in primary culture: Association of mammary fibroblasts with estradiol regulation of progesterone receptors. *Endocrinology (Baltimore)* **116,** 1835–1844.
31. Haslam, S. Z. (1986). Mammary fibroblast influence on normal mouse mammary epithelial cell responses to estrogen in vitro *Cancer Res.* **46,** 310–316.
32. Petersen, D. W., Hoyer, P. E., and Van Deurs, P. (1987). Frequency and distribution of estrogen receptor positive cells in normal non-lactating human breast tissue. *Cancer Res.* **47,** 5748–5751.
33. King, W. J., DeSombre, E. R., Jensen, E. V., and Greene, G. L. (1985). Comparison of immunocytochemical and steroid-binding assays for estrogen receptor in human breast tumors. *Cancer Res.* **45,** 293–304.
34. Silberstein, G. B., and Daniel, C. W. (1987). Reversible inhibition of mammary gland growth by transforming growth factor beta. *Science* **237,** 291–293.
35. Bolander, F. F., and Topper, Y. J. (1979). Stimulation of lactose synthetase activity in casein synthesis in mice mammary explants by estradiol. *Endocrinology (Baltimore)* **106,** 490–495.
36. Kleinberg, D., Todd, G., Babitsky, G., and Greising, J. (1981). Evidence that estradiol inhibits prolactin-induced milk protein production in primate mammary tissue organ cultures. *Clin. Res.* **29,** 506A.

37. Jensen, E. V. (1960). Studies of growth phenomenon using tritium labelled steroids. *Proc. Int. Congr. Biochem., 4th, 1958* Vol. 15, p. 119.
38. Toft, D., and Gorski, J. (1966). A receptor molecule for estrogens: Isolation from the rat uterus and preliminary characterization. *Proc. Natl. Acad. Sci. U.S.A.* **55,** 1574.
39. Jensen, E. V., Suzuki, T., Kawashima, T., Stumpf, W. E., Jungblut, P. W., and DeSombre, E. R. (1968). A two-step mechanism for the interaction of estradiol with rat uterus. *Proc. Natl. Acad. Sci. U.S.A.* **59,** 632–638.
40. O'Malley, B. W., and Means, A. R. (1974). Female steroid hormones and target cell nuclei. *Science* **183,** 610–620.
41. King, W. J., and Greene, G. L. (1984). Monoclonal antibodies localized oestrogen receptor in the nuclei of target cells. *Nature (London)* **307,** 745–747.
42. Welshons, W. V., Lieberman, M. E., and Gorski, J. (1984). Nuclear localization of unoccupied oestrogen receptors. *Nature (London)* **307,** 747–749.
43. Schuh, S., Yamamoto, W., Brügge, J., Bauer, V. H., Riehl, R. M., Sullivan, W. P., and Toft, D. O. (1985). A 90,000 dalton binding protein common to both steroid receptors and the Rous sarcoma transforming protein pp60^{v-src}. *J. Biol. Chem.* **260,** 14292–14296.
44. Cano, A., Coffey, A. I., Adatia, R., Willis, R. R., Rubens, R. D., and King, R. J. B. (1986). Histochemical studies with an estrogen receptor related protein in human breast tumors. *Cancer Res.* **46,** 6475–6480.
45. Puca, G. A., Sica, V., and Nola, E. (1974). Identification of a high affinity nuclear acceptor site for estrogen receptor of calf uterus. *Proc. Natl. Acad. Sci. U.S.A.* **171,** 979–983.
46. Spelsberg, T. C., Webster, R. A., and Pikler, G. M. (1976). Chromosomal proteins regulate steroid binding to chromatin. *Nature (London)* **262,** 65–67.
47. Green, S., Walter, P., Kumar, V., Krust, A., Bornert, J., Argos, P., and Chambon, P. (1986). Human oestrogen receptor cDNA: Sequence, expression and homology to v-erb-A. *Nature (London)* **320,** 134–139.
48. Evans, R. M. (1988). The steroid and thyroid hormone receptor superfamily. *Science* **240,** 887–895.
49. Kumar, V., Green, S., Staub, A., and Chambon, P. (1986). Localization of oestradiol binding and putative DNA binding domains of the human oestrogen receptor. *EMBO J.* **5,** 2231–2236.
50. Jost, J. P., Giser, M., and Seldran, M. (1985). Specific modulation of the transcription of cloned avian vitellogenin II gene by estradiol–receptor complex in vitro. *Proc. Natl. Acad. Sci. U.S.A.* **82,** 988–991.
51. Miller, J., McLachlan, A. D., and Klug, A. (1985). Repetitive zinc-binding domains in the protein transcription factor IIIA from *Xenopus* oocytes. *EMBO J.* **4,** 1609–1614.
52. Adler, S., Waterman, M. L., Phe, X., and Rosenfeld, N. G. (1988). Steroid receptor mediated inhibition of rat prolactin gene expression does not require the receptor DNA-binding domain. *Cell (Cambridge, Mass.)* **52,** 685–695.
53. Maurer, R. A. and Notides, A. C. (1987). Identification of an estrogen responsive element from the 5'-flanking region of the rat prolactin gene. *Mol. Cell. Biol.* **7,** 4247–4254.
54. Jost, J. P., Seldran, M., and Geiser, M. (1984). Preferential binding of estrogen receptor complex to a region containing the estrogen dependent hypomethylation site preceding the chicken vitellogenin II gene. *Proc. Natl. Acad. Sci. U.S.A.* **81,** 429–433.
55. Klein-Hitpass, L., Schorpp, M., Wagner, U., and Ryffel, G. U. (1986). An estrogen-responsive element derived from the 5'-flanking region of the *Xenopus* vitellogenin gene functions in transfected human cells. *Cell (Cambridge, Mass.)* **46,** 1053–1061.

56. Briand, P. (1983). Hormone-dependent mammary tumors in mice and rats as a model for human breast cancer. *Anticancer Res.* 3, 273–282.
57. Brunner, N., Osborne, C. K., and Spang-Thomsen, M. (1987). Endocrine therapy of human breast cancer grown in nude mice. *Breast Cancer Res. Treat.* 10, 229–242.
58. Osborne, C. K., Hobbs, K., and Trent, J. M. (1987). Biological differences among MCF-7 human breast cancer cell lines from different laboratories. *Breast Cancer Res. Treat.* 9, 22–121.
59. Jensen, E. V., and Jacobson, H. I. (1962). Basic guide to the mechanisms estrogen action. *Recent Prog. Horm. Res.* 18, 387–414.
60. Mueller, G. C., Vonderhaar, B., Kim, U. H., and LeMahieu, M. (1972). Estrogen action: An inroad to cell biology. *Recent Prog. Horm. Res.* 28, 1–48.
61. Soule, H. D., and McGrath, C. M. (1980). Estrogen responsive proliferation of clonal human breast carcinoma cells in athymic mice. *Cancer Lett.* 10, 177–189.
62. Engle, L. W., and Young, N. W. (1978). Human breast carcinoma cells in continuous culture: A review. *Cancer Res.* 38, 4327–4339.
63. Lippman, M., Bolan, G., and Huff, K. (1976). The effects of estrogens and anti-estrogens on hormone responsive human breast cancer in long-term tissue culture. *Cancer Res.* 36, 4595–4601.
64. Lippman, M., and Bolan, G. (1975). Oestrogen responsive human breast cancer in long term tissue culture. *Nature (London)* 256, 592–593.
65. Page, M. J., Field, J. K., Everett, N. P., and Green, C. D. (1983). Serum regulation of the estrogen responsiveness of the human breast cancer cell line MCF-7. *Cancer Res.* 43, 1244–1249.
66. Darbre, P., Yates, J., Curtis, S., and King, R. J. B. (1983). Effect of estradiol on human breast cancer cells in culture. *Cancer Res.* 43, 349–354.
67. Chalbos, D., Vignon, F., Keydar, I., and Rochefort, H. (1982). Estrogens stimulate cell proliferation and induce secretory proteins in a human breast cancer cell line (T47D). *J. Clin. Endocrinol. Metab.* 55, 276–283.
68. Leung, B. S., Qureshi, S., and Leung, J. S. (1982). Response to estrogen by the human mammary carcinoma cell line CAMA-1. *Cancer Res.* 43, 5060–5066.
69. Katzenellenbogen, B. S., Norman, M. J., Eckert, R. L., Peltz, S. W., and Mangel, W. F. (1983). Bioactivities, estrogen receptor interactions, and plasminogen activator-inducing activities of tamoxifen and hydroxy-tamoxifen isomers in MCF-7 human breast cancer cells. *Cancer Res.* 44, 112–119.
70. Weichselbaum, R. W., Hellman, S., Piro, A., Nove, J. J., and Little, J. B. (1978). Proliferation kinetics of a human breast cancer cell line in vitro following treatment with 17betaestradiol and 1-β-o-arabinofuranasylcytosine. *Cancer Res.* 38, 2239–2342.
71. Sonnenschein, C., and Soto, A. M. (1980). But are estrogens per se growth promoting hormones? *JNCL, J. Natl. Cancer Inst.* 64, 211–215.
72. Lykkesfeldt, A. E., and Briand, P. (1986). Indirect mechanism of estradiol stimulation of cell proliferation of human breast cancer cell line. *Br. J. Cancer* 53, 29–35.
73. Berthois, Y., Katzenellenbogen, J. A., and Katzenellenbogen, B. S. (1986). Phenol red in tissue culture media is a weak estrogen: Implications concerning the study of estrogen-responsive cells in culture. *Proc. Natl. Acad. Sci. U.S.A.* 83, 2496–2500.
74. Yee, D., Cullen, K. J., Paik, S., Perdue, J. F., Hampton, B., Schwartz, A., Lippman, M. E., and Rosen, N. (1988). Insulin-like growth factor II expression in human breast cancer. *Cancer Res.* 48, 6691–6696.
75. Huff, K. K., Kaufman, B., Gabbay, K. H., Spencer, E. M., Lippman, M. E., and Dickson, R. B. (1986). Human breast cancer cells secrete an insulin-like growth factor I related polypeptide. *Cancer Res.* 46, 4613–4619.

76. Aitken, S. C., and Lippman, M. E. (1982). Hormonal regulation of net DNA synthesis in MCF-7 human breast cancer cells in tissue culture. *Cancer Res.* **42,** 1727–1735.
77. Edwards, D. P., Murphy, S. R., and McGuire, W. L. (1980). Effects of estrogen and antiestrogen on DNA polymerase in human breast cancer. *Cancer Res.* **40,** 1722–1726.
78. Bronzert, D. A., Monaco, M. E., Pinkus, L., Aitken, S., and Lippman, M. E. (1981). Purification and properties of estrogen responsive cytoplasmic thymidine kinase from human breast cancer. *Cancer Res.* **41,** 604–610.
79. Kasid, A., Davidson, N. E., Gelmann, E. P., and Lippman, M. E. (1986). Transcriptional control of thymidine kinase gene expression by estrogen and antiestrogens in MCF-7 human breast cancer cells. *J. Biol. Chem.* **261,** 5562–5567.
80. Groudine, M., and Casimir, C. (1984). Post-transcriptional regulation of the chicken thymidine kinase gene. *Nucleic Acids Res.* **12,** 1427–1435.
81. Aitken, S. C., and Lippman, M. E. (1983). Hormonal regulation of *de novo* pyrimidine synthesis and utilization in human breast cancer cells in tissue culture. *Cancer Res.* **43,** 4681–4690.
82. Cowan, K. H., Goldsmith, M. E., Levine, R. M., Aitken, S. C., Douglass, E., Clendeninn, N., Nienhuis, A. W., and Lippman, M. E. (1982). Dihydrofolate reductase gene amplification and possible rearrangement in estrogen responsive methotrexate resistant human breast cancer cells. *J. Biol. Chem.* **257,** 15079–15086.
83. Levine, R. M., Rubalcaba, E., Lippman, M. E., and Cowan, K. (1985). Effects of estrogen and tamoxifen on the regulation of dihydrofolate reductase gene expression in a human breast cancer cell line. *Cancer Res.* **45,** 1644–1650.
84. Roesler, W. J., Vandenbark, G. R., and Hanson, R. W. (1988). Cyclic AMP in the induction of eukaryotic gene transcription. *J. Biol. Chem.* **263,** 9033–9066.
85. Keuhl, F. A., Ham, E. A., Zanetti, M. E., Sanford, C. H., Nicol, S. E., and Goldberg, N. D. (1974). Estrogen related increases in uterine guanosine cycle monophosphate levels. *Proc. Natl. Acad. Sci. U.S.A.* **71,** 1866–1870.
86. Pastan, I., Johnson, G. S., and Anderson, W. V. (1975). Role of cyclic nucleotides in growth control. *Annu. Rev. Biochem.* **44,** 491–522.
87. Shafie, S., and Brooks, S. C. (1977). Effects of prolactin on growth in the estrogen receptor level of human breast cancer cells (MCF-7). *Cancer Res.* **37,** 792–799.
88. Cho-Chung, Y. S., Clair, T., Shepherd, C., and Berghoffer, B. (1983). Arrest of hormone dependent mammary cancer growth *in vivo* and *in vitro* by cholera toxin. *Cancer Res.* **43,** 1473–1476.
89. Cho-Chung, Y. S. (1974). *In vivo* inhibition of tumor growth by cyclic AMP derivatives. *Cancer Res.* **34,** 3492–3496.
90. Matusik, R. J., and Hilf, R. (1976). Relationship of c-AMP and guanosine cyclic monophosphate to growth of DMBA-induced mammary tumors in rats. *J. Natl. Cancer Inst. (U.S.)* **56,** 659–661.
91. Bowin, J. S., Hirayama, P. H., Rego, J. A., and Cho-Chung, Y. S. (1981). Regression of hormone dependent mammary tumors in Sprague–Dawley rats as a result of tamoxifen or pharmacologic doses of 17 beta-estradiol: Cyclic AMP mediated events. *JNCI, J. Natl. Cancer Inst.* **66,** 321–326.
92. Handschin, J. C., Handloser, K., Takahashi, A., and Eppenberger, U. (1983). Cyclic AMP receptor proteins in dysplastic and neoplastic human breast tissue cytosol and their inverse relationship with estrogen receptors. *Cancer Res.* **43,** 2947–2954.
93. Cho-Chung, Y. S., Freesia, L. H., and Kapoor, C. L. (1985). Role of cyclic AMP in modifying the growth of mammary carcinomas. *Biol. Responses Cancer* **4,** 161–182.
94. Clair, T., and Cho-Chung, Y. S. (1984). Suppression of v-ras[H] oncogene linked to the

mouse mammary tumor virus promoter by cyclic AMP. *Proc. Annu. Meet. AACR* **25**, A67.

95. Sheffield, L. G., and Welch, C. W. (1985). Cholera toxin enhanced growth of human breast cancer cell lines *in vitro* and *in vivo:* Interaction with estrogen. *Int. J. Cancer* **36**, 479–483.

96. Kung, W., Roos, W., and Eppenberger, U. (1983). Growth stimulation of human breast cancer MCF-7 cells by dibutyryl cyclic AMP. *Cell Biol. Int. Rep.* **7**, 345–351.

97. Bringman, T. S., Lindquist, P. B., and Derynck, R. (1987). Different TGF-alpha species are derived from a glycosylated and palmitoylated precursor. *Cell (Cambridge, Mass.)* **48**, 429–440.

98. Gentry, L. E., Twardzik, D. R., Lim, G. J., Ranchalis, J. E., and Lee, D. C. (1987). Expression and characterization of TGF-alpha precursor protein in transfected mammalian cells. *Mol. Cell. Biol.* **7**, 1585–1591.

99. Ignotz, R. A., Kelly, B., Davis, R. J., and Massague, J. (1986). Biologically active precursor for transforming growth factor type alpha released by retrovirally transformed cells. *Proc. Natl. Acad. Sci. U.S.A.* **83**, 6307–6311.

100. Marquardt, H., and Todaro, G. J. (1982). Human transforming growth factor. Production by a melanoma cell line, purification and initial characterization. *J. Biol. Chem.* **257**, 5220–5225.

101. Marquardt, H., Hunkapiller, M. W., Hood, L. E., Twardzik, D. R., DeLarco, J. E., Stephenson, J. R., and Todaro, G. J. (1983). Transforming growth factors produced by retrovirus-transformed rodent fibroblasts in human melanoma cells: Amino acid sequence homology with epidermal growth factor. *Proc. Natl. Acad. Sci. U.S.A.* **80**, 4684–4688.

102. DeLarco, J. E., and Todaro, G. J. (1978). Growth factors from murine sarcoma virus transformed cells. *Proc. Natl. Acad. Sci. U.S.A.* **75**, 4001–4005.

103. Downward, J., Yarden, Y., Mayes, E., Scrace, G., Totty, N., Stockwell, P., Ullrich, A., Schlessinger, J., and Waterfield, M. D. (1984). Close similarity of epidermal growth factor receptor and v-erb-B oncogene protein sequences. *Nature (London)* **307**, 521–527.

104. Marquardt, H., Hunkapiller, M. W., Hood, L. E., and Todaro, G. J. (1984). Rat transforming growth factor type I: Structure and relation to epidermal growth factor. *Science* **223**, 1079–1083.

105. DeLarco, J. E., Reynolds, R., Carlberg, K., Engle, C., and Todaro, G. J. (1980). Sarcoma growth factor from mouse sarcoma virus-transformed cells. Purification by binding and elution from epidermal growth factor-receptor rich cells. *J. Biol. Chem.* **255**, 3685–3690.

106. Schreiber, A. B., Winkler, M. E., and Derynck, R. (1986). Transforming growth factor alpha: A more potent angiogenic mediator than epidermal growth factor. *Science* **232**, 1250–1253.

107. Imai, Y., Leung, C. K. H., Friesen, H. G., and Shiu, R. P. (1982). Epidermal growth factor receptors and effect of epidermal growth factor on growth of human breast cancer cells in long term tissue culture. *Cancer Res.* **42**, 4394–4398.

108. Karey, K. P., and Sirbasku, D. A. (1988). Responses of MCF-7 and T-47D human breast cancer cell lines to growth factors, estrogen, attachment factors and secreted/autocrine IGF-I in serum-free defined media. *Proc. Annu. Meet. AACR* **29**, A178.

109. Osborne, C. K., Hamilton, B., Titus, G., and Livingston, R. B. (1980). Epidermal growth factor stimulation of human breast cancer cells in culture. *Cancer Res.* **40**, 2361–2366.

110. Goustin, A. S., Leof, E. B., Shipley, G. D., and Moses, H. L. (1986). Growth factors and cancer. *Cancer Res.* **46**, 1015–1029.
111. Murphy, L. C., and Bell, G. I. (1988). Epidermal growth factor and transforming growth factor alpha expression in human breast cancer is associated with reduced sensitivity to the antiproliferative effects of progestins and antiestrogens. *Proc. Annu. Meet. AACR* **29**, A943.
112. Dickson, R. B., Bates, S. E., McManaway, M. E., and Lippman, M. E. (1986). Characterization of estrogen responsive transforming activity in human breast cancer cell lines. *Cancer Res.* **46**, 1707–1713.
113. Dickson, R. B., Huff, K., Spencer, E. M., and Lippman, M. E. (1986). Induction of epidermal growth factor related polypeptides by 17beta-estradiol in MCF-7 human breast cancer cells. *Endocrinology (Baltimore)* **118**, 138–142.
114. Bates, S. E., Davidson, N. E., Valverius, E. M., Freter, C. E., Dickson, R. B., Tam, J. P., Kudlow, J. E., Lippman, M. E., and Salomon, D. S. (1988). Expression of transforming growth factor alpha and its messenger ribonucleic acid in human breast cancer: Its regulation by estrogen and its possible functional significance. *Mol. Endocrinol.* **2**, 543–555.
115. Salomon, D. S., Kim, N., Ciardiello, F., Bates, S., Valverius, E., Dickson, R., Kidwell, W. R., Callahan, R., Ali, T., Merlo, G., Liscia, D., and Lippman, M. (1988). Expression of transforming growth factor alpha in human mammary epithelial cells. *Proc. Annu. Meet. AACR* **29**, A936.
116. Shafie, M. (1980). Estrogen in the growth of breast cancer: New evidence suggests indirect action. *Science* **209**, 701.
117. Arteaga, C. L., and Osborne, C. K. (1988). Blockade of the epidermal growth factor receptor inhibits transforming growth factor alpha induced but not estrogen induced growth of hormone dependent human breast cancer. *Proc. Annu. Meet. AACR* **29**, A946.
118. Pekonen, F., Partanen, S., Makinen, T., and Rutanen, E. M. (1988). Receptors for epidermal growth factor and insulin-like growth factor-I and their relation to steroid receptors in human breast cancer. *Cancer Res.* **48**, 1343–1347.
119. Davidson, N. E., Gelmann, E. P., Lippman, M. E., and Dickson, R. B. (1987). EGF receptor gene expression and its relation to the estrogen receptor in human breast cancer cell lines. *Mol. Endocrinol.* **1**, 216–233.
120. Filmus, J., Trent, J. M., Polak, M. N., and Buick, R. N. (1987). Epidermal gene-amplified MDA-468 cell line and its nonamplified varients. *Mol. Cell. Biol.* **7**, 251–257.
121. Velu, T. J., Bequinot, L., Vass, W. C., Willingham, M. C., Merlino, G. T., Pastan, I., and Lowy, D. R. (1987). Epidermal growth factor-dependent transformation by a human EGF receptor proto-oncogene. *Science* **238**, 1048–1050.
122. Rosenthal, A., Lindquist, P. B., Bringman, T. S., Goeddel, D. V., and Derynck, R. (1986). Expression in rat fibroblasts of a human transforming growth factor alpha results in transformation. *Cell (Cambridge, Mass.)* **46**, 301–309.
123. Watanabe, S., Lazar, E., and Sporn, M. B. (1987). Transformation of normal rat kidney (NRK) cells by an infectious retrovirus carrying a synthetic rat type alpha transforming growth factor gene. *Proc. Natl. Acad. Sci. U.S.A.* **84**, 1258–1262.
124. Finzi, E., Fleming, T., Segatto, O., Pennington, C. Y., Bringman, T. S., Derynck, R., and Aaronson, S. A. (1987). The human transforming growth factor alpha coding sequence is not a direct-acting oncogene when overexpressed in NIH-3T3 cells. *Proc. Natl. Acad. Sci. U.S.A.* **84**, 3733–3737.

125. Greenberg, M. E., and Ziff, E. B. (1983). Stimulation of 3T3 cells induces transcription of the c-fos proto-oncogene. *Nature (London)* **311**, 433–438.
126. Ross, R., and Vogel, A. (1978). The platelet derived growth factor. *Cell* **14**, 203–210.
127. Deuel, T. F., Huang, J. S., Proffitt, R. T., Baenziger, J. U., Chang, D., and Kennedy, B. B. (1981). Human platelet derived growth factor. Purification and resolution into active protein fractions. *J. Biol. Chem.* **256**, 8896.
128. Deuel, T. F. (1987). Polypeptide growth factors: Roles in normal and abnormal cell growth. *Annu. Rev. Cell Biol.* **3**, 443–492.
129. Dalla-Favera, R., Gallo, R. C., Giallongo, A., and Croce, C. M. (1982). Chromosomal localization of the human homolog (c-sis) of the simian sarcoma virus oncogene. *Science* **218**, 686–688.
130. Betsholtz, C., Johnson, A., Heldin, C. H., Westermark, R., Lind, P., Urdea, M. S., Eddy, R., Shows, T. B., Philpott, K., Mellor, A. L., Knott, A. L., and Scott, J. (1986). cDNA sequence and chromosomal localization of human PDGF A chain and its expression in tumor cell lines. *Nature (London)* **320**, 695–699.
131. Antoniades, H. N., Pantzis, P., and Owen, A. J. (1987). Human platelet-derived growth factor and the sis-PDGF-2 gene. *In* "Oncogenes, Genes, and Growth Factors" (G. Guroff, ed.). Wiley, New York.
132. Glenn, K., Bowen-Pope, D. F., and Ross, R. (1982). Platelet derived growth factor. III. Identification of a PDGF receptor by affinity labelling. *J. Biol. Chem.* **257**, 5172–5176.
133. Williams, L. T., Tremble, P. M., Lavin, M. F., and Sunday, M. E. (1984). Platelet-derived growth factor receptors form a high affinity state in membrane preparations. *J. Biol. Chem.* **259**, 5287.
134. Escobedo, J. A., Navankasatussas, S., Cousens, L. S., Coughlin, S. R., Bell, G. I., and Williams, L. T. (1988). A common PDGF receptor is activated by homodimeric A and B forms of PDGF. *Science* **240**, 1532–1534.
135. Hart, C. E., Forstrom, J. W., Kelly, J. D., Seifert, R. A., Smith, R. A., Ross, R., Murray, N. J., and Bowen-Pope, D. F. (1988). Two classes of PDGF receptor recognized different isoforms of PDGF. *Science* **240**, 1529–1531.
136. Peres, R., Betsholtz, C., Westermark, B., and Heldin, C. (1987). Frequent expression of growth factors for mesenchymal cells in human mammary carcinoma cell lines. *Cancer Res.* **47**, 3425–3429.
137. Bronzert, D. A., Pantazis, P., Antoniades, H. N., Kasid, A., Davidson, N., Dickson, R. B., and Lippman, M. E. (1987). Synthesis and secretion of platelet derived growth factor by human breast cancer cell lines. *Proc. Natl. Acad. Sci. U.S.A.* **84**, 5763–5767.
138. Bronzert, D. A., Valverius, E., Bates, S., Stampfer, M., and Dickson, R. B. (1988). Production of alpha and beta chains of platelet derived growth factor by human mammary epithelial cells. *Proc. 70th Annu. Meet., Am. Endocr. Soc.* Abstr. No. 1219.
139. Sariban, E., Sitaras, N., Antoniades, H., Kufe, D., and Pantazis, P. (1988). Expression of PDGF related transcripts and synthesis of biologically active PDGF-like proteins by human malignant epithelial cell lines. *Proc. Annu. Meet. AACR* **29**, A1774.
140. van der Burg, B., Rutteman, G. R., Blankenstein, M. A., de Latt, S. W., and van Zoelen, E. J. (1988). Mitogenic stimulation of human breast cancer cells in a growth factor defined medium: Synergistic action of insulin and estrogen. *J. Cell. Physiol.* **134**, 101–108.
141. Clemmons, D. R., Underwood, L. E., and Van Wyck, J. J. (1981). Hormonal control

of immunoreactive somatomedin production by cultured human fibroblasts. *J. Clin. Invest.* **67,** 10–16.

142. Westley, B., and Rochefort, H. (1979). Estradiol induced proteins in the MCF-7 human breast cancer cell line. *Biochem. Biophys. Res. Commun.* **90,** 410–416.

143. Westley, B., and Rochefort, H. (1980). A secreted glycoprotein induced by estrogen induced in human cancer cell lines. *Cell (Cambridge, Mass.)* **20,** 353–362.

144. Vignon, V. P., Derocq, F., and Rochefort, D. H. (1982). Effect of estradiol on the ultrastructure of MCF-7 human breast cancer cells in culture. *Cancer Res.* **42,** 667–673.

145. Veith, F. O., Capony, F., Garcia, M., Chantelard, J., Pujol, H., Veith, F., Zajvela, A., and Rochefort, H. (1983). Release of estrogen induced glycoprotein with a molecular weight of 52,000 by breast cancer cells in primary culture. *Cancer Res.* **43,** 1861–1868.

146. Vignon, F., Capony, F., Chambon, M., Fress, G., Garcia, M., and Rochefort, H. (1986). Autocrine growth stimulation of the MCF-7 breast cancer cells by the estrogen-regulated 52K protein. *Endocrinology (Baltimore)* **118,** 1537–1545.

147. Vignon, F., Bardon, S., Chalbos, D., Derocq, D., Gill, P., and Rochefort, H. (1987). Antiproliferative effect of progestins and antiprogestins in human breast cancer cells. *Monogr. Ser. Eur. Organ. Res. Treat. Cancer* **18,** 47–54.

148. Rochefort, H., Capony, F., Cavalie-Barthez, G., Chambon, M., Garcia, M., Massot, O., Morisset, M., Touitou, I., Vignon, F., and Westley, B. (1986). Estrogen-regulated proteins and autocrine control of cell growth in breast cancer. *Dev. Oncol.* **43,** 57–68.

149. Roth, R. A. (1988). Structure of the receptor for insulin-like growth factor II: The puzzle amplified. *Science* **239,** 1269–1271.

150. Cullen, K. J., Yee, D., Perdue, J. F., Hampton, B., Sly, W. S., Lippman, M. E., and Rosen, N. (1989). Type I and Type II IGF receptor expression and function in human breast cancer. *J. Cell. Biochem.* **13B,** E315.

151. Rochefort, H., Capony, F., Garcia, M., Cavailles, V., Fress, G., Chambon, M., Morisset, M., and Vignon, F. (1987). Estrogen-induced lysosomal proteases secreted by breast cancer cells: A role in carcinogenesis? *J. Cell. Biochem.* **35,** 17–29.

152. Morisset, M., Capony, F., and Rochefort, H. (1986). The 52-kD estrogen-induced protein secreted by MCF-7 cells is a lysosomal acidic protease. *Biochem. Biophys. Res. Commun.* **138,** 102–109.

153. Capony, F., Morisset, M., Barrett, A. J., Capony, J. P., Broquet, P., Vignon, F., Chambon, M., Louisot, P., and Rochefort, H. (1987). Phosphorylation, glycosylation, and proteolytic activity of the 52-kD estrogen-induced protein secreted by MCF-7 cells. *J. Cell Biol.* **104,** 253–262.

154. Augereau, P., Garcia, M., Mettei, M. G., Cavailles, V., Depadova, F., Derocq, D., Capony, F., Ferrara, P., and Rochefort, H. (1988). Cloning and sequencing of the 52K/cathepsin D complimentary dioxyribonucleic acid of MCF-7 breast cancer cells and mapping on chromosome 11. *Mol. Endocrinol.* **2,** 186–192.

155. Boundell, T. L., and Humbel, R. V. (1980). Hormone families: Pancreatic hormones and homologous growth factors. *Nature (London)* **287,** 781–787.

156. Baxter, R. C. (1986). The somatomedins: Insulin-like growth factors. *Adv. Clin. Chem.* **25,** 49–115.

157. Nissley, S. P., and Rechler, M. M. (1986). Insulin-like growth factors: Biosynthesis, receptors, and carrier proteins. *Horm. Proteins Pept.* **12,** 127–203.

158. Zapf, J., and Froesch, V. R. (1986). Insulin-like growth factors/somatomedins: Structure, secretion, biological actions and physiological roles. *Horm. Res.* **24,** 121–130.

159. Ullrich, A., Bell, J. R., Chen, F. Y., Herrera, R., Petrozelli, M., Dull, T. J., Gray, *et al.* (1985). Human insulin receptor and its relation to the tyrosine kinase family of oncogenes. *Nature (London)* **313**, 756–761.
160. Massague, J., and Czech, M. P. (1982). The subunit structures of two distinct receptors for insulin like growth factors I and II and their relationship to the insulin receptor. *J. Biol. Chem.* **257**, 5038–5045.
161. Morgan, D. O., Edman, J. C., Standring, D. N., Fried, V. A., Smith, M. C., Roth, R. A., and Rutter, W. J. (1987). Insulin-like growth factor II receptor as a multifunctional binding protein. *Nature (London)* **329**, 301–307.
162. Lobel, P., Dahms, N. M., Breitmeyer, J., Chirgwin, J. M., and Kornfeld, S. (1987). Cloning of the bovine 215-kDa cation-independent mannose-six-phosphate receptor. *Proc. Natl. Acad. Sci. U.S.A.* **84**, 2233.
163. Waheed, A., Braulke, T., Junghans, U., and von Figura, K. (1988). Mannose 6-phosphate/insulin-like growth factor II receptor: The two types of ligand bind simultaneously to one receptor at different sites. *Biochem. Biophys. Res. Commun.* **152**, 1248–1254.
164. Guler, H. P., Zapf, J., and Froesch, E. R. (1987). Short-term metabolic effect of recombinant human insulin-like growth factor I in healthy adults. *N. Engl. J. Med.* **317**, 137–140.
165. Ewton, B. Z., Falen, S. L., and Florini, J. R. (1987). The type II insulin-like growth factor (IGF) receptor has low affinity for IGF-I analogs: Pleiotropic action of IGF's on myoblasts are apparently mediated via the type I receptor. *Endocrinology (Baltimore)* **120**, 115–123.
166. Rosenfeld, R. G., Conover, C. A., Hodges, D., Lee, P. D., Misra, P., Hintz, R. L., and Li, C. A. (1987). Heterogeneity of insulin like growth factor-I affinity for the insulin-like growth factor II receptor: Comparison of natural, synthetic and recombinant DNA-derived insulin-like growth factor I. *Biochem. Biophys. Res. Commun.* **143**, 199.
167. Froesch, E. R., Schmid, C., Schwander, J., and Zapf, J. (1985). Actions of the insulin like growth factors. *Annu. Rev. Physiol.* **47**, 443–467.
168. Rechler, M. M., and Nissley, S. P. (1985). The nature and regulation of the receptors for the insulin-like growth factors. *Annu. Rev. Physiol.* **47**, 425–442.
169. De Leon, D. D., Bakker, B., Wilson, B. M., Hintz, R. L., and Rosenfeld, R. G. (1988). Demonstration of insulin-like growth factor (IGF-I and II) receptors and binding protein in human breast cancer cell lines. *Biochem. Biophys. Res. Commun.* **152**, 398–405.
170. Daughaday, W. H., Kapadia, M., and Mariz, I. (1987). Serum somatomedin binding proteins: Physiologic significance and interference in radioligand assay. *J. Lab. Clin. Med.* **109**, 355–363.
171. Rutanen, E. M., Pekonen, F., and Makinen, T. (1988). Soluble 34K binding protein inhibits the binding of insulin-like growth factor I to its cell receptors in human secretory phase endometrium: Evidence for autocrine/paracrine regulation of growth factor action. *J. Clin. Endocrinol. Metab.* **66**, 173–180.
172. Gowan, L. K., Hampton, B., Hill, D. J., Schlueter, R J., and Perdue, J. F. (1987). Purification and characterization of a unique high molecular weight form of insulin-like growth factor II. *Endocrinology (Baltimore)* **121**, 449–458.
173. Lee, P. K., Powell, D. R., Li, C. H., Bohn, H., Liu, F., and Hintz, R. L. (1988). High molecular weight forms of insulin-like growth factor II and its binding protein identified by protein immunoblotting. *Biochem. Biophys. Res. Commun.* **152**, 1131–1137.
174. Melton, V. A., Krieg, P. A., Rebagliati, M. R., and Maniatis, T. (1984). Efficient *in*

vitro synthesis of biologically active RNA and RNA hybridization probes on plasmids containing a bacteriophage SP6 promoter. *Nucleic Acids Res.* **25**, 7035–7056.

175. Yee, D., Favoni, R. E., Huff, K. K., Paik, S., Dickson, R. B., Lebovic, G. S., Schwartz, A., Lippman, M. E., and Rosen, N. (1988). Insulin-like growth factor I expression and a novel IGF-I related activity in human malignancy. *Proc. Annu. Meet. AACR* **29**, A216.

176. Ogasawara, M., Karey, K. P., and Sirbasku, D. A. (1988). Insulin-like growth factor I: Relationship between plasma and tissue sources, biological potency and N alpha truncation. *Proc. Annu. Meet. AACR* **29**, A207.

177. Rohlik, Q. T., Adams, B., Kull, F. C., and Jacobs, S. An antibody to the receptor for insulin-like growth factor I inhibits the growth of MCF-7 cells in tissue culture. *Biochem. Biophys. Res. Commun.* **149**, 276–281.

178. Artega, C. L., Kitten, L., Coronado, E., Jacobs, S., Kull, F., and Osborne, C. K. (1988). Blockade of the type I somatomedin receptor inhibits growth of estrogen receptor negative human breast cancer cells in athymic mice. *Proc. 70th Annu. Meet., Am. Endocr. Soc.* Abstr. No. 683.

179. Huff, K. K., Knabbe, C., Lindsey, R., Kaufman, B., Bronzert, V., Lippman, M. E., and Dickson, R. B. (1988). Multihormonal regulation of insulin-like growth factor I related protein in MCF-7 human breast cancer cells. *Mol. Endocrinol.* **2**, 200–208.

180. Mathews, L. S., Norstedt, G., and Palmiter, R. D. (1986). Regulation of insulin-like growth factor I gene expression by growth hormone. *Proc. Natl. Acad. Sci. U.S.A.* **83**, 9343–9347.

181. Yee, D., Cullen, K. J., Paik, S., Schwartz, A., Veillette, A., Foss, F., Bates, S., Favoni, R., Lippman, M., and Rosen, N. (1988). Expression of insulin-like growth factor mRNAs in human breast cancer. *J. Cell Biochem.* **12**, C127.

182. Coronado, E., Ramasharma, K., Li, C. H., Kitten, L., Marshall, M., Fuqua, S., and Osborne, K. (1988). Insulin-like growth factor II: A potential autocrine growth factor for human breast cancer. *Proc. Annu. Meet. AACR* **29**, A942.

183. Paik, S. Unpublished data.

184. Cullen, K. J., Yee, D., Paik, S., Hampton, B., Perdue, J. F., Lippman, M. E., and Rosen, N. (1988). Insulin like growth factor II expression and function in human breast cancer. *Proc. Annu. Meet. AACR* **29**, A947.

185. Knabbe, C., Lippman, M. E., Wakefield, L. M., Flanders, K. C., Kasid, A., Derynck, R., and Dickson, R. B. (1987). Evidence that transforming growth factor beta is a hormonally regulated negative growth factor in human breast cancer cells. *Cell (Cambridge, Mass.)* **48**, 417–428.

186. Sporn, M. B., Roberts, A. B., Wakefield, L. M., and Assoian, R. K. (1986). Transforming growth factor beta: Biological function in chemical structure. *Science* **233**, 532–534.

187. Tucker, R. F., Shipley, G. D., Moses, H. L., and Holley, R. W. (1984). Growth inhibitor from BCS-I cells closely related to platelet type beta transforming growth factor. *Science* **226**, 705–707.

188. Roberts, A. B., Anzano, M. A., Wakefield, L. M., Roche, N. S., Stern, D. F., and Sporn, M. B. (1985). Type of beta transforming growth factor: A bifunctional regulator of cellular growth. *Proc. Natl. Acad. Sci. U.S.A.* **82**, 119–123.

189. Vonderhaar, B. K. (1988). Regulation of development in the normal mammary glands by hormones and growth factors. *In* "Breast Cancer: Cellular and Molecular Biology" (M. E. Lippman and R. B. Dickson, eds.). Martinus Nijhoff, Boston, Massachusetts.

190. Cheifetz, S., Like, B., and Massague, J. (1982). Cellular distribution of type I and type II receptors for transforming growth factor-beta. *J. Biol. Chem.* **261**, 9972.

191. Goustin, A. S., Leof, E. B., Shipley, G. D., and Moses, H. L. (1986). Growth factors in cancer. *Cancer Res.* **46**, 1015.

192. Derynck, R., Goeddel, D. B., Ullrich, A., Gutterman, J. U., Williams, R. D., Bringman, T. S., and Berger, W. H. (1987). Synthesis of messenger RNAs for transforming growth factor alpha and beta in the epidermal growth factor receptor by human tumors. *Cancer Res.* **47**, 707–712.

193. Lyons, R. M., Keski-Oja, J., and Moses, H. L. (1986). Cleavage of a transforming growth factor beta-immunoreactive 62kDa polypeptide by plasmin yields a TGF-beta-like 25kDa polypeptide. *Proc. Annu. Meet. Am. Soc. Chem. Biol.* Abstr. No. 1652.

194. O'Connor-McCourt, M. D., and Wakefield, L. M. (1987). Latent transforming growth factor beta in serum. *J. Biol. Chem.* **262**, 14090–14099.

195. Huang, S. S., O'Grady, P., and Huang, J. S. (1985). Human transforming growth factor beta/alpha 2-macroglobulin complex is a latent form of transforming growth factor beta. *J. Biol. Chem.* **263**, 1535–1538.

196. Hagino, Y., Mawatari, M., Yoshimura, A., Kohno, K., Kobawashi, M., and Kuwano, M. (1988). Estrogen inhibits the growth of MCF-7 cell variants resistant to transforming growth factor beta. *Jpn. J. Cancer Res.* **79**, 74–81.

197. Zugmaier, G., Knabbe, C., Deschauer, B., Lippman, M. E., and Dickson, R. B. (1988). Response of estrogen receptor negative and estrogen receptor positive human breast cancer cell lines to TGF-beta I and TGF-beta II in anchorage independent growth. *Proc. Annu. Meet. AACR* **29**, A232.

198. Sirbasku, D. A., Ogasawara, M., and Karey, K. P. (1988). Roles of endocrine and autocrine growth factors and inhibitors in human breast cancer cell growth. *Proc. Annu. Meet. AACR* **29**, A949.

199. Laug, W. E., Jones, P. A., and Benedict, W. F. (1975). Relationship between fibrinolysis of cultured cells and malignancy. *J. Natl. Cancer Inst. (U.S.)* **54**, 173–179.

200. Butler, W. B., Kirkland, W. L., and Jorgenson, T. L. (1979). Induction of plasminogen activator by estrogen in a human breast cancer cell line MCF-7. *Biochem. Biophys. Res. Commun.* **90**, 1328–1334.

201. Ryan, T. J., Seeger, J. I., Kumar, A., and Dickerman, H. W. (1984). Estradiol preferentially enhances extracellular tissue plasminogen activators of MCF-7 breast cancer cells. *J. Biol. Chem.* **259**, 14324–14327.

202. Mira-y-Lopez, R., and Ossowski, L. (1987). Hormonal modulation of plasminogen activator: An approach to the prediction of human breast tumor responsiveness. *Cancer Res.* **47**, 3558–3564.

203. Duffy, M. J., O'Grady, P., Simon, J., Rose, M., and Lijnen, H. R. (1986). Tissue-type plasminogen activator in breast cancer: Relationship with estradiol and progesterone receptors. *JNCI, J. Natl. Cancer Inst.* **77**, 621–623.

204. Shafie, S. M., and Liotta, L. A. (1980). Formation of metastasis by human breast carcinoma cells in nude mice. *Cancer Lett.* **11**, 81–87.

205. Kao, R. T., and Stern, R. (1986). Collagenases in human breast carcinoma cell lines. *Cancer Res.* **46**, 1349–1354.

206. Paranjpe, M., Engel, L., Young, N., and Liotta, L. A. (1980). Activation of human breast carcinoma collagenase through plasminogen activator. *Life Sci.* **26**, 1223–1231.

207. Barsky, S. H., Togo, S., Spiridione, G., and Liotta, L. (1983). Type IV collagenase immunoreactivity in invasive breast carcinoma. *Lancet* **1**, 296–297.

208. Ogilvie, D. J., Hailey, J. A., Juacaba, S. F., Lee, E., and Tarin, D. (1985). Col-

lagenase secretion by human breast neoplasms: A clinicopathologic investigation. *JNCI, J. Natl. Cancer Inst.* **74,** 19–27.

209. Pucci-Minafra, I., Luparello, C., Schillaci, R. and Sciarrino, S. (1987). Ultrastructural evidence of collagenolytic activity in ductal infiltrating carcinoma of the human breast. *Int. J. Cancer* **39,** 599–603.

210. Easty, G. C., Dowsett, M., Powles, T. J., Easty, D. M., Gazet, J. C., and Neville, A. M. (1977). In vitro osteolysis by human breast tumors. *Proc. R. Soc. Med.* **70,** 191–195.

211. Horwitz, K. B., and McGuire, W. L. (1975). Specific progesterone receptors in human breast cancer. *Steroids* **25,** 497–550.

212. Bayard, F., Damilano, S, Robel, P., and Baulieu, E. E. (1975). Estradiol and progesterone receptors in human endometrium during the menstrual cycle. *C. R. Hebd. Seances Acad. Sci.* **281,** 1341–1344.

213. Horwitz, K. B., and McGuire, W. L. (1978). Estrogen control of progesterone receptor in human breast cancer. *J. Biol. Chem.* **253,** 2223–2228.

214. Eckert, R. L., and Katzenellenbogen, B. S. (1982). Effects of estrogens and antiestrogens on estrogen receptor dynamics and the induction of progesterone receptor in MCF-7 breast cancer cells. *Cancer Res.* **42,** 139.

215. Nardulli, A. N., Green, G. L., O'Malley, B. W., and Katzenellenbogen, B. S. (1988). Regulation of progesterone receptor messenger ribonucleic acid and protein levels in MCF-7 cells by estradiol: Analysis of estrogen's effect on progesterone receptor synthesis and degradation. *Endocrinology (Baltimore)* **122,** 935–944.

216. Edwards, D. P., Chamness, G. C., and McGuire, W. L. (1979). Estrogen and progesterone receptor proteins in breast cancer. *Biochim. Biophys. Acta* **560,** 457–486.

217. Chalbos, D., and Rochefort, H. (1984). Dual effects of the progestin R-5020 on proteins released by the T-47-D human breast cancer cells. *J. Biol. Chem.* **259,** 1231–1238.

218. Liotta, L. A., Rao, C. N., and Weiner, U. M. (1986). Biochemical interactions of tumor cells with the basement membrane. *Annu. Rev. Biochem.* **55,** 1037.

219. Barsky, S. H., Rao, C. N., Hyams, D., and Liotta, L. A. (1984). Identification of a laminin receptor in human breast cancer tissue. *Breast Cancer Res. Treat.* **4,** 181–188.

220. Albini, A., Graf, J. O., Kitten, T., Kleinman, H. K., Martin, G. R., Veillete, A., and Lippman, M. E. (1986). Estrogen and v-ras[H] transfection regulate the interactions of MCF-7 breast carcinoma cells to basement membrane. *Proc. Natl. Acad. Sci. U.S.A.* **83,** 8182.

221. Edwards, D. P., Adams, D. J., Savage, N., and McGuire, W. L. (1980). Estrogen-induced synthesis of specific proteins in human breast cancer cells. *Biochem. Biophys. Res. Commun.* **93,** 804–812.

222. Fuqua, S. A., Richards, D., Moretti-Rojs, I., Blum, M., and McGuire, W. L. (1988). Heat shock protein 27 is estrogen regulated in MCF-7 human breast cancer cells. *Proc. Annu. Meet. AACR* **29,** A973.

223. Burke, R. E., Harris, S. C., and McGuire, W. L. (1978). Lactate dehydrogenase in estrogen responsive human breast cancer cells. *Cancer Res.* **38,** 2773–2776.

224. Masiakowski, P., Breathnach, R., Bloch, J., Gannon, F., Krust, A., and Chambon, P. (1982). Cloning of cDNA sequences of hormone-regulated genes from the MCF-7 human breast cancer cell line. *Nucleic Acids Res.* **10,** 7895–7903.

225. Flamm, S. L., Wellstein, A., Kern, F., Lippman, M. E., and Gelmann, E. P. (1988). Expression of FGF peptides in normal and malignant human mammary epithelial cells. *Cold Spring Harbor Meet. Cancer Cells* Meet. Abstr., p. 33.

226. Kasid, A., Lippman, M. E., Papageorge, A. G., Lowy, D. R., and Gelmann, E. P. (1985). Transfection of v-ras^H DNA into MCF-7 human breast cancer cells bypasses dependence on estrogen for tumorigenicity. *Science* **228,** 725–728.

227. Dickson, R. B., Kasid, A., Huff, K. K., Bates, S. E., Knabbe, C., Bronzert, D., Gelmann, E. P., and Lippman, M. E. (1987). Activation of growth factor secretion in tumorigenic state of breast cancer induced by 17 beta-estradiol or v-Ha-ras oncogene. *Proc. Natl. Acad. Sci. U.S.A.* **84,** 837–841.

228. Katzenellenbogen, B. S., Kendra, K. L., Norman, M. J., and Berthois, Y. (1987). Proliferation, hormonal responsiveness and estrogen receptor content of MCF-7 human breast cancer cells grown in the short-term and long-term absence of estrogens. *Cancer Res.* **47,** 4355–4360.

Calcium Homeostasis in Birds

SHMUEL HURWITZ

Institute of Animal Science,
Agricultural Research Organization
The Volcani Center
Bet Dagan, Israel

I. INTRODUCTION

The importance of Ca^{2+} in controlling a variety of metabolic functions in the body, ranging from muscle contraction to blood coagulation, has been recognized for many years. More recently, the role of calcium in cellular information transfer became recognized. In this capacity, Ca^{2+} participates together with inositol phosphates in the mediation of hormone action in the target cell, including the regulation of secretion of several hormones (Downes and Michell, 1985; Kojima *et al.*, 1985). Although over 99% of body calcium is contained in the skeleton, the metabolic priority of the organism is the maintenance of a constant concentration of calcium in plasma and extracellular fluids, at the expense of bone calcification and in extreme conditions by the net breakdown of skeletal material. Thus, the relatively insoluble calcium phosphates of bone serve as a calcium reservoir to be utilized during need. This function of bone is particularly prominent in female birds during reproduction as will be discussed (Section VI).

The plasma calcium concentration in growing and male birds is maintained at approximately 2.5 mM (10 mg/dl), of which about 60%

is ionic, typical of land vertebrates including mammals. During reproduction, the plasma calcium concentration in female birds may reach 8 mM, due to the appearance in the plasma of specific protein-bound calcium. The significance of this and other aspects of calcium metabolism during reproduction is discussed in Section VI.

The regulation of Ca^{2+} concentration in body fluids is achieved through the action of a complex feedback-control system which includes several subsystems and regulating hormones. A perturbation in plasma calcium or in any of the control subsystems usually results in a cascade of events with an often obscure temporal hierarchy. For this reason, it is difficult to obtain detailed information on the behavior of individual subsystems by *in vivo* experimentation. In the last three decades, *in vitro* techniques have been widely used in order to isolate single components of the calcium-regulating system. Initially, isolated organs such as the everted gut sac (T. H. Wilson and Wiseman, 1954), isolated bone (Raisz, 1963), and kidney slices (Chase and Aurbach, 1967) have been studied. Isolated organs were also studied *in situ,* including intestinal loops (Wasserman, 1963) and perfused endocrine glands (Copp *et al.,* 1972). With the development of culture techniques, cellular and subcellular preparations have been applied to study components of the calcium control systems. These include bone cells (Rodan and Rodan, 1974), cartilage cells (Pines and Hurwitz, 1988), parathyroid cells (Brown *et al.,* 1976), kidney cells (Bar and Hurwitz, 1980), and intestinal cells or brush border vesicles (Rasmussen *et al.,* 1979). Some information acquired by *in vitro* techniques can be implemented as such, especially that related to diagnosis of pathological states. However, for full physiological comprehension of the control system, the mosaic of information obtained by *in vitro* experimentation ought to be assembled in the context of the entire organism. Models of simulation, activated by the computer, provide means for the required integration. In general, models of simulation must be more comprehensive than others designed to describe empirical observations (Aubert *et al.,* 1963; Staub *et al.,* 1988), although some components of the descriptive models can be utilized in the simulation framework.

Physiological simulation models can be constructed at different levels of detail, ranging from the molecular through subcellular and cellular levels up to the level of the entire organism. The selection of the appropriate level depends on the level of the available information and on the required answers which are functions of the expected inputs and outputs. When validated, a model can be used to predict the responses of the control subsystems to various perturbations. The scope of a metabolic model is limited depending on its level of detail and the number of factors included.

Early attempts to formulate models simulating calcium metabolism were made by Bonnier and Cabanac (1970) for the analog computer and by Jaros *et al.* (1979). In this review, calcium metabolism of birds is described within the framework of a more recent simulation model (Hurwitz *et al.*, 1987a,b). The review includes basic information at greater detail than applied so far in the simulation model, with special emphasis on results with avian tissues. Further information on calcium metabolism in birds may be found in previous reviews (Simkiss, 1961; Hurwitz, 1978).

II. The Conceptual Model

The model of regulation of plasma calcium (Hurwitz *et al.*, 1987a,b) is schematically represented in Fig. 1. The control system consists of three main subsystems: intestine, bone, and kidney. The net transport of calcium through the intestinal epithelium (F_i) is the only route of entry of calcium from the exterior. The net transport of calcium by the kidney (F_k) is the means of calcium removal to the exterior. Bone may remove calcium from the central plasma pool, by the process loosely defined as bone formation, and return calcium to the system by bone resorption. F_b defines the net calcium flow to this tissue. The change in total plasma calcium (M) is then given by the sum of the flows:

$$dM/dt = F_i - F_k - F_b - k\Delta C$$

which, upon integration and division by the blood volume (V_b), results in the plasma calcium concentration (C). In addition, plasma calcium equilibrates rapidly (k) with extracellular calcium (M_e). The rate of equilibration is driven by the difference in calcium concentration between plasma and the extracellular fluid (ΔC). When integrated and divided by the volume of extracellular fluid (V_e), the concentration of calcium in the extracellular fluid (C_e) is obtained. Plasma calcium concentration is "sensed" by the kidney, which responds directly by modulating the excretion of calcium (F_k); by the ultimobranchial gland (UB), which, in response, may vary its calcitonin (CT) secretion; by bone, which modifies its calcium flow (F_b); by the parathyroid gland (PT) with secretion of parathyroid hormone (PTH); and by the kidney hydroxylase enzyme system (OH-ase), which is responsible for the production of 1,25-dihydroxycholecalciferol [1,25$(OH)_2D_3$]. PTH regulates bone calcium flow (F_b) and the production of 1,25$(OH)_2D_3$ and

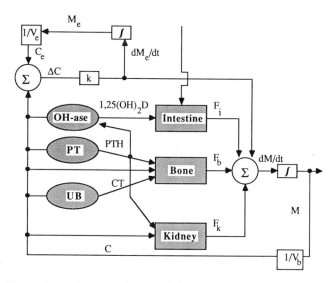

Fig. 1. Feedback regulation of plasma calcium concentration. The sum (Σ) of the net calcium flows from intestine (F_i), bone (F_b), and kidney (F_k), is the change in total plasma calcium (dM/dt) which, when added ($\int$) to existing plasma calcium and divided by the blood volume (V_b), yields the plasma calcium concentration (C). Plasma calcium then undergoes a rapid exchange with extracellular calcium (M_e) which, upon division by the extracellular volume (V_e), yields extracellular calcium concentration (C_e). Plasma calcium concentration determines kidney calcium excretion (F_k), bone calcium flow (F_b), calcitonin (CT) secretion by the ultimobranchial gland (UB), parathyroid hormone (PTH) from the parathyroid gland (PT), and production of 1,25(OH)$_2$D by the kidney 25-hydroxycholecalciferol-1-hydroxylase system (OH-ase). Bone flow and 1,25(OH)$_2$D production are also controlled by PTH.

affects urinary calcium excretion. Bone calcium flow may also be influenced by CT.

The concentration of each of the hormones and other biochemicals that participate in calcium transfer is governed by first-order kinetics: the synthesis of each is a function of the activity of the stimulant, while its transfer, including its degradation, is determined by its own concentration.

The model was initially developed (Hurwitz *et al.*, 1983, 1984) without considering the direct effects of growth, and could therefore be applied only to animals in which the change in body weight during simulation time was negligible and not to young chicks, which more than double their body weight during a single week. By modification of the model to include growth, its scope has been considerably enhanced (Hurwitz *et al.*, 1987a). In addition to various adjustments to

TABLE I
EQUATIONS DESCRIBING GROWTH AND DEVELOPMENT[a]

No.	Equation	Description	Unit
1	$BW = W_1\exp[-W_2\exp(-W_3t)]$	Body weight	g
1a	$G = dBW/dt$	Weight gain	g/sec
2	$C_f = Q_1\exp[-Q_2\exp(-Q_3t)]$	Carcass fat	—
3	$V_b = V_1BW$	Blood volume	ml
4	$V_e = V_2BW$	Interstitial volume	ml
5	$V_{IN} = h_t(t)BW$	Intestinal pool	ml
6	$Ca_c = U_1 + t/(U_2 + U_3t)$	Normal carcass calcium	—
7	$E_I = h_2(T)BW^{2/3} + E_gG$	Energy intake	kcal/sec
8	$E_g = F_m + F_fF_g$	Energy for growth	kcal/g
9	$F_{in} = (E_t/E_f)Ca_f$	Calcium intake	mg/sec

[a] Parameters and variables with values: W_1, Gompertz coefficient, 4081 g; W_2, Gompertz coefficient, 4.612; $W3$, Gompertz coefficient, 4.31×10^{-7}/sec; Q_1, Gompertz coefficient, 0.265; Q_2, Gompertz coefficient, 1.018; Q_3, Gompertz coefficient, 8.7×10^{-8}/sec; V_1, proportionality coefficient, 0.04; V_2, proportionality coefficient, 0.25; $h_1(t)$, age function, proportion of intestinal pool, variable; U_1, parameter of carcass calcium, 2.72×10^{-3}; U_2, parameter of carcass calcium, 1.01×10^{-8}; U_3, parameter of carcass calcium, 206/sec; $h_2(T)$, energy for maintenance as a function of temperature, variable, kcal/(sec $\times$ g$^{2/3}$); F_m, energy for gain, 0.6 kcal/g; F_f, energy for gain in fat, 9.2 kcal/g; F_g, ratio of gained fat/weight, variable; E_f, energy of feed, variable, kcal/g; Ca_f, feed calcium, variable, mg/g.

accommodate changes in pool size and in the activity of the control systems due to growth, the Gompertz growth equation, which is a genetic determinant, was included. By calculation of the energy needs of growing birds (Hurwitz et al., 1980), feed intake and hence calcium intake could be calculated. The equations describing growth and feed intake are given in Table I. The detailed equations describing the hormone concentrations, their actions on the target tissues, and the various calcium flows are given in Table II.

III. THE REGULATING HORMONES

In the context of a metabolic system, a quantitative relationship exists between the rate of secretion of the regulating hormone and the controlled entity and between the response of the control system and the concentration of the regulating hormone, resulting in a proportional control. The response to a hormone may be modified by modulation of receptor number or affinity (up- or down-regulation). This more sluggish control may provide a means of adaptation to chronic pertur-

TABLE II
EQUATIONS FOR CALCIUM HOMEOSTASIS[a]

No.	Equation	Description	Units
10	$dCa_p/dt = F_i + F_k - K\Delta C$	Plasma calcium	mg
11	$dCa_e/dt = K\Delta C$	Interstitial calcium	mg
12	$G_p = S_1 + S_2/[1 + (C/S_3)S_4]$	PTH secretion	sec^{-1}
13	$dP/dt = G_p - B_p P$	Plasma PTH level	Arbitrary
14	$G_E = [h_3(P)]BW$	Hydroxylase formation	pmol/sec
15	$dE/dt = G_E - B_E \bar{E}$	1-Hydroxylase	pmol/sec
16	$dD_{TB}/dt = V_T(-R_2 D_b + R_1 D_1 - BD_B) + E$	Pool 1,25(OH)$_2$D$_3$	pmol
16a	$D_B = D_{TB}/(V_b + V_e)$	Pool concentration	pmol/ml
17	$dD_{TI}/dt = V_{IN}(R_4 D_8 - R_3 D_1)$	Intestinal 1,25(OH)$_2$D$_3$	pmol
17b	$D_1 = D_{TI}/V_{IN}$	Concentration	pmol/ml
18	$F_b = F_p - F_r$	Bone flow	mg/sec
19	$F_p = A_3 C_b + C_g$	Bone formation	mg/sec
20	$C_g = dC_b/dt = 1000(GCa_c + BWdCa_c/dt)$	Bone growth	mg/sec
21	$F_r = P_b PC_b$	Bone resorption	mg/sec
22	$F_k = (X_1 + X_2 C + X_3 C^2 + X_4 C^3)BW$	Kidney calcium flow	mg/sec
23	$dL/dt = \rho DI - \beta L$	Fractional absorption	
24	$F_i = (A_1 + A_2 L)F_{in}$	Calcium absorption	mg/sec
25	$C = 100 Ca_p/V_b$	Plasma calcium	mg/dl

[a] Parameters, description, and values: K, plasma–interstitial fluid exchange, 9×10^{-3} ml/sec; S_1, parameter of PTH secretion, 5.5×10^{-3}; S_2, parameter of PTH secretion, 11.0×10^{-3}/sec; S_3, parameter of PTH secretion, 3.55 mg/dl; S_4, parameter of PTH secretion, 5.71; B_p, coefficient of PTH inactivation, 2.3×10^{-3}/sec; B_E, coefficient of 1-hydroxylase decay, 1.5×10^{-5}/sec; B, coefficient of 1,25(OH)$_2$D$_3$ decay, 6×10^{-5}/sec; R_1, 1,25(OH)$_2$D$_3$ entry from intestine, 3.5×10^{-5}/sec; R_2, 1,25(OH)$_2$D$_3$ exit from plasma, 1.05×10^{-4}/sec; R_3, 1,25(OH)$_2$D$_3$ exit to plasma, 2.4×10^{-4}/sec; R_4, 1,25(OH)$_2$D$_3$ entry from plasma, 7.2×10^{-4}/sec; A_3, coefficient of bone formation, 7×10^{-7}; P_b, coefficient of bone resorption, 2.5×10^{-7} mg/sec; X_1, parameter of kidney calcium flow, 4.4×10^{-7} mg/sec; X_2, parameter of kidney calcium excretion, 3.11×10^{-8} dl/sec; X_3, parameter of kidney calcium excretion, 7.1×10^{-8} dl²/sec × mg; X_4, parameter of kidney calcium excretion, 1.4×10^{-8} dl³/sec × mg; β, coefficient of absorption decay, 1.2×10^{-5}/sec; ρ, absorption dependence on 1,25(OH)$_2$D$_3$, 3.8×10^{-6}/g(sec × pmol); A_1, vitamin D-independent calcium absorption, 0.1286; A_2, proportionality coefficient, 0.87. Other variables are defined in Table I.

bations and may be part of an anticipatory control (Moore-Ede, 1986). Similar to other control systems, calcium metabolism is regulated by peptide and steroid hormones. The secretion of the peptide hormones—PTH and CT—responds to plasma calcium concentration within minutes. The peptide hormones have a short half-life and deal with acute perturbations by transient actions (in the time range of minutes to hours), although they may also have long-term effects through activating other regulating hormones with slower response times. The immediate target for the action of either PTH or CT is bone. PTH stimulates bone resorption, thereby increasing calcium flow from bone to circulation. CT presumably acts in the opposite direction by inhibiting bone resorption. This action of PTH may be considered from the nutritional viewpoint as noneconomical, since it involves a loss of calcium from bone. The reduction in bone resorption by CT is also not desirable, since it can result in a decrease in bone turnover and a diminution of the calcium-regulating capacity of bone and in a decrease in the plasma concentration of phosphate, which may impede bone formation.

Under conditions of a sustained perturbation, the steroid hormone $1,25(OH)_2D_3$, with its slower response time, assumes domination in the control of calcium metabolism. The secretion of the hormone responds to perturbation through PTH mediation only within hours, and its half-life is also in the range of hours. Furthermore, the physiological action of the hormone occurs only after a lag time of 1–2 hours. Similar to PTH, the hormone acts by increasing the flow of calcium into the circulation. However, $1,25(OH)_2D_3$ increases the flow of calcium from the exterior by stimulating calcium absorption from the intestine, hence its action may be considered beneficial to the calcium economy of the body. In addition, this steroid hormone may also act on bone and kidney. These and other aspects of the biochemical and physiological actions of the calcium-regulating hormones will be discussed.

A. PARATHYROID HORMONE

1. *Parathyroid glands*

Two pairs of parathyroid glands are found in the thoracic cavity of birds, just caudal to the thyroid gland. Another parathyroid gland may be enclosed by the ultimobranchial body. The glands develop from the third, fourth, and fifth embryonic pharyngeal pouches. The size of the gland in the domestic fowl may vary from less than 1 mg in a normal growing bird to 30–40 mg in a vitamin D-deficient chick or a calcium-deficient laying hen.

2. *Structure of PTH*

PTH has been isolated and its amino acid sequence was determined in the bovine (Niall *et al.,* 1970; Brewer and Ronan, 1970), the human (Keutman *et al.,* 1978), and the pig (Sauer *et al.,* 1974). The amino acid sequence of rat preproPTH was deduced from the nucleotide sequence (Heinrich *et al.,* 1984). Details of PTH synthesis at the molecular biology level were reviewed by Kemper (1986) and by Kronenberg (1986). Avian PTH was the first nonmammalian PTH to be isolated (MacGregor *et al.,* 1976; Pines *et al.,* 1984). Recently, the hormone has also been cloned and its amino acid sequence was determined (Khosla *et al.,* 1988; Russell and Sherwood, 1989). Whereas the mammalian parathyroid peptides are 84 amino acids in length, the avian hormone contains 88 amino acids (Fig. 2). In comparison with human PTH, several deletions and insertions are observed in the avian sequence. About 60% homology between the human and avian is found in the 1–34 amino-terminal sequence, with the 1–14 sequence containing only two substitutions. This is important in view of the essentiality of this sequence to biological activity (Khosla *et al.,* 1988). The avian hormone contains four substitutions within the 25–34 sequence, considered important for receptor binding and hence conserved in the several mammalian PTHs (Rosenblatt, 1982). In the mammalian hormone, the 33–44 sequence contains three cleavage sites. This sequence is missing in the avian hormone and is replaced by an insertion of a four-amino acid sequence. Another deletion of amino acids 62–70 is replaced in the avian hormone by an insertion of a distinct 22-amino acid sequence.

3. *Hormone Secretion and Metabolism*

Similar to the mammalian hormones, the avian preproPTH is the complete translation product of the specific mRNA. As reviewed by Hurwitz (1989) the Met–Met residue of the amino terminus of the preproPTH is cleaved soon after emergence on the ribosome. The leader sequence of 23 amino acids is cleaved probably during insertion into the membrane of the endoplastic reticulum and the pro sequence of six amino acids is cleaved after transport to the Golgi apparatus. The hormone is then enveloped in secretory granules contained in the cytoplasm, ready for exocytosis.

Ambient calcium is the classic modulator of PTH secretion. Brown *et al.* (1976) observed in isolated bovine parathyroid cells *in vitro* a sigmoidal relationship between PTH secretion and ambient calcium. Mayer *et al.* (1979) found in calves *in vivo* a similar relationship between the active parathyroid peptide secretion and the plasma calcium

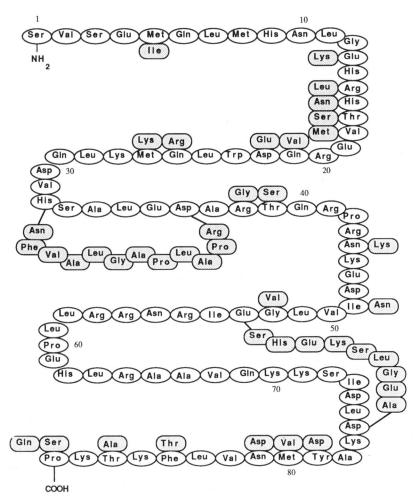

FIG. 2. Amino acid sequence of chicken PTH (Khosla *et al.*, 1988). Dotted boxes represent substitutions in human PTH. The numbers refer to the avian peptide. Note the large substitution at positions 32 and 53 and the corresponding deletions.

concentration. Secretion of PTH has not been studied in detail in birds due to the lack of a suitable assay, but Feinblatt *et al.* (1974) using a bioassay confirmed in organ culture the reciprocal relationship between ambient calcium and PTH secretion.

A dependence was found between intra- and extracellular calcium concentration (Brown and Shoback, 1984), and a reciprocal relationship was found between intracellular calcium concentration and hormone secretion. However, extracellular calcium and magnesium evoked rapid transient increases in intracellular calcium concentration, which involved mobilization of cellular Ca^{2+} (Nemeth and Scarpa, 1986, 1987). Furthermore, the impermeable cation La^{3+} also inhibited PTH secretion, suggesting that the effects of extracellular calcium on hormone secretion are offset by its binding to cell membrane receptors. The binding of calcium to its receptor was found to increase cell permeability to calcium (Gylfe et al., 1986). The action of a guanine nucleotide regulatory protein (Fitzpatrick et al., 1986) or a calcium–calmodulin-dependent protein kinase (Kinder et al., 1987) has also been implicated in the suppression of PTH secretion by the glandular cells.

The four-compartment model by Brown (1983), incorporating a sigmoidal relationship between ambient calcium and PTH secretion, was adopted for simulation (Hurwitz et al., 1987a), as given in Table II. Arbitrary units are assigned to PTH concentration until physiological concentrations can be accurately assessed in the plasma of birds. The relationship between PTH secretion and ambient calcium is not symmetrical, since the plasma ionic calcium concentration is 1.2–1.5 mM, higher than the calculated midpoint of response corresponding to 0.95 mM of calcium. The rate of increase in PTH secretion when plasma calcium decreases below normal values is much greater than the decrease in hormone secretion when plasma calcium increases. Thus, the PTH mechanism is more effective in dealing with a calcium deficiency than with an excess of calcium.

Several hormones were found to stimulate PTH secretion, apparently through cyclic adenosine monophosphate (cAMP) mediation. These included catecholamines (Brown et al., 1977), dopamine (Attie et al., 1980), and secretin (Windeck et al., 1978). The physiological significance of the action of these hormones has not been elucidated and therefore is not included in the present model.

In view of the vitamin D–parathyroid interactions, a direct action of the $1,25(OH)_2D_3$ in the parathyroid gland could be expected. In vitamin D deficiency, the parathyroid glands of chicks become grossly hypertrophied (Bar et al., 1972). A 3.3 S receptor for $1,25(OH)_2D_3$ was identified in the parathyroid glands (Pike et al., 1980), suggesting that the gland was a target organ for the hormone. However, in short-term incubation of parathyroid cells, contradictory results were obtained on the effect of $1,25(OH)_2D_3$ on PTH secretion. After 24–48 hours of incubation of parathyroid cells with the hormone, PTH secretion decreased as a consequence of the reduction in specific mRNA synthesis

(Cantly *et al.*, 1985), suggesting that $1,25(OH)_2D_3$ suppresses synthesis of PTH.

The metabolic fate of the avian PTH in birds has not been studied. Results with mammalian PTH indicate that some of the hormone is cleaved within the parathyroid cells (Cohn *et al.*, 1986) and that this breakdown is a function of plasma calcium (Mayer *et al.*, 1979). Once secreted, the hormone is taken up by the liver, where it is broken down into carboxy-terminal fragments similar to those found in the circulation (Canterbury *et al.*, 1975). The fragments are finally degraded by renal tubular cells (Hesch *et al.*, 1978). The half-life of the intact hormone is 10 minutes and that of the 1–34 PTH is 2 minutes (Schneider *et al.*, 1980). On the basis of additional literature (Neumann *et al.*, 1979), an approximated half-life of 5 minutes was taken for PTH in the chicken (Table II).

4. *Action of PTH*

Kidney and bone are the classical target organs for PTH. Similar to the response of the mammalian kidney, PTH in birds stimulates phosphate and sodium excretion but augments calcium reabsorption, as reviewed by Wideman (1987). In bone, PTH stimulates resorption but also induces anabolic effects. The hormone causes smooth muscle relaxation in the vascular bed of birds, and consequently a reduction in blood pressure (Pang *et al.*, 1984). In adrenocortical cells, PTH stimulates corticosterone and aldosterone secretion (Rosenberg *et al.*, 1987).

Similar to other peptide hormones, the action of PTH is initiated by binding to specific receptors, leading to synthesis of the secondary messenger. In the chick, Nissenson and Arnaud (1979) and McKee and Murray (1985) found a high-affinity PTH receptor coupled to adenylate cyclase. McKee and Murray also suggested the presence of a low-affinity receptor not coupled to this enzyme system. Down-regulation of PTH action is manifested by the decrease in the number of receptors in the chicken kidney during vitamin D deficiency (Carnes *et al.*, 1980; Forte *et al.*, 1982; Forte, 1983), leading to a refractoriness to PTH with regard to its calcemic (Harrison and Harrison, 1963; Gonnerman *et al.*, 1975) or 25-hydroxycholecalciferol-1-hydroxylase (1-hydroxylase) responses (Booth *et al.*, 1985). However, according to Liang *et al.* (1984), the decrease in the number of receptors cannot explain the entire refractoriness of phosphate excretion to PTH during a vitamin D deficiency. An up-regulation of the PTH receptors, observed in the kidneys of egg-laying hens was attributed by Forte *et al.* (1983) to the action of estrogen. The concept of down- and up-regulation of the PTH response has at the present not been introduced into the simulation model due to lack of quantitative information on receptor turnover.

Considerable evidence suggests that cAMP is the messenger of PTH action on target cells (Aurbach and Heath, 1974; Aurbach, 1982), although the involvement of inositol phosphate has been suggested (Rappaport and Stern, 1986). The stimulation by PTH of cAMP production by the kidney tubular cells (Chase and Aurbach, 1967) results in excretion of this cyclic nucleotide in the urine (Broadus, 1981). In the chicken, urinary cAMP was stimulated by a single dose of PTH, as well as by chronic hyperparathyroidism induced by feeding of a low-calcium diet (Pines et al., 1983)

PTH inhibits phosphate resorption by the renal tubular cell and, in various species of birds, also increases tubular phosphate secretion (Levinski and Davidson, 1957; Clark et al., 1976; Clark and Wideman, 1977; Clark and Sasayama, 1981). Also in birds, PTH augments renal tubular resorption of calcium, as reviewed by Wideman (1987), and suppresses reabsorption of sodium and water (Wideman and Youtz, 1985).

Rapid (10- to 30-minute) morphological changes were observed in osteoclasts of quail medullary bone following in vivo PTH administration. These changes included the appearance of ruffled borders, which serve as the resorptive surfaces (Miller et al., 1984; Miller and Kenny, 1985). However, no response to PTH could be obtained in a pure culture of osteoclasts (Chambers et al., 1985), suggesting that osteoclasts do not bear receptors for PTH. Osteoblasts indeed harbor PTH receptors (Rodan and Rodan, 1983; Hermann-Erlee et al. 1983) and may be required for the activation of the osteoclasts (McSheehy and Chambers, 1986). Osteoblasts may act as intermediates by releasing osteoclast-activating factors in response to PTH (Gowen and Mundy, 1986). Several paracrine factors, including interleukin I, have been implicated in the control of bone resorption together with PTH (Dewhirst et al., 1987).

Receptors for PTH are found in chondrocytes or chondroprogenitor cells (Pines and Hurwitz, 1988). In these cells, PTH activates adenylate cyclase (Kawashima et al., 1980) and stimulates cell proliferation (Chin et al., 1986; Pines and Hurwitz, 1988). The physiological significance of the responses to PTH by the different bone cells is not clear. Chronic PTH administration in some mammalian species causes increased bone mass (Tam et al., 1982). It may be speculated that cellular PTH responses are aimed at a preparation of bone infrastructure in anticipation of the expected increase in influx of calcium secondary to PTH stimulation of $1,25(OH)_2D_3$ release; this would compensate for loss of bone material by PTH–stimulated resorption. Since these responses have not been absolutely conceptualized and their kinetics have not been investigated, they have not been included in the simulation model of calcium metabolism (Hurwitz *et al.*, 1987a).

B. CALCITONIN

Copp *et al.* (1972) showed that perfusion of the parathyroid–thyroid complex of birds with hypercalcemic blood caused release of calcitonin, which lowered plasma calcium. Tauber (1967) identified the ultimobranchial origin of this substance in birds. As mentioned, this gland is positioned caudal to the main parathyroid glands and may engulf a third parathyroid.

1. *Structure and Biosynthesis*

Avian calcitonin has been purified by Nieto *et al.* (1973). and sequenced by Homma *et al.* (1986) and Lasmoles *et al.* (1985). The avian peptide consists of a 32-amino acid sequence and shows a high degree of homology with eel (94%) and salmon (84%) calcitonin (Lasmoles *et al.*, 1985). The avian hormone is also similar to the eel and salmon hormones in its immunological and biological activity. The hormone mRNA was cloned (Lasmoles *et al.*, 1985) and its gene was isolated and sequenced. Two mRNAs are expressed by tissue-specific alternate splicing, encoding calcitonin and calcitonin gene-related peptide, in the ultimobranchial gland and brain, respectively (Minvielle *et al.*, 1986).

2. *Calcitonin Action*

In mammals, calcitonin (thyrocalcitonin) lowers plasma calcium by inhibition of bone resorption. The action of the hormone in bone appears to be mediated by cAMP (Chase and Aurbach, 1970; Nicholson *et al.*, 1986). Calcitonin also stimulates adenylate cyclase of some renal tubular cells. *In vitro,* calcitonin causes the disappearance of the ruffled border of the osteoclasts and inhibits their motility, thereby inhibiting their bone-resorbing activity (Arnett and Dempster, 1987), regardless of its source (Dempster *et al.*, 1987). In birds, neither ultimobranchiectomy nor exogenous calcitonin affected plasma calcium (Kraintz and Intcher, 1969). Reports are conflicting about its action in the osteoclasts. Cao and Gay (1985) and de Vernejoul *et al.* (1988) observed in chickens inhibition of bone resorption by calcitonin and the expected morphological changes in the osteoclast. In contrast, Nicholson *et al.* (1987) and Dempster *et al.* (1987) found no calcitonin binding and no calcitonin stimulation of cAMP production in chicken osteoclasts. Receptors for calcitonin may also be lacking in the chicken kidney, since the hormone neither induced cAMP formation (Dousa, 1974) nor influenced calcium or phosphorus excretion (Clark and Wideman, 1980). These findings are also in agreement with the lack of significant effect of ultimobranchiectomy in chickens on plasma calcium or bone calcification. Thus, although circulating levels of calcitonin in the avian are even higher than in the mammal and respond to plasma calcium (Copp et al., 1972), calcitonin does not appear in birds to elicit any calcium response and its importance as a calcium-regulating hormone has not been elucidated. We have therefore omitted any formal description of calcitonin effect in the simulation model of calcium homeostasis given in Table II.

C. 1,25-DIHYDROXYCHOLECALCIFEROL

$1,25(OH)_2D_3$ was discovered in the early 1970s (Fraser and Kodicek, 1970; Norman et al., 1971; Holick et al., 1971), and since that time has been studied extensively. Much of the information on the hormone, such as regulation by PTH (Fraser and Kodicek, 1973) and expression of its action in the intestine with induction of calbindin [(CaBP) Wasserman and Taylor, 1966] synthesis, derives from studies of chicks. In addition to its role in calcium metabolism, the hormone has been found to be important in regulating cell proliferation and differentiation in diverse cellular systems such as the immune system and skin. The present discussion of its metabolism and physiological effects is restricted to the framework of calcium homeostasis. For more comprehensive reviews on vitamin D in birds, see Norman et al. 1982; Norman, 1987.

1. Biosynthesis and Secretion

The precursor for synthesis of the hormone, cholecalciferol (vitamin D_3), is obtained from diet or is synthesized endogenously in the skin. Vitamin D_3 is found only in foods derived from animal sources. The existence of intact or glycosylated $1,25(OH)_2D_3$ in some plants, such as Solanum or Cestrum species (reviewed by Boland, 1986), is an exception. Artificially produced feed supplements, such as irradiated yeast, contain vitamin D_2 (ergocalciferol), which may function equally as well as vitamin D_3 in most mammalian species. Birds (and some New World monkeys), however, hardly respond to vitamin D_2 (Steenbock et al., 1932) for reasons yet to be elucidated. No differences were found in the intestinal uptake of the two forms of the vitamin from food (Hurwitz *et al.*, 1967) or in the capacity of the chicken liver to hydroxylate the vitamin (Jones *et al.*, 1976). Recent evidence suggests a greater clearance of vitamin D_2 than that of vitamin D_3 in the chicken (Hoy *et al.*, 1988) or a poorer binding of 25-hydroxyvitamin D_2 to the plasma-binding protein and hence a reduced mobility (DeLuca *et al.*, 1988); the dihydroxy metabolites bind to the intestinal receptor equally well. It has been known for over 60 years that vitamin D_3 is synthesized from 7-dehydrocholesterol in skin under the influence of ultraviolet radiation. In birds, a vitamin D deficiency can be induced by feeding vitamin D-free diets in environments lacking ultraviolet irradiation. Since most of the skin of birds is covered by feathers and the legs are covered by thick scales, the main site of vitamin D synthesis must be the head region. Due to the hydrophobicity of the vitamin, its concentration in central compartments of the body is low, and the synthesized or absorbed vitamin is stored in the adipose tissue, from which it can be released only at a very slow rate. Water solubility is enhanced by hydroxylation of the vitamin at position 25 in the liver. 25-Hydroxycholecalciferol represented the first (Blunt *et al.*, 1968) in a long list of discoveries of naturally occurring and synthetic vitamin D derivatives. Synthesis of $25(OH)D_3$ is apparently regulated by product inhibition (Omdahl and DeLuca, 1973) rather than by factors associated with calcium metabolism and may therefore be considered external to calcium homeostasis. Relatively to other vitamin D metabolites, high concentrations of $25(OH)D_3$ are found in the circulation, mostly bound to specific transport proteins (DeLuca *et al.*, 1988). The compound is distributed in many tissues, most importantly in muscle, and is therefore considerably more available for further processing than vitamin D_3 itself.

The regulatory step in the calcium control system is the synthesis of $1,25(OH)_2D_3$ from $25(OH)D_3$ in the proximal renal tubular cells (Akiba *et al.*, 1980). The hydroxylation, carried out by the 1-hydroxylase enzyme system, involves cytochrome P-450. As depicted in Fig. 1, the synthesis and secretion of $1,25(OH)_2D_3$ are regulated by PTH (Fraser and Kodicek, 1973). A direct stimulation by PTH of 1-hydroxylase was observed in isolated renal tubular cells *in vitro* (Bar and Hurwitz, 1980) or in culture, where it requires insulin for maximal expression (Henry, 1981; Armbrecht *et al.*, 1984). Forskolin, which stimulates cAMP production, mimics the effect of PTH on the 1-hydroxylase (Henry, 1985). Thus, cAMP appears to mediate also the 1-hydroxylase response to PTH. The level of $1,25(OH)_2D_3$ (Omdahl *et al.*, 1980) and plasma calcium and plasma phosphate (as reviewed by Omdahl and DeLuca, 1973) have also been implicated in regulation of the enzyme activity. Since the separation between the direct action of calcium from that of PTH is rather difficult, the simulation model considers the modulation of the 1-hydroxylase enzyme as entirely due to PTH.

Hormones such as growth hormone (Spanos et $al.$, 1978), prolactin (Spanos et $al.$, 1981), or estrogen in birds (Tanaka et $al.$, 1976) were implicated as $1,25(OH)_2D_3$ secretagogues. However, no direct effect of estrogen on cultured chick kidney cells was found (Henry, 1981). Since the estrogen effect could be blunted by feeding of a high-calcium diet, it was suggested (Bar and Hurwitz, 1979) that the increase in 1-hydroxylase activity was secondary to the primary responses to the gonadal hormones, such as vitellogenesis (see Section VI, 3) and induction of medullary bone formation (see Section VI, 3), which cause a drain of calcium from circulation and a consequent increase in parathyroid activity. The up-regulation of PTH kidney receptors by estrogen (Forte et $al.$, 1983) could potentiate the response of the 1-hydroxylase system to PTH. Since the activity of 1-hydroxylase was found in chicks to be proportional to the rate of growth (Bar and Hurwitz, 1981), which also involves a drain on the calcium pool, restoration of the enzyme activity after pituitary ablation by replacement therapy with growth hormone (Spanos et $al.$, 1978) could also have been secondary to restoration of growth, rather than to direct stimulation by growth hormone. The relationship between growth and activity of the calcium control system is discussed in Section V.

Several additional hydroxylated vitamin D metabolites are produced in the kidney. From a quantitative viewpoint, $24,25(OH)_2D_3$ is the most important. This metabolite is considered by some (Ornoy et $al.$, 1978) to be important in the proper structural development of bone, whereas others discount the biological importance of this metabolite and consider $1,25(OH)_2D_3$ to be the sole physiologically active metabolite (Brommage and DeLuca, 1985). $24,25(OH)_2D_3$ can elicit responses of the calcium-mobilizing system, such as calcium absorption, but its affinity for intestinal receptors and its potency are considerably lower than those of $1,25(OH)_2D_3$ (Proscal et $al.$, 1975).

$1,25(OH)_2D_3$ is degraded probably through 24-hydroxylation and elimination through biliary excretion, with a half-life determined in the chick to be 14 hours (Hurwitz et $al.$, 1983).

2. $Action$ of $1,25(OH)_2D_3$

Classically, vitamin D_3 or its metabolites prevent and cure rickets. The intestine, bone, and kidney are main target tissues for $1,25(OH)_2D_3$. Receptors for the hormone were located in the epithelial cells of the intestine and the kidney, in osteoblasts (but not osteoclasts),

and in the reticuloendothelial system in bone (Haussler, 19.
tors for the hormone have also been found in many othe
including endocrine organs. Notably in birds, $1,25(OH)_2D_3$
were found in the shell gland and the parathyroid cells (Taka   ᴧᵢ
al., 1980; Coty, 1980). The chick intestinal $1,25(OH)_2D_3$ receptor has
been the most extensively studied (Haussler, 1986). The avian receptor
was purified and its cDNA was cloned (McDonnell et al., 1987). The
receptor is an acidic protein with a molecular weight of 63,000–64,000.
It contains high-affinity (K_d 10^{-10} to 10^{-11} M) binding domains for
$1,25(OH)_2D_3$ and for association with DNA (Haussler, 1986). The DNA-
binding domain is similar in configuration to that of other steroid
receptors, supporting the classification of $1,25(OH)_2D_3$ as a steroid
hormone. The receptor is mostly localized at the cell nucleus, but some
of the unoccupied receptor may also reside in the cytoplasm.

The biological potency of various di- and trihydroxyvitamin D metabolites correlates well with receptor affinity, with $1,25(OH)_2D_3$
being most active (Proscal et al., 1975). The appearance of the intestinal receptor in the developing embryo also correlates well with a
large increase in calcium transport capacity (Seino et al., 1982). Thus,
receptor binding appears to mediates the action of $1,25(OH)_2D_3$.

After a single intravenous administration of $1,25(OH)_2D_3$ in chicks,
peak concentrations are found in the intestine 1–2 hours later (Hurwitz et al., 1983). At that time, the concentration of the hormone in the
intestinal mucosa is about three times as high as that in the blood.
Within minutes after entry into the cell, the hormone becomes associated with the nuclear receptor (Wecksler and Norman, 1980; Fishman
et al., 1986). Receptor binding is therefore responsible for the preferential uptake of the hormone into the mucosal cell. The kinetics of intestinal uptake and release of $1,25(OH)_2D_3$ in the intestine, together with
its disappearance rate (Hurwitz et al., 1983), are used in the simulation
of the intestinal action of the hormone (Table II).

3. Vitamin D and Protein Synthesis

Uptake of $1,25(OH)_2D_3$ into the cell nucleus and binding of the
receptor to DNA are followed by formation of mRNA and specific
protein synthesis. The dependence of the physiological action of vitamin D on protein synthesis was suggested by early studies which
showed a lag period of several hours in the response to vitamin D and
that actinomycin D administration prevented the action of the vitamin
(Zull et al., 1956). This concept was questioned by Bikle et al. (1978),
who found that cycloheximide or actinomycin D treatment did not
inhibit the early response of calcium absorption in chicks to vitamin D,

while syntheses of calbindin and alkaline phosphatase were significantly inhibited. Moreover, a single dose of $1,25(OH)D_3$ causes increased calcium absorption (Wasserman and Fullmer, 1983) and enhanced calcium transport observed in brush border vesicles isolated from intestinal mucosa (Rasmussen et al., 1979; Bikle et al., 1983) before there are any detectable changes in calbindin concentration. Vitamin D also induces changes in the lipids of the brush border membrane (reviewed by Wasserman and Corradino, 1973).

Of the proteins considered to be induced by $1,25(OH)_2D_3$, such as alkaline phosphatase (Haussler et al., 1970), actin (Wilson and Lawson, 1977, 1978), and tubulin (Nemere et al., 1987), synthesis of calbindin [calcium-binding protein (CaBP)] has been most extensively studied since its discovery by Wasserman and Taylor (1966). The molecular weight of this vitamin D-dependent protein was determined to be 28,000 (Wasserman and Fullmer, 1983). The protein contains four repeating calcium-binding domains with an apparent K_a of 2×10^6 M^{-1} and is distinguished by a high content of dicarboxylic amino acids with an isoelectric point of pH 4.2–4.3. The amino acid sequence was established from the cDNA sequence and chemical mapping (Hunziker, 1986; Wilson et al., 1985, 1988).

Calbindin has been identified in the avian intestine, kidney, and eggshell gland (Jand et al., 1981), which transport massive quantities of calcium, especially during reproduction. The protein was also localized in other tissues such as brain, pancreas, and the parathyroid gland. In the intestine, a linear relationship was found between the concentration of $1,25(OH)_2D_3$ and calbindin (A. Bar, unpulished observations), which suggested that synthesis of this protein was modulated by the hormone. Furthermore, concentration of calbindin is linearly related to permeability of the intestine to calcium, as indicated by fractional transport (Bar and Hurwitz, 1979). In embryonic intestine, verapamil, a calcium antagonist, suppressed the induction of calbindin by $1,25(OH)_2D_3$ (Corradino, 1985). Calbindin content in the kidney decreased during calcium deficiency, although $1,25(OH)_2D_3$ concentration increased (Bar et al., 1975). No correlation could be established between the concentration of $1,25(OH)_2D_3$ and that of calbindin, although the appearance of the protein and its maintenance in the tissue were vitamin D dependent (Rosenberg et al., 1986), as was also demonstrated in kidney cells in vitro (Cravisio et al., 1987). A positive correlation was found in birds between kidney CaBP and calcium excretion or plasma calcium concentration, rather than with the rate of calcium reabsorption (Rosenberg et al., 1986). A similar correlation was also found for humans (Jacob and Chan, 1987). In the shell gland, calbindin remains undetectable so long as the gland is inactive and appears during the calcification of the first shell (Bar and Hurwitz, 1973). Sex steroid appears to be involved in the induction of shell gland calbindin (Navickis et al., 1979). Furthermore, calbindin concentration is not proportional to the tissue concentration of 1,25-$(OH)_2D_3$ but is positively correlated with egg shell calcium deposition (Bar et al., 1984).

Calbindin mRNA appeared after a single dose of $1,25(OH)_2D_3$ in the intestine of rachitic chicks, and its concentration was proportional to the dose of the hormone (Wilson et al., 1985; Hall et al., 1988). However, an increase in intestinal $1,25(OH)_2D_3$ by feeding of low-calcium or low-phosphate diets did not affect calbindin mRNA, although the concentration of calbindin itself increased (Theofan et al., 1987), leading to the suggestion that the hormone affects posttranscriptional mechanisms in addition to the initiation of mRNA synthesis. Theofan et al. (1987) and Mayel-Afsar et al. (1988) suggested that posttranscriptional mechanisms are also responsive to plasma calcium and phosphate. It is therefore not unlikely that the induction of calbindin synthesis requires $1,25(OH)_2D_3$ but its concentration in the epithelial cells is modulated by other factors such as calcium.

Early after its discovery, calbindin was considered to be the calcium carrier molecule participating in active transport of the cation or in its facilitated diffusion. It became clear, however, that calbindin was localized in the cytoplasm rather than in the brush border and could therefore not act as a membrane carrier. Bronner et al. (1986) hypothesized that calbindin acted to ferry calcium across the cell since, according to their calculation, the mobility of calcium was too slow to explain its flux across the entire length of the epithelial cell. This hypothesis is supported by Feher (1983), who found facilitated calcium diffusion through a series of two membranes upon addition of calbindin to the central compartment. Wasserman and Fullmer (1983) favor the theory that calbindin sequesters calcium in the epithelial cell in order to avoid excessively high intracellular calcium concentration and uptake of calcium by cellular organelles.

4. Vitamin D and Calcium Homeostasis

Some controversy exists with regard to the role of vitamin D and its active metabolite $1,25(OH)_2D_3$ in calcium homeostasis. In vitamin deficiency the capacity of the control system of chicks to maintain normal plasma calcium concentration is overcome, and total plasma calcium may decline to 5 mg/100 ml, about 50% of normal. Treatment with hormone causes plasma calcium to increase gradually back to normal. According to Garabedian *et al.* (1974), based on results obtained with the rat, the initial response to the hormone is due to bone calcium mobilization. Since the blood calcium response requires parathyroid function (see Section III, A, 4), the bone calcium-mobilizing action of $1,25(OH)_2D_3$ appears to be indirect.

Most of the studies on vitamin D action were made on D-deficient rachitic birds. The participation of $1,25(OH)_2D_3$ in calcium homeostasis could also be studied by providing the hormone from an exogenous source, such as diet, on a steady-state basis. This procedure bypasses the regulatory activity of the $1,25(OH)_2D_3$ intestinal axis, allowing the evaluation of its importance in animals with a normal plasma calcium and normal bone. The synthetic derivative 1α-hydroxycholecalciferol [$1\alpha(OH)D_3$] was also used in this capacity, since it is rapidly metabolized to $1,25(OH)_2D_3$ (Holick *et al.*, 1976). Data given in Table III (Hurwitz *et al.*, 1984) show that the normal homeostatic decrease in calcium absorption during challenge with a high calcium intake is overcome when $1\alpha(OH)D_3$ is given in the diet, with remarkable agreement between the experimental results and those predicted by computer simulation. When calcium intake was changed, plasma calcium concentrations of the $1\alpha(OH)D_3$-fed birds, initially the same as those of the normal animals, rapidly increased to extremely high levels as calcium intake exceeded a normal level of 10 g/kg (Fig. 3). Vitamin D-fed birds showed only small changes in plasma calcium, with intakes of calcium between 7 and 18 g/kg. This suggested that the response of the intestine, mediated by $1,25(OH)_2D_3$, was essential in avoiding the hypercalcemia associated with high dietary intakes of calcium. This study again demonstrated a remarkable agreement between simulated and experimental results. Since simula-

TABLE III

RESPONSE OF CALCIUM ABSORPTION TO DIETARY CALCIUM:
SIMULATED VERSUS EXPERIMENTAL RESULTS

Dietary calcium (g/kg)	Dietary hormone[a]	Calcium absorption (% of intake)	
		Predicted	Experimental
5	−	51	55 ± 2[b]
17	−	25	19 ± 2
5	+	78	66 ± 2
17	+	61	73 ± 5

[a] $1,25(OH)_2D_3$ and $1\alpha(OH)D_3$, in the simulated and experimental results, respectively.
[b] Values are expressed as means $\pm$ SE.

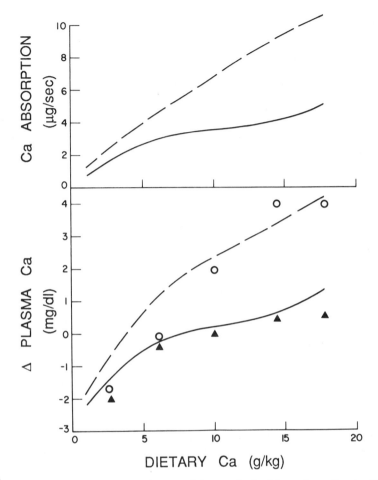

FIG. 3. Simulated response of plasma calcium and of calcium absorption to dietary calcium. Solid lines, normal chickens; broken lines, chickens fed 1,25(OH)$_2$D$_3$; triangles and circles, experimental results of normal and 1α(OH)$_3$, respectively. (From Hurwitz *et al.*, 1984.)

tion describes only the intestinal and not any skeletal action of the hormone, the results suggest that the hormone participation in calcium homeostasis may by fully explained by its intestinal action. The results also demonstrate the utmost importance of the intestine in the control of calcium homeostasis in the chick.

1,25(OH)$_2$D$_3$ is the active principle in the process of adaptation of the bird to low calcium intake, as demonstrated experimentally (Edelstein *et al.*, 1975; Bar *et al.*, 1976) and by computer simulation (Hurwitz *et al.*, 1983). The consumption of a low-calcium diet results in a decrease in plasma calcium concentration followed immediately by an increase in plasma PTH. PTH stimulates bone resorption, which corrects some of the hypocalcemia, and facilitates the production of the kidney 1-hydroxylase enzyme, with a resulting increase in the release of $1,25(OH)_2D_3$ into the circulation. The accumulation of $1,25(OH)_2D_3$ in the intestinal mucosa is followed by an increase in the fractional absorption of calcium. A lag time of a few hours in the absorption response is due to the delay caused by the limited synthesis and first-order disappearance rate of the participating agents—the 1-hydroxylase enzyme, $1,25(OH)_2D_3$, and the absorptive mechanism.

IV. The Controlling Systems

A. Bone

The skeleton may be considered a large internal calcium reservoir which contains about 99% of the body calcium, from which calcium can be drawn during need or stored when in excess. In the rat, bone was considered to be the most important calcium-controlling system, since the kidney handled only a small fraction of the calcium load (Bronner and Aubert, 1965). In chickens and humans, the kidney handles a significant part of any calcium load and the relative homeostatic importance of bone is not so great as in the rat. The processes of bone calcium removal may be rapidly activated and sustained for long periods of time. Bone undergoes a constant turnover due to formation and resorption, which constitute the remodeling process. Since bone flows are modulated by plasma calcium and phosphorus and regulated by hormones, they may be part of the calcium control system. Parfitt (1987), however, considered the system participating in calcium homeostasis to be independent of bone formation and resorption and carried out by different bone cell populations.

An important determinant of bone calcium flow is the process of growth. Growth causes a flow of calcium into bone, which is determined to a large extent by processes external to calcium metabolism and may therefore be considered a steady-state perturbation of calcium homeostasis.

The metabolism of bone has been studied by two entirely different approaches which are not directly reconcilable. The *in vivo* approach considers inflow and outflow of calcium from bone as governed by physiochemical processes of transport among different pools, which can be studied with calcium isotopes. This approach used compartmental analysis, which describes calcium movements among the compartments as following linear (Aubert *et al.*, 1963) or nonlinear (Staub *et al.*, 1988) kinetics. Furthermore, calcium was considered to move to bone mineral directly from the extracellular space, which is an "extension" of the central calcium pool. The other approach investigated bone cell biology by histological techniques or *in vitro* cultures (Nijweide *et al.*, 1986). Some conceptual attempt was made to describe the bone extracellular matrix, including the mineral phase, as separated from circulation by the various bone cells (Talmage *et al.*, 1975). Calcium movement in and out of the mineral phase of the bone is then governed by the metabolism of bone cells, which in turn is affected by the calcium-regulating hormones.

Since most approaches concerning the homeostatic action of bone are based on unifying concepts, validation of theories regarding calcium flows is complicated by the heterogeneity of bone with regard to morphological organization and cellular populations, composition of the organic matrix, proportion between mineral and organic matrix, and the different chemical forms of calcium phosphate.

1. *Morphological Organization*

Bone structure varies among different bones and in different locations in the same bone and is influenced by many physiological and nutritional factors. In macroscopic terms, the skeleton contains elements of cartilage located mostly in the growth plate, trabecular or spongy bone found, for example, in the epiphyses of the long bones, and compact or cortical bone of the shafts. Bones of female birds during reproduction also contain a gonadal hormone-induced medullary bone, with a morphology quite distinct from other types of bone, (Section VI,3). Calcium turnover rate, as measured with the aid of ^{45}Ca, varies widely among the various bone types, with half-lives ranging from several months in cortical bone to several weeks in trabecular bone to 1–2 days in medullary bone (Hurwitz, 1965). Under conditions of calcium deficiency, trabecular bone is depleted the most and cortical bone the least (Hurwitz and Bar, 1966). Thus, any measured differences in parameters of calcium metabolism by the whole-body kinetic approach, are complicated by changes in bone morphology.

2. *Cellular Populations*

Bone contains five important cell populations (not including bone marrow): (1) cartilage cells, (2) bone-forming cells, osteoblasts, (3) bone-resorbing cells, osteoclasts, (4) mature bone cells, osteocytes, and (5) bone-lining cells.

Bone elongation is dependent on proliferation of the chondroprogenitor cells within the growth plate. The thickness of the growth plate is proportional to the rate of growth as determined by age and genetics (LeBlanc et al., 1986; Leach and Gay, 1987). Rate of proliferation of chondroprogenitor cells can be enhanced by somatomedins and other growth factors (Isaksson et al., 1987) and cAMP activators, such as PTH, and suppressed by cGMP (Pines and Hurwitz, 1988). After cartilage formation, endochondral calcification and cartilage cell atrophy precede the invasion by bone cells and formation of osseous tissues (Leach and Gay, 1987). Thus, cartilage formation during growth which is controlled by factors external to calcium metabolism (the growth curve) determines the consequent flow of calcium into bone. Some feedback to calcium metabolism of this system may be related to PTH action and may be part of the anabolic effect of PTH.

Osteoblasts take over bone formation from chondrocytes, and are primary bone-forming cells in the process of the radial increase in bone mass. These cells are equipped with receptors for both PTH and $1,25(OH)_2D_3$ (Rodan and Rodan, 1983; Stern, 1980), which modulate the activities of several enzyme systems such as alkaline phosphatase and probably also modify some calcium transport characteristics. Osteoblasts differentiate into osteocytes, once embedded in the osteoid tissue.

Osteoclasts are polynucleated cells which probably originate from cells of the reticuloendothelial system. Cells such as macrophages may differentiate into osteoclasts under the influence of $1,25(OH)_2D_3$, losing their $1,25(OH)_2D_3$ receptors at the end of differentiation (Miyaura et al., 1986; Haussler, 1986). As noted above, osteoclasts are devoid of PTH receptors, and their response to the hormone is mediated by other cells, probably osteoblasts (McSheehy and Chambers, 1986). Osteoclasts in mammals (see Section III,B,2) bear calcitonin receptors and their activity is inhibited by calcitonin, whereas in birds this mechanism appears to be lacking. The stimulation of the osteoclast formation by $1,25(OH)_2D_3$ may provide the mechanism for the bone-resorbing action of this hormone on the one hand, and the basis for its interaction with PTH on the other. (Section II,A,3).

Osteoclasts cause bone resorption by attachment to the surface of bone and the actual removal of the entire osseous mass including both matrix and mineral. A prolonged action of these cells leads to osteoporosis. Through the action of osteoclasts, laying hens which deposit in the egg shell about 10% of their body calcium within less than

1 day, may lose up to 40% of their carcass osseous material, if deprived of dietary calcium, and may become extremely osteoporotic (Hurwitz and Bar, 1966).

Flat, elongated bone-lining cells cover the nonremodeling endosteal surfaces of bone, and are thus not involved in remodeling. They were, however, implicated in the control of bone ionic fluxes (Bowman and Miller, 1986), including those involved in calcium homeostasis (Parfitt, 1987).

3. Bone Mineral

The association between calcium and phosphate, the two main inorganic constituents of bone, yields a diversity of salts in a complex phase transition, depending on the conditions prevailing during precipitation, such as calcium and phosphate concentration, concentration of other cations and anions, pH, pCO_2, temperature, etc. There are also transitions from one calcium phosphate to another. Hydroxyapatite is the major bone salt, but early during calcification other salts may precipitate. These calcium phosphate intermediates may be stabilized under some conditions (Parfitt, 1987). The various salts have different solubility products and different isotope exchangeability characteristics and hence different homeostatic implications.

4. Homeostatic Considerations

Due to the heterogeneity of bone turnover processes, construction of a detailed model of the involvement of the various bone elements in calcium homeostasis is at the present not feasible, and one has to rely on simplified information derived from whole-animal experiments. This would certainly limit the applicability of the models to conditions close to those under which the information was collected. In the rat, two- (Bronner and Aubert, 1965) or six-compartment models (Staub *et al.*, 1988) were evaluated by whole-body calcium kinetics. Since similar kinetic experiments have not been conducted in chickens, the simulation model considered only two processes of inflow of calcium into bone—one related to growth, driven by the rate of growth and normative calcification (Hurwitz and Plavnik, 1986). Another route of entry of calcium into bone is part of bone remodeling and is dependent on the size of the skeleton. Calcium removal processes were grouped as dependent on PTH concentration which, in turn, rapidly responds to changes in plasma calcium concentration. The parameters for the respective equations were obtained by subjecting the entire model to a curve-fitting procedure against results of plasma calcium in chicks which had received bolus injections of calcium (Hurwitz *et al.*, 1983).

The validity of the model and determined parameters were tested by comparing model predictions to results of the inverse treatment of injecting ethylenediaminetetraacetic acid (EDTA) (Hurwitz et al., 1983) and by evaluating bone calcium as a function of calcium intake (Hurwitz et al., 1987b).

Bones of birds undergo important changes in preparation for the large increase of calcium turnover during reproduction. These changes will be discussed in Section VI.

B. Intestinal Absorption

Intestinal absorption provides the means for entry of calcium from the environment, and is determined by the supply of calcium in the diet. Bronner and Aubert (1965) considered intestinal absorption to be a "disturbing signal" in the context of calcium homeostasis. Nicolayesen et al. (1953) observed an increase in calcium absorption of rats, to satisfy the increased demands during low calcium intakes. The adaptation of animals to low calcium intakes was later linked to increased synthesis of $1,25(OH)_2D_3$ (Edelstein et al., 1975; Ribovich and DeLuca, 1976), providing the feedback link between intestinal calcium absorption and calcium homeostasis. A large diurnal increase in calcium absorption was observed in laying hens during the hours of egg shell formation, as was a subsequent return to low levels once calcification of the egg shell had been completed (Hurwitz and Bar, 1965; Hurwitz et al., 1973). Thus, the intestine is not a simple gateway for calcium entry but rather an important control system in calcium homeostasis.

Early studies used balance techniques to estimate calcium absorption. In vitro techniques (Wilson and Wiseman, 1954) were applied to the study of calcium absorption (Harrison and Harrison, 1960; Schachter et al., 1960). These techniques and variants of the in situ loop (Wasserman, 1963) have provided the major portion of the detailed information on calcium absorption and most importantly on its dependence on vitamin D metabolites. The disadvantage of these techniques is that they regard only mucosal and transmucosal transfer of calcium out of artificially defined media and ignore other processes which may be important in vivo determinants of calcium absorption, such as concentration of ionic calcium in the intestinal content and differences in sites of absorption and of transit time along the intestine. Although a large active in vitro transport of calcium was observed in the duodenum of the rat, a rapid transit of digesta results in a small contribution of this intestinal segment to the overall absorption of calcium, casting doubt as to the relevance of many *in vitro* observations to the *in vivo* process. In the chick, the major areas for calcium absorption are the duodenum and the jejunum (Hurwitz and Bar, 1972; Hurwitz *et al.*, 1973). Vitamin D stimulates calcium absorption in these segments, while it reduces net secretion in the ileum.

In the diets of birds as well as in mammals after weaning, calcium is provided as poorly soluble salts, such as calcium carbonate and several calcium phosphates. These are solubilized in the stomach and are made available for absorption. However, upon entry of the digesta into the duodenum and titration of the acidity by pancreatic bicarbonate, calcium reprecipitates, leaving in the solution only a fraction of the amount entered. The activity of calcium in the duodenum of the chicken depends on the dietary calcium concentration and source (Hurwitz and Bar, 1968), and possibly on some metabolic factors such as acid–base balance (Sauveur and Mongin, 1983). However, within a wide range of calcium intakes, the activity of ionic calcium in the intestinal contents is sufficiently high to maintain a positive electrochemical potential gradient of calcium and to allow a transmembrane diffusion. A need for active calcium transport arises only under extreme conditions of calcium deficiency (Hurwitz and Bar, 1968).

Early disagreements concerning the mechanism of calcium absorption and of its control by vitamin D have still not been settled. Schachter *et al.* (1960), based on *in vitro* experiments with the rat duodenum, suggested that vitamin D acted by promoting active calcium transport. Bronner (1987) concluded, on the basis of experimentation with intestinal loop *in situ* and *in vitro*, that in the rat $1,25(OH)_2D_3$ regulated the saturable calcium translocation, consistent with the active transport hypothesis. Harrison and Harrison (1960) observed that vitamin D promoted transfer of calcium down an almost infinite transmucosal gradient, when active transport was inhibited by N-methylmaleimide. These authors suggested that vitamin D increased the "diffusibility" of calcium across the intestinal mucosa (Harrison and Harrison, 1963). In the chick intestine *in situ* Wasserman (1963), using the criterion of flux ratio, concluded that primary calcium transfer was by passive diffusion at least at higher calcium concentrations. The slope of the plot of transmembrane calcium flux on calcium concentration was higher in vitamin D replete than in rachitic birds, suggesting that vitamin D increased the permeability of the intestine to calcium. A similar analysis of calcium absorption *in vivo* (Hurwitz *et al.*, 1973) supported this hypothesis.

The effect of $1,25(OH)_2D_3$ can be examined in greater detail at the cellular level. Calcium absorption may be effected through paracellular and cellular routes. Paracellular transport proceeds through intercellular junctions, apparently by diffusion. Transcellular transport involves transfer through the brush border membrane, passage through the cytoplasm, and transport across the basolateral membrane. Due to the relatively low intracellular calcium concentration and the negative electrical potential difference between the lumen and the exterior, the transport of calcium across the brush border is a downhill process. Transport in isolated brush border vesicles is stimulated by vitamin D in both the chick and the rat (Rasmussen et al., 1979; Bikle et al., 1983). The movement of calcium through the cytoplasm may be facilitated by the vitamin D-dependent calbindin (Bronner et al., 1986) and hence may also be controlled by $1,25(OH)_2D_3$. Finally, calcium is transported uphill across the basolateral membrane. This translocation is mediated by a adenosine triphosphate (ATP)-activated calcium pump which is probably identical to the high affinity, calcium-dependent ATPase (as reviewed by Wasserman and Fullmer, 1983). There is some evidence that the basolateral process is stimulated by vitamin D or $1,25(OH)_2D_3$ but Bronner (1987) calculated that it was not limiting under normal nutritional conditions.

The fractional calcium absorption in vivo, analogous to the average permeability of the intestine, was calculated as a function of intestinal $1,25(OH)_2D_3$ by combining the linear relationship between calbindin and $1,25(OH)_2D_3$ (A. Bar, unpublished observations) with the linear relationship between calbindin and fractional absorption (Bar and Hurwitz, 1979). This linear relationship (Hurwitz et al., 1983) was then used in the simulation model (Table II). The intercept of the function represents the vitamin D-independent calcium absorption, which is only about 10% in the chick, about one quarter of the value for vitamin D-fed chicks consuming normal calcium diets.

A special regulatory response of calcium absorption to the increased calcium needs during reproduction is discussed in Section VI.

C. The Renal Calcium Flow

The avian renal system differs from the mammalian kidney in several anatomical and physiological aspects. Urine empties into the cloaca and is voided together the the fecal material, but some may reach the upper colon. Both the colon and the lower ileum are capable of transporting water and electrolytes, under the influence of pituitary as well as adrenal hormones (as reviewed by Arad and Skadhauge, 1984). Thus, the final regulatory changes in water and electrolyte balance are made on the combined excretory products. This fact impeded research on renal (and intestinal) physiology in the fowl and also limits conclusions based on surgical approaches such as colostomy (Hurwitz and Griminger, 1961) or installation of cloacal cannulae (Clark and Wideman, 1977; Pines et al., 1983).

In addition to the arterial blood supply, the avian kidney is equipped with an afferent portal system through which blood is shunted from the femoral vein into the kidney. The portal flow of blood is regulated by a complex valvular system. Unilateral infusion into this portal system can be utilized to apply materials directly to the renal tubule, without undergoing filtration (Wideman and Braun, 1981; Kissell and Wideman, 1985). From an anatomical viewpoint, the avian kidney consists of a mixture of reptilian- and mammalian-type nephrons (Braun and Dantzler, 1984). The major urinary catabolic product of nitrogen metabolism is uric acid, which is excreted mostly in a solid form. Although the avian kidney handles minerals in a way similar to the mammalian kidney, secretion of phosphate, augmented by PTH, was observed in birds (Levinski and Davidson, 1957).

In contrast to rat or bovine species in which only a small fraction of the absorbed calcium load (0.5–2%) is handled by urinary excretion but similar to the human, close to 10% of an absorbed calcium load is excreted in the urine of birds (Hurwitz and Griminger, 1961). Furthermore, urinary calcium excretion is proportional to calcium intake and is reduced during egg shell formation (Fussell, 1960), suggesting that in the bird renal transport is important in calcium homeostasis.

The proportion between glomerular filtration rate and calcium reabsorption in birds is similar to that observed in mammals (96–99%). Parathyroidectomy substantially reduces calcium reabsorption and enhances calcium excretion (Clark and Wideman, 1977). During a $CaCl_2$ infusion into parathyroidectomized starlings, a net secretion of calcium was observed (Wideman, 1987). Exogenous PTH can restore the normal calcium reabsorption, but in normal birds it causes an increase in calcium excretion, probably due to the elevation of plasma calcium and the increased filtered load. PTH regulates phosphorus excretion by depressing phosphate resorption and by stimulating phosphate secretion and is the main regulator of the enzyme 1-hydroxylase, responsible for the production of $1,25(OH)_2D_3$. Calcitonin hardly affects calcium excretion, and $1,25(OH)_2D_3$ does not significantly influence renal calcium flux (Wideman, 1987).

According to Wideman (1987), the kidney in normal birds operates close to the maximal tubular reabsorption capacity for calcium $(T_mR\ Ca)$, and therefore does not respond to exogenous PTH. The simulation model, aimed mainly at normal animals, does not include any control of kidney calcium flow by calcium-regulating hormone. Since a detailed relationship between plasma calcium and kidney excretion was not available, the Nordin plot was adopted for use in the chicken. The curve was normalized by using the values for urinary calcium excretion observed by Hurwitz and Griminger (1961) and was fitted with a polynomial function (Table II).

V. Calcium Homeostasis System: Simulated Oscillatory Behavior

The equations described in Tables I and II can be integrated using numerical procedures with the aid of the computer operating at small increments of time, Δt. The results, which are discussed below, are obtained by simulation rather than by experimental procedures, although the validity of some was confirmed experimentally.

Simulation along $t = 168$ hours for chicks between 1 and 2 weeks of age demonstrated an oscillatory behavior of plasma calcium (amplitude of about 0.5 mg/100 ml) as well as of other components of the calcium-regulating system (Fig. 4). Oscillations are known in most of the physiological systems, as discussed in detail by Moore-Ede (1986). Goodwin (1963) even considered oscillations to be desirable is some control systems. Oscillations were observed in the plasma calcium of rats (Milhaud *et al.*, 1972) and humans (Jubitz *et al.*, 1972), in calcium absorption (Wrobel and Nagel, 1979), and in the 1-hydroxylase system in chicks (Miller and Norman, 1979). In the rat, the oscillations in plasma calcium were initially believed to reflect calcitonin action but more recently were related to a temporal self-organization of bone mineral (Staub *et al.*, 1988). The present simulated oscillations seem to be due to the dual effect of PTH in stimulation of the two control systems—bone resorption and intestinal absorption—each with a characteristic delay caused by the the sequences of events in the expression of the hormone (Hurwitz *et al.*, 1987a). An initial fall in plasma calcium is probably due to calcium removal from the central compartment into bone, driven by the growth process. Phase shifts are apparent among the oscillations of each of the subsystems, depending on the magnitude of stimulation and the decay rates. The negative feedback between plasma calcium and PTH is manifested by the opposing direction of the oscillations in both. There is hardly a noticeable phase shift between the two, due to the rapid decay rate of PTH. A larger phase shift is observed between the oscillation of PTH and that of the 1-hydroxylase enzyme, mostly due to the longer decay rate of the

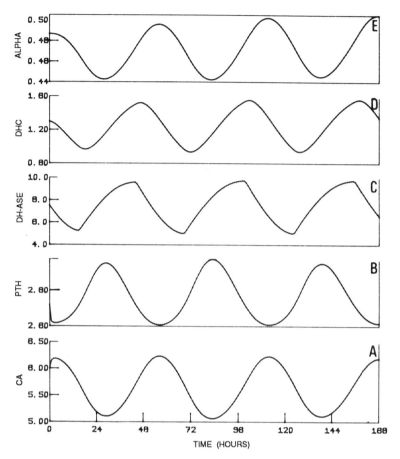

FIG. 4. Simulated oscillations in plasma calcium [(A) mg/dl], plasma PTH (B), kidney 1-hydroxylase [(C) pmol $\times$ 10^{-4}/sec], intestinal 1,25(OH)$_2$D$_3$ [(D) pmol/g], and fractional calcium absorption (E). Note the phase shift from (B) to (E). (From Hurwitz *et al.*, 1987a.)

enzyme. The change in the activity of the 1-hydroxylase enzyme results in secretion of 1,25(OH)$_2$D$_3$ into the circulation and accumulation of the hormone in the intestine. The delay in the appearance of hormone in the intestine, following an increase in the production of the hormone, is due to the decay of the hormone and the rates of transfer into and out of the mucosal cell, which in turn is dependent on the association with the intestinal receptor for the hormone (see Section III,C). Finally, the rate of calcium absorption is increased, by which means additional calcium flows into circulation at a time when

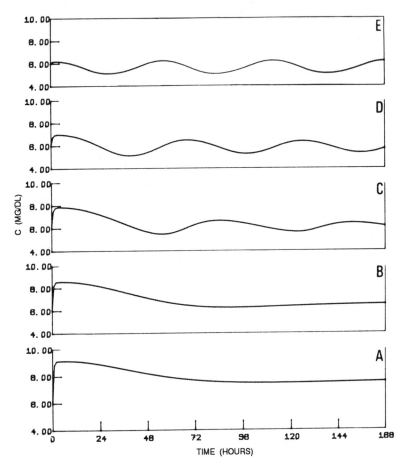

F$_{\text{IG}}$. 5. Dependence of oscillations in plasma calcium concentration (C) of chicks on their growth rate (simulated results). Fraction of maximal growth: (A) 0, (B) 0.25, (C) 0.5, (D) 0.75, (E) 1.00. (From Hurwitz *et al.*, 1987a.)

previous hypocalcemia had already been corrected by the action of PTH on bone. The additional calcium flow results in an overshoot in plasma calcium concentration, which in turn depresses PTH, followed by a decrease in bone resorption, leading to another decrease in plasma calcium and continued oscillatory behavior. The periodicity of the oscillation is about 55 hours.

The process of growth causes two major perturbations in the system of calcium homeostasis. First, it produces volume expansion, which by itself results in a reduction in plasma calcium. Second, bone growth driven by genetic factors (given by the growth equation and genotypic

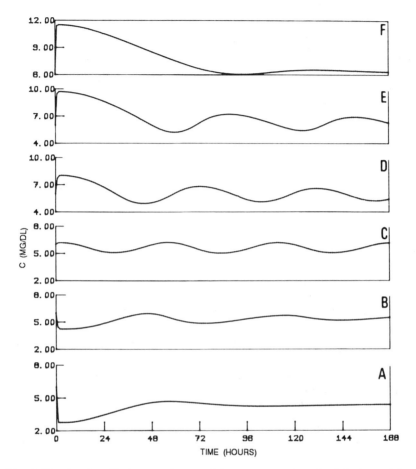

FIG. 6. Simulated oscillations in plasma calcium concentration (C) of chicks on different dietary calcium intakes: (A) 0.5%, (B) 0.7%, (C) 0.8%, (D) 1.2%, (E) 1.5%, (F) 2% Ca. (From Hurwitz *et al.*, 1987b.)

calcification) represents an important drain of calcium from the central pool. The implication of growth on the oscillatory behavior was studied by changing the parameters of the growth equation (Table I). The model itself then calculated the appropriate feed intake. As shown in Fig. 5, the periodicity of oscillation was gradually increased and its magnitude was diminished as growth was reduced, until oscillations virtually disappeared when growth was made equal to zero. The average plasma calcium concentration increased as growth was reduced, in agreement with experimental results (Bar and Hurwitz, 1981).

In another simulation study (Fig. 6), oscillations in plasma calcium were found to be dependent on calcium intake (Hurwitz *et al.*, 1987b). Oscillations at the high and low levels of dietary calcium disappear as the control system is overcome. The low intake of calcium cannot maintain any significant oscillation in the rate of calcium absorption, although the absorption mechanism operates at a maximal capacity. At high calcium concentrations, the system operates at minimal concentrations of PTH and $1,25(OH)_2D_3$, and their regulatory action is overcome, leading to loss of oscillations.

VI. Calcium Metabolism and Avian Reproduction

1. *General*

In the chicken, the ovary commences activity due to the action of gonadotropins, about 3 weeks prior to the onset of egg production. Morphologically, this activity is characterized by the hypertrophy of the ovary and the appearance of macroscopic yolk follicles. At the appropriate stage of development, the first ovulation occurs. During the 3-week prelaying period, the concentration of estrogen (and androgen) increases due to the secretory activity of the ovary, reaching a peak at the onset of egg laying (Bar *et al.*, 1978). This leads to the hypertrophy of the oviduct, which reaches a length of about 40 cm, and several other secondary morphological changes.

Each egg-laying cycle, initiated by ovulation, is completed after 24–27 hours. A rupture of the follicle results in the release of the ovum. The ovum is taken up by the upper part of the oviduct, the infundibulum. While moving down the oviduct, the ovum obtains its albumin coat in the magnum during about 4 hours, its two membranes in the isthmus within about 1 hour when it arrives at the shell gland. The forming egg remains in the shell gland for 17–19 hours. The first 2 hours are characterized by large movement of sodium and water into the egg and initiation of calcification. During the remaining time, the organic matrix and egg shell are deposited. Oviposition occurs at the end of this period. The initiation of ovary development and ovulation are sensitive to photoperiod.

The egg shell is made of about 5% organic collagen-like matrix, small concentrations of various inorganic ions, and close to 95% calcium carbonate (calcite). In the domestic chicken, the egg shell contains approximately 2 g of calcium, as compared with 20 g of calcium in its carcass. During deposition of the shell, the turnover rate of the central calcium pool is therefore extremely high. This rate of calcium turnover in the bird is considerably higher than that of female mammals during reproduction (Garel, 1987).

2. Calcium Transport in the Shell Gland

The mechanism of the transepithelial transport of calcium and its deposition in the egg shell is poorly understood. Ehrnspeck *et al.* (1971) concluded on the basis of *in vitro* experimentation that calcium was actively transported by the shell gland. However, the rates of calcium transport in this *in vitro* study and in others (Pearson and Goldner, 1973); Easten and Spaziani, 1978) were lower by several orders of magnitude than the *in vivo* transport.

The presence of receptors for $1,25(OH)_2D_3$ in the shell gland and the appearance of calbindin (see Section III,C,3) during shell calcification suggest that calbindin participates in calcium transport in the shell gland. Further support for the role of calbindin is supplied by the significant quantitative correlation between calbindin concentration and shell deposition (Bar *et al.*, 1984). The process, however, appears not to be regulated by $1,25(OH)_2D_3$, since the level of the hormone is not correlated with calbindin.

3. Calcium Metabolism during the Preovulatory and Early Egg-Laying Periods

The striking changes in calcium metabolism during the 3 weeks preceding egg laying are a most remarkable example of predictive or anticipatory regulation. These changes are consequences of the increase in the concentration of the gonadal hormones estrogen and androgen. In liver cells gonadal hormones induce vitellogenesis. The resulting protein, vitellogenin, is a 480-kDa dimer (Deely *et al.*, 1975; Tata and Smith, 1979). During transfer of the protein through the follicular membrane, each monomer is cleaved into one lipovitellin and two phosvitin molecules, which are the main egg yolk proteins. Similar proteins are involved in yolk formation in amphibia and reptiles.

The appearance of vitellogenin, a lipophosphoprotein with a high calcium-binding capacity, results in a large increase in the plasma calcium concentration from about 10 to 30 mg/dl. The entire calcium increment is due to bound calcium, with little change in the concentration of ionic calcium. Since vitellogenin is the precursor for yolk formation, the increase in plasma calcium prior to egg laying is not related to egg shell formation, as is sometimes erroneously assumed.

Two weeks prior to the onset of egg production (Hurwitz, 1964), medullary bone appears in the lumen of the long bones. The appearance of this osseous material was found to be a primary action of gonadal hormones and is initiated by DNA synthesis, and organic matrix synthesis and followed by calcification (Turner and Schraer, 1977; Kushuhara and Schraer, 1982).

Medullary bone is rich in cellular components, especially osteoclasts. In egg-laying hens, calcium is turned over in this bone extremely rapidly with a half-life of less than 2 days compared with months in cortical bone (Hurwitz, 1965). Birds are given a low-calcium diet or, during the hours of eggshell formation, form medullary bone (Benoit and Clavert, 1945). The high turnover rate and persistence during low calcium intakes may qualify this bone as a calcium "buffer" to be used during any temporary disruption of the calcium supply during shell formation, rather than being a simple calcium store.

Another important change during the preovulatory period is a small increase in circulating levels of $1,25(OH)_2D_3$ caused by the increase in the activity of the 1-hydroxylase enzyme (Bar $et\ al.$, 1978; Castillo $et\ al.$, 1979). Bar and Hurwitz (1979) suggested that this estrogen-induced increase in $1,25(OH)_2D_3$ was mediated by PTH, which increases due to calcium deficiency conditions created by vitellogenesis and medullary bone formation. Up-regulation of the PTH receptor by estrogen (Forte $et\ al.$, 1983) may also contribute to the increase in $1,25(OH)_2D_3$ production. $1,25(OH)_2D_3$ induces the increase in calcium absorption noted in early studies (Common, 1932). Some of the absorbed calcium flows into the forming medullary bone or is stored in trabecular bone and in cortical bone. As a result of this storage, the amount of body calcium approximately doubles. There is a further increase in $1,25(OH)_2D_3$ concentration after calcification of the first few shells (Montecuccoli $et\ al.$, 1977; Bar $et\ al.$, 1978). At the onset of production, energy (feed) intake is slow to respond to the increased energy demands, resulting in a temporary calcium deficiency. During this time, use is made of the prelaying calcium storage. Even given a virtually calcium-free diet, birds can continue egg-laying, although with a reduced rate of shell calcium deposition, for a period of 7–14 days, depending on the amount of calcium stored in bone.

4. Calcium Metabolism during the Laying Cycle

The short-term response of calcium absorption to shell formation (Hurwitz $et\ al.$ 1973) provides a powerful regulatory tool. Shell calcification imposes a calcium drain from body pools of about 150 mg/hr, when the average calcium intake is about 180 mg/hr. This calcium loss occurs only during 17 hours of residence in the shell gland and not during the 5- to 6-hour period when no shell is formed. The diurnal increase in calcium demand during shell formation is met by a regulatory increase in calcium absorption from 30 to 80% of dietary calcium. The supply of calcium through the night as the egg shell is formed reflects increased intake of feed late in the afternoon (Sauveur and Mongin, 1974) and storage of the food in the crop (esophagus), again in anticipation of the future short-term needs. The mechanism of the increase in calcium absorbability during egg shell calcification remains unknown. Kenny (1976) attempted to explain this short-term response by a corresponding change in the activity of 1-hydroyxlase and the production of $1,25(OH)_2D_3$. This observation was not confirmed by Montecuccoli et al. (1977). Moreover, the regulatory absorption response persisted even when the $1,25(OH)_2D_3$ intestinal axis was bypassed by feeding 1α-hydroxycholecalciferol (Bar et al., 1976), also indicating that the hormone was not responsible for the modulation of calcium absorption during the egg-laying cycle, in agreement with the conclusion by Nys et al. (1984). Calcium absorptive capacity, as measured by ^{45}Ca transport by duodenal loops in situ, did not increase during shell formation (Wasserman and Combs, 1978; S. Hurwitz, unpublished observations), arguing against the involvement of cellular processes in the regulation of absorption. A possible explanation, in line with the increase in calcium diffusibility, may be provided by the increase in the concentration of intestinal soluble calcium during shell formation (Sauver and Mongin, 1983). This increase, probably caused by the prevailing metabolic acidosis, raises the lumen–blood concentration gradient of calcium.

REFERENCES

Akiba, T., Endou, H., Koseki, C., Sakai, F., Horiuchi, N., and Suda, T. (1980). Localization of 25-hydroxyvitamin D_3-1α-hydroxylase activity in mammalian kidney. Biochem. Biophys. Res. Commun. **94**, 313–318.

Arad, Z., and Skadhauge, E. (1984). Plasma hormones (arginine vasotocin, prolactin, aldosterone and corticosterone) in relation to hydration state, NaCl intake and egg laying in fowls. J. Exp. Zool. **232**, 707–714.

Armbrecht, H. J., Wongsurawat, N., Zenser, T. V., and Davis, B. B. (1984). Effect of PTH and $1,25(OH)_2D_3$ on renal $25(OH)D_3$ metabolism, adenylate cyclase and protein kinase. Am. J. Physiol. **246**, E102–E107.

Arnett, T. R., and Dempster, D. W. (1987). A comparative study of disaggregated chick and rat osteoclasts in in vitro: Effects of calcitonin and prostaglandins. Endocrinology (Baltimore) **120**, 602–608.

Attie, M. F., Brown, E. M., Gardner, D. G., Spiegel, A. M., and Aurbach, G. D. (1980). Characterization of the dopamine-responsive adenylate cyclase of bovine parathyroid cells and its relationship to parathyroid hormone secretion. Endocrinology (Baltimore) **107**, 1776–1781.

Aubert, J.-P., Bronner, F., and Richelle, L. (1963). Quantitation of calcium metabolism theory. *J. Clin. Invest.* **42,** 885–897.

Aurbach, G. D. (1982). Polypeptide and amine hormone regulation of adenylate cyclase. *Annu. Rev. Physiol.* **44,** 653–666.

Aurbach, G. D., and Heath, D. A. (1974). Parathyroid hormone and calcitonin regulation of renal function. *Kidney Int.* **6,** 331–345.

Bar, A., and Hurwitz, S. (1973). Uterine valcium-binding protein in the laying fowl. *Comp. Biochem. Physiol.* A **45A,** 579–586.

Bar, A., and Hurwitz, S. (1979). The interaction between dietary calcium and gonadal hormones in their effect on plasma calcium, bone, 25-hydroxycholecalciferol-1-hydroxylase, and duodenal calcium-binding protein, measured by a radioimmunoassay in chicks. *Endocrinology (Baltimore)* **104,** 1455–1460.

Bar, A., and Hurwitz, S. (1980). The 25-hydroxycholecalciferol-1-hydroxylase activity of chicks' kidney cells: Direct effect of parathyroid. *FEBS Lett.* **113,** 328–330.

Bar, A., and Hurwitz, S. (1981). Relationship between cholecalciferol metabolism and growth in chicks as modified by age, breed and diet. *J. Nutr.* **11,** 399–404.

Bar, A., Hurwitz, S., and Cohen, I. (1972). Relationship between duodenal calcium-binding protein, parathyroid activity and various parameters of mineral metabolism in the rachitic and vitamin D-treated chick. *Comp. Biochem. Physiol. A.* **43A,** 519–526.

Bar, A., Hurwitz, S., and Edelstein, S. (1975). Response of renal calcium-binding protein: Independence of kidney vitamin D hydroxylation. *Biochim. Biophys. Acta* **411,** 106–112.

Bar, A., Eisner, U., Montecuccoli, G., and Hurwitz, S. (1976). Regulation of intestinal calcium absorption in the laying quail: Independent of kidney vitamin D hydroxylation. *J. Nutr.* **106,** 1336–1342.

Bar, A., Cohen, A., Edelstein, S., Shemesh, M., Montecuccoli, G., and Hurwitz, S. (1978). Involvement of cholecalciferol metablism in birds in the adaptation of calcium absorption to the needs during reproduction. *Comp. Biochem. Physiol. B* **59B,** 245–249.

Bar, A., Rosenberg, J., and Hurwitz, S. (1984). The lack of relationships between vitamin D_3 metabolites and Calcium-binding protein in the egg shell gland of laying birds. *Comp. Biochem. Physiol.* **78B,** 75–79.

Benoit, J., and Clavert, J. (1945). Hypercalcemia et ostéogènes medullair folliculinique chez la canard domestique soumis à regime à calcique. *C.R. Seances Soc. Biol. Ses Fil.* **139,** 737–742.

Bikle, D. D., Zolok, D. T., Morrissey, R. L., and Herman, R. H. (1978). Independence of 1,25-dihydroxyvitamin D_3-mediated calcium transport from *de novo* RNA and protein synthesis. *J. Biol. Chem.* **253,** 484–488.

Bikle, D. D., Munson, S., and Zolok, D. T. (1983). Calcium flux across chick duodenal brush border membrane vesicles: Regulation by 1,25-dihydroxyvitamin D. *Endocrinology (Baltimore)* **113,** 2072–2080.

Blunt, J. W., DeLuca, H. F., and Schmoes, H. K. (1968). 25-hydroxycholecalciferol. A biologically active metabolite of vitamin D_3. *Biochemistry* **7,** 3317–3322.

Boland, R. L. B. (1986). Plants as a source of vitamin D_3 metabolites. *Nutr. Rev.* **44,** 1–8.

Bonnier, G., and Cabanac, M. (1970). Régulation de la calcémie. Étude analogique. *Rev. Eur. Étud. Clin. Biol.* **15,** 551–557.

Booth, B. E., Tsai, H. C., and Morris, R. C., Jr. (1985). Vitamin D status regulates 25-hydroxyvitamin D_3-1-α-hydroxylase and its responsiveness to parathyroid hormone in the chick. *J. Clin. Invest.* **75,** 155–161.

Bowman, B. M., and Miller, S. C. (1986). The proliferation and differentiation of the bone-lining cell in estrogen-induced osteogenesis. *Bone* **7**, 351–357.

Braun, E. J., and Dantzler, W. H. (1984). Endocrine regulation of avian renal function. *J. Exp. Zool.* **232**, 715–723.

Brewer, H. B., and Ronan, R. (1970). Bovine parathyroid hormone: Amino acid sequence. *Proc. Natl. Acad. Sci. U.S.A.* **67**, 1862–1869..

Broadus, A. E. (1981). Nephrogenous cyclic AMP. *Recent Prog. Horm. Res.* **37**, 667–701.

Brommage, R., and DeLuca, H. F. (1985). Evidence that 1,25-dihydroxyvitamin D_3 is the physiologically active metabolite of vitamin D_3. *Endoc. Rev.* **6**, 491–511.

Bronner, F. (1987). Intestinal calcium absorption: Mechanisms and applications. *J. Nutr.* **117**, 1347–1352.

Bronner, F., and Aubert, J. P. (1965). Bone metabolism and regulation of blood calcium level in rats. *Am. J. Physiol.* **209**, 887–890.

Bronner, F., Pansu, D., and Stein, W. D. (1986). An analysis of intestinal calcium transport across the rat intestine. *Am. J. Physiol.* **250**, G561–G569.

Brown, E. M. (1983). Four-parameter model of the sigmoidal relationship between parathyroid hormone release and extracellular calcium concentration in normal and abnormal parathyroid tissue. *J. Clin. Endocrinol. Metab.* **56**, 572–581.

Brown, E. M., and Shoback, D. (1984). The relationship between PTH secretion and cytosolic calcium concentration in bovine parathyroid cells. *In* "Epithelial Calcium and Phosphorus Transport: Molecular and Cellular Aspects" (F. Bronner and M. Peterlik, eds.), pp. 139–144. Liss, New York.

Brown, E. M., Hurwitz, S., and Aurbach, G. D. (1976). Preparation of viable isolated bovine parathyroid cells. *Endocrinology (Baltimore)* **99**, 1582–1588.

Brown, E. M., Hurwitz, S., and Aurbach, G. D. (1977). Beta-adrenergic stimulation of cyclic AMP content and parathyroid hormone release from isolated parathyroid cells. *Endocrinology (Baltimore)* **100**, 1696–1702.

Canterbury, J. M., Bricker, L. A., Levy, G. S., Kozlovkis, P. L., Ruiz, E., Zull, J. E., and Reiss, E. (1975). Metabolism of bovine parathyroid hormone: Immunological and biological characteristics of fragments generated by liver perfusion. *J. Clin. Invest.* **55**, 1245–1253.

Cantley, L. K., Russell, J., Lettieri, D., and Sherwood, L. M. (1985). 1,25-Dihydroxyvitamin D_3 suppresses parathyroid hormone secretion from bovine parathyroid cells in tissue culture. *Endocrinology (Baltimore)* **117**, 2114–2119.

Cao, H., and Gay, C. V. (1985). Effects of parathyroid hormone and calcitonin on carbonic anhydrase location in osteoclasts of cultured embryonic chick bone. *Experientia* **41**, 1472–1474.

Carnes, D. L., Nickols, G. A., Anast, C. S., and Forte, L. R. (1980). Regulation of renal adenylate cyclase by parathyroid hormone. *Am. J. Physiol.* **239**, E396–E400.

Castillo, L., Tanaka, Y., Wineland, M. J., Jowsey, J. O., and DeLuca, H. F. (1979). Production of 1,25-dihydroxyvitamin D_3 and formation of medullary bone in the egg-laying hen. *Endocrinology (Baltimore)* **104**, 1598–1601.

Chambers, T. J., McSheehy, P. M. J., Thomson, B. M., and Fuller, K. (1985). The effect of calcium-regulating hormones and prostaglandins on bone resorption by osteoclasts disaggregated from neonatal rabbit bone. *Endocrinology (Baltimore)* **116**, 234–239. 234–239.

Chase, L. R., and Aurbach, G. D. (1967). Parathyroid function of the renal excretion of 3',5-adenylic acid. *Proc. Natl. Acad. Sci. U.S.A.* **58**, 518–525.

Chase, L. R., and Aurbach, G. D. (1970). The effect of parathyroid hormone on the concentration of adenosine $3',5'$-monophosphate in skeletal tissue, *in vitro. J. Biol. Chem.* **245**, 1520–1526.

Chin, J. E., Schalk, E. M., Kemic, M. L. S., and Wuthier, R. E. (1986). Effect of synthetic human parathyroid hormone on the levels of alkaline phosphatase activity and formation of alkaline phosphatase-rich matrix vesicles by primary cultures of chicken epiphyseal growth plate chondrocytes. *Bone Miner.* **1**, 421–436.

Clark, N. B., and Sasayama, Y. (1981). The role of parathyroid hormone in renal excretion of calcium and phosphate in the Japanese quail. *Gen. Comp. Endocrinol.* **45**, 234–241.

Clark, N. B., and Wideman, R. F., Jr. (1977). Renal excretion of phosphate and calcium in parathyroidectomized starlings. *Am. J. Physiol.* **233**, F138–F144.

Clark, N. B., and Wideman, R. F., Jr. (1980). Calcitonin stimulation of urine flow and sodium excretion in the starling. *Am. J. Physiol.* **238**, R406–R412.

Clark, N. B., Braun, E. J., and Wideman, R. F. (1976). Parathyroid hormone and renal excretion of phosphate and calcium in normal starlings. *Am. J. Physiol.* **231**, 1152–1158.

Cohn, D. V., Kumarasamy, R., and Ramp, W. K. (1986). Intracellular processing and secretion of parathyroid gland proteins. *Vitam. Horm. (N.Y.)* **43**, 283–316.

Common, R. H. (1932). Mineral balance studies in poultry. *J. Agric. Sci.* **22**, 576–594.

Copp, H. D., Byfield, P. G. H., Kerr, C. R., Newsome, F., Walker, V., and Watts, E. G. (1972). Calcitonin and ultimobranchial function in fishes and birds. *Int. Cong. Ser.—Excerpta Med.* **243**, 12–20.

Corradino, R. A. (1985). Effects of verapamil and dexamethasone on the 1,25-dihydroxy-vitamin D_3-mediated calcium absorptive mechanism in the organ cultured embryonic chick duodenum. *Biochem. Pharmacol.* **34**, 1971–1974.

Coty, W. A. (1980). A specific, high affinity binding protein for $1\alpha,25$ dihydroxy vitamin D in the chick oviduct shell gland. *Biochem. Biophys. Res. Commun.* **93**, 285–292.

Cravisio, G. L., Garrett, K. P., and Clemens, T. L. (1987). 1,25-dihydroxyvitamin D_3 induces the synthesis of vitamin D-dependent calcium-binding protein in cultured chick kidney cells. *Endocrinology (Baltimore)* **120**, 894–902.

Deely, R. G., Mullinix, K. P., Wetekam, W., Kronenberg, H. M., Meyers, M., Eldridge, J. D., and Goldhaber, R. F. (1975). Vitellogenin synthesis in the avian liver. *J. Biol. Chem.* **250**, 9060–9066.

DeLuca, H. F., Nakada, M., Tanaka, Y., Scinski, R., and Phelps, M. (1988). The plasma binding protein for vitamin D is a site of discrimination against vitamin D-2 compounds by the chick. *Biochim. Biophys. Acta* **965**, 16–21.

Dempster, D. W., Murills, R. J., Herbert, W. R., and Arnett, T. R. (1987). Biological activity of chicken calcitonin: Effects on neonatal rat and embryonic chick osteoclasts. *J. Bone Miner. Res.* **2**, 443–448.

de Vernejoul, M.-C., Horowitz, M., Demignon, J., Neff, L., and Baron, R. (1988). Bone resorption by isolated chick osteoclasts in culture is stimulated by murine spleen cell supernatant fluids (osteoclast activating factor) and inhibited by calcitonin and prostaglandin E_2 *J. Bone Miner. Res.* **3**, 69–80.

Dewhirst, F. E., Ago, J. M., Peros, W. J., and Stashenko, P. (1987). Synergism between parathyroid hormone and interleukin I in stimulating bone resorption in organ culture. *J. Bone Miner. Res.* **2**, 127–134.

Dousa, T. P. (1974). Effects of hormones on cyclic AMP formation in kidneys of non-mammalian vertebrates. *Am. J. Physiol.* **226**, 1193–1197.

Downes, C. P., and Michell, R. (1985). Inositol phospholipid breakdown as a receptor controlled generator of second messengers. *In* "Molecular Mechanisms of Transmembrane Signalling" (P. Cohen and M. D. Houslay, eds.), pp. 3–56. Elsevier, Amsterdam.

Easten, W. C., Jr., and Spaziani, E. (1978). On the control of calcium secretion in the avian shell gland (uterus). *Biol. Reprod.* **19**, 493–504.

Edelstein, S., Harell, A., Bar, A., and Hurwitz, S. (1975). The functional metabolism of vitamin D in chicks fed low-calcium and low-phosphorus diets. *Biochim. Biophys. Acta* **385**, 438–442.

Ehrenspeck, G., Schraer, H., and Schraer, R. (1971). Calcium transfer across isolated avian shell gland. *Am. J. Physiol.* **220**, 967–972.

Feher, J. J. (1983). Facilitated calcium diffusion by intestinal calcium-binding protein. *Am. J. Physiol.* **244**, C303–C307.

Feinblatt, J. D., Tai, L. R., and Kenny, A. D. (1974). Avian parathyroid glands in organ culture: Secretion of parathyroid hormone and calcitonin. *Endocrinology (Baltimore)* **96**, 282–288.

Fishman, S., Talpaz, H., Bar, A., and Hurwitz, S. (1986). Parameter estimation for ligand binding systems kinetics applied to 1,25-dihydroxycholecalciferol. *Anal. Biochem.* **154**, 144–151.

Fitzpatrick, L. A., Brandi, M. L., and Aurbach, G. D. (1986). Calcium-controlled secretion is effected through a guanine nucleotide regulatory protein in parathyroid cells. *Endocrinology (Baltimore)* **119**, 2700–2703.

Forte, L. R. (1983). Activation of renal adenylate cyclase by forskolin: Assessment of enzymatic activity in animal models of the secondary hyperparathyroid state. *Arch. Biochem. Biophys.* **225**, 898–905.

Forte, L. R., Langeluttig, S. G., Poelling, R. E., and Thomas, M. L. (1982). Renal parathyroid hormone receptor in the chick: Downregulation in secondary hyperparathyroid animal models. *Am. J. Physiol.* **242**, E154–E163.

Forte, L. R., Langeluttig, S. G., Biellier, H. V., Poelling, R. E., Magiola, L., and Thomas, M. L. (1983). Upregulation of kidney adenylate cyclase in the egg-laying hen: Role of estrogen. *Am. J. Physiol.* **245**, E273–280.

Fraser, D. R., and Kodicek, E. (1970). Unique biosynthesis by kidney of a biologically active vitamin D metabolite. *Nature (London)* **228**, 764–766.

Fraser, D. R., and Kodicek, E. S. (1973). Regulation of 25-hydroxycholecalciferol-1-hydroxylase by parathyroid hormone. *Nature (London), New Biol.* **241**, 163–166.

Fussell, M. H. (1960). Studies on the calcium and phosphorus metabolism in the hen with particular reference to absorption and excretion. Ph.D. Dissertation, Cambridge University.

Garabedian, M., Tanaka, Y., Holick, M. F., and DeLuca, H. F. (1974). Response of intestinal calcium transport and bone calcium mobilization to 1,25-dyhydroxyvitamin D_3 in thyroparathyroidectomized rats. *Endocrinology (Baltimore)* **94**, 1022–1027.

Garel, J.-M. (1987). Hormonal control of calcium metabolism during reproductive cycle in mammals. *Physiol. Rev.* **67**, 1–66.

Gonnerman, W. A., Ramp, W. K., and Toverud, S. U. (1975). Vitamin D, dietary calcium and parathyroid interactions in chicks. *Endocrinology (Baltimore)* **96**, 275–281.

Goodwin, B. C. (1963). "Temporal Organization in Cells." Academic Press, New York.

Gowen, M., and Mundy, G. R. (1986). Actions of recombinant interleukin 1, interleukin 2, and interferon-gamma on bone resorption *in vitro*. *J. Immunol.* **136**, 2478–2482.

Gylfe, E., Larsson, R., Johansson, H., Nygren, P., Rastad, J., Wallfelt, C., and

Akerström, G. (1986). Calcium-activated calcium permeability in parathyroid cells. *FEBS Lett.* **205**, 132–136.

Hall, A. K., Reichel, H., and Norman, A. W. (1988). Differential effects of 1,25-dihydroxyvitamin D_3 upon intestinal vitamin D_3-dependent calbindin (a 28,000-dalton calcium binding protein) and its mRNA in D-replete and D-deficient chickens. *Arch. Biochem. Biophys.* **260**, 645–652.

Harrison, H. E., and Harrison, H. C. (1960). Transfer of Ca^{45} across intestinal wall *in vitro* in relation to vitamin D and cortisol. *Am. J. Physiol.* **199**, 265–271.

Harrison, H. E., and Harrison, H. C. (1963). Theories of vitamin D action. *In* "Transfer of Calcium and Strontium Across Biological Membranes" (R. H. Wasserman, ed.), pp. 229–251. Academic Press, New York.

Haussler, M. R. (1986). Vitamin D receptors: Nature and function. *Annu. Rev. Nutr.* **6**, 527–562.

Haussler, M. R., Nagode, L. A., and Rasmussen, H. (1970). Induction of intestinal brush border alkaline phosphatase by vitamin D and its identity with CaATPase. *Nature (London)* **228**, 1199–1201.

Heinrich, G., Kronenberg, H. M., Potts, J. T., Jr., and Habener, J. F. (1984). Gene encoding parathyroid hormone: Nucleotide sequence of the rat gene and deduced amino acid sequence of rat preproparathyroid hormone. *J. Biol. Chem.* **259**, 3320–3329.

Henry, H. L. (1981). 25(OH)D_3 metabolism in kidney cell cultures: Lack of direct effect of estradiol. *Am. J. Physiol.* **240**, E119–E124.

Henry, H. L. (1985). Parathyroid hormone modulation of 25-hydroxyvitamin D_3 metabolism by cultured chick kidney cells is mimicked and enhanced by forskolin. *Endocrinology (Baltimore)* **116**, 503–510.

Hermann-Erlee, M. P. M., Nijweide, P. J., van der Meer, J. M., and Ooms, M. A. C. (1983). Action of bPTH and bPTH fragments on embryonic bone, *in vitro:* Dissociation of the cAMP and bone resorbing response. *Calcif. Tissue Int.* **35**, 70–77.

Hesch, R. D., Ebel, H., Hhrmann, R., and Jueppner, H. (1978). Endocrinological aspects of PTH metabolism in the kidney. *Contrib. Nephrol.* **13**, 104–114.

Holick, M. F., Schnoes, H. K., and DeLuca, H. F. (1971). Identification of 1,25-dehydroxycholecalciferol. A metabolite of vitamin D_3 metabolically active in the intestine. *Proc. Natl. Acad. Sci. U.S.A.* **68**, 803–804.

Holick, S. A., Holick, M. F., Tavela, T. E., Schnoes, H. K., and DeLuca, H. F. (1976). Metabolism of 1 α-hydroxyvitamin D_3 in the chick. *J. Biol. Chem.* **251**, 1025–1028.

Homma, T., Watanabe, M., Hirose, S., Kanai, A., Kangawa, K., and Matsuo, H. (1986). Isolation and determination of the amino acid sequence of chicken calcitonin I from chicken ultimobranchial glands. *J. Biochem. (Tokyo)* **100**, 459–467.

Hoy, D. A., Ramberg, C. F., Jr., and Horst, R. L. (1988). Evidence that discrimination against ergocalciferol by the chick is the result of enhanced metabolic clearance rates for its mono- and dihydroxylated metabolites. *J. Nutr.* **118**, 633–638.

Hunziker, W. (1986). The 28-kDa vitamin D-dependent calcium-binding protein has a six-domain structure. *Proc. Natl. Acad. Sci. U.S.A.* **83**, 7578–7582.

Hurwitz, S. (1964). Calcium metabolism of pullets at the onset of egg production, as influenced by dietary calcium level. *Poult. Sci.* **43**, 1462–1472.

Hurwitz, S. (1965). Calcium turnover in different bone segments of laying fowl. *Am. J. Physiol.* **208**, 203–207.

Hurwitz, S. (1978). Calcium metabolism in birds. *In* "Chemical Zoology" (M. Florkin and B. T. Scheer, eds.), Vol. 10, pp. 273–306. Academic Press, New York.

Hurwitz, S. (1989). Parathyroid hormone. *In* "Vertebrate Endocrinology: Fundumentals and Biomedical Implications" (P. K. T. Pang and M. P. Schreibman, eds.), Vol. 3. Academic Press, San Diego, California, in press.

Hurwitz, S., and Bar, A. (1965). Absorption of calcium and phosphorus along the gastrointestinal tract of the laying fowl as influenced by dietary calcium and egg shell formation. *J. Nutr.* **86**, 433–438.

Hurwitz, S., and Bar, A. (1966). Calcium depletion and repletion in laying hens. 1. Effect on calcium in various bone segments, in egg shells in plasma, and on calcium balance. *Poult. Sci.* **45**, 345–352.

Hurwitz, S., and Bar, A. (1968). Activity, concentration, and lumen–blood electrochemical potential difference of calcium in the intestine of the laying hen. *J. Nutr.* **95**, 647–654.

Hurwitz, S., and Bar, A. (1972). Site of vitamin D action in chick intestine. *Am. J. Physiol.* **222**, 761–767.

Hurwitz, S., and Griminger, P. (1961). Partition of calcium and phosphorus excretion in the laying hen. *Nature (London)* **180**, 759–760.

Hurwitz, S., and Plavnik, I. (1986). Carcass minerals in chickens (*Gallus domesticus*) during growth. *Comp. Biochem. Physiol. A* **83A**, 225–227.

Hurwitz, S., Harrison, H. C., and Harrison, H. E. (1967). Comparison of the actions of vitamin D_2 and D_3 in the chick with their retention in serum, liver and intestinal mucosa. *J. Nutr.* **91**, 208–212.

Hurwitz, S., Bar, A., and Cohen, I. (1973). Regulation of calcium absorption by fowl intestine. *Am. J. Physiol.* **225**, 150–154.

Hurwitz, S., Weiselberg, M., Eisner, U., Bartov, I., Riesenfeld, G., Sharvit, M., Niv, A., and Bornstein, S. (1980). The energy requirements and performance of growing chickens and turkeys as affected by environmental temperature. *Poult. Sci.* **59**, 2290–2299.

Hurwitz, S., Fishman, S., Bar, A., Pines, M., Riesenfeld, G., and Talpaz, H. (1983). Simulation of calcium homeostasis: Modeling and parameter estimation. *Am. J. Physiol.* **245**, R664–R672.

Hurwitz, S., Fishman, S., Bar, A., and Talpaz, H. (1984). Role of the 1,25-dihydroxycholecalciferol-regulated component of calcium absorption in calcium homeostasis. *In* "Epithelial Calcium and Phosphate Transport: Molecular and Cellular Aspects" (F. Bronner and M. Peterlik, eds.), pp. 357–362. Liss, New York.

Hurwitz, S., Fishman, S., and Talpaz, H. (1987a). Model of plasma calcium regulation: System oscillations induced by growth. *Am. J. Physiol.* **252**, R1173–R1181.

Hurwitz, S., Fishman, S., and Talpaz, H. (1987b). Calcium dynamics: A model system approach. *J. Nutr.* **73**, 177–185.

Isaksson, O. G. P., Lindahl, A., Nilsson, A., and Isgaard, J. (1987). Mechanism of the stimulatory effect of growth hormone on longitudinal bone growth. *Endocr. Rev.* **8**, 426–438.

Jacob, M., and Chan, C. M. (1987). Effect of variations in dietary calcium on renal and intestinal calcium-binding proteins. *Pediatr. Res.* **22**, 518–523.

Jand, S. S., Tolnai, S., and Lawson, D. E. M. (1981). Immunohistochemical localization of vitamin D-dependent calcium-binding protein in duodenum, kidney, uterus and cerebellum of chickens. *Histochemistry* **71**, 99–116.

Jaros, G. G., Coleman, T. G., and Guyton, A. C. (1979). Model of short-term regulation of calcium ion concentration. *Simulation* **32**, 193–204.

Jones, G., Schnoes, H. K., and DeLuca, H. F. (1976). An *in vitro* study of vitamin D_2 hydroxylases in the chick. *J. Biol. Chem.* **251**, 24–28.

Jubitz, W. J., Canterbury, M., Reiss, E., and Tyler, F. H. (1972). Circadian rhythm in serum parathyroid hormone concentration in human subjects: Correlation with serum calcium, phosphate, albumen and growth hormone levels. *J. Clin. Invest.* **51,** 2040–2046.

Kawashima, K., Iwata, S., and Endo, H. (1980). Selective activation of diaphyseal chondrocytes by parathyroid hormone, calcitonin and N^6,O^2-dibutyryl adenosine $3'5'$-cyclic monophosphoric acid in proteoglycan synthesis of chick embryonic femur cultivated *in vitro*. *Endocrinol. Jpn.* **27,** 357–361.

Kemper, B. (1986). Molecular biology of parathyroid hormone. *CRC Crit. Rev. Biochem.* **19,** 353–379.

Kenny, A. D. (1976). Vitamin D metabolism: Physiological regulation in egg laying Japanese quail. *Am. J. Physiol.* **230,** 1609–1615.

Keutman, H. T., Sauer, M. M., Hendy, G. N., O'Riordan, J. L. H., and Potts, J. T., Jr. (1978). Complete amino acid sequence of human parathyroid hormone. *Biochemistry* **17,** 5723–5729.

Khosla, S., Demay, M., Pines, M., Hurwitz, S., Potts, J. T., Jr., and Kronenberg, H. M. (1988). Nucleotide sequence of cloned cDNAs encoding chicken preproparathyroid hormone. *J. Bone Miner. Res.* **3,** 689–698.

Kinder, B. K., Delahunt, N. G., Jamiesen, J. D., and Gorelick, F. S. (1987). Calcium-calmolulin-dependent protein kinase in hyperplastic human parathyroid glands. *Endocrinology (Baltimore)* **120,** 170–177.

Kissell, R. E., and Wideman, R. F., Jr. (1985). Parathyroid transplants and unilateral renal delivery of parathyroid hormone in domestic fowl. *Am. J. Physiol.* **249,** R732–R739.

Kojima, I., Kojima, K., and Rasmussen, H. (1985). Role of calcium fluxes in the sustained phase of angiotensin II-mediated aldosterone secretion from adrenal glomerulosa cells. *J. Biol. Chem.* **260,** 9177–9184.

Kraintz, L., and Intcher, K. (1969). Effect of calcitonin on the domestic fowl. *Can J. Physiol. Pharmacol.* **47,** 313–315.

Kronenberg, H. M. (1986). The human parathyroid hormone gene: Regulation of transcription and function of the precursor protein. *In* "Advances in Skeletogenesis/3" (S. Hurwitz and J. Sela, eds.), pp. 213–217. Heiliger Publ. Co., Jerusalem.

Kushuhara, S., and Schraer, H. (1982). Cytology and autoradiography of estrogen-induced differentiation of avian endosteal cells. *Calcif. Tissue Int.* **34,** 352–358.

Lasmoles, F., Jullienne, A., Desplan, C., Milhaud, G., and Moukhtar, M. S. (1985). Structure of chicken calcitonin predicted by partial nucleotide sequence of its precursor. *FEBS Lett.* **180,** 113–116.

Leach, R. M., Jr., and Gay, C. V. (1987). Role of epiphyseal cartilage in endrochondral bone formation. *J. Nutr.* **117,** 784–790.

LeBlanc, B., Wyers, M., Cohn-Bendit, F., Legall, J. M., and Thibault, E. (1986). Histology and histomorphometry of the tibia growth in two turkey strains. *Poult. Sci.* **65,** 1787–1795.

Levinski, N. G., and Davidson, D. G. (1957). Renal action of parathyroid hormone in the chicken. *Am. J. Physiol.* **191,** 530–536.

Liang, C. T., Balakir, R. A., Barnes, J., and Sacktor, B. (1984). Responses of chick renal cell to parathyroid hormone: Effect of vitamin D. *Am. J. Physiol.* **246,** C401–C406.

MacGregor, R. R., Chu, L. L. H., Hamilton, J. W., and Cohn, D. V. (1976). Partial purification of parathyroid hormone from chicken parathyroid glands. *Endocrinology (Baltimore)* **92,** 1312–1317.

Mayel-Afshar, S., Lane, S. M., and Lawson, D. E. M. (1988). Relationship between the levels of calbindin and calbindin mRNA in chick intestine. *J. Biol. Chem.* **263**, 4355–4361.

Mayer, G. P., Keaton, J. A., Hurst, J. G., and Habener, J. F. (1979). Effect of plasma calcium concentration on the relative proportion of hormone and carboxyl fragments in parathyroid venous blood. *Endocrinology (Baltimore)* **104**, 1778–1784.

McDonnell, D. P., Mangelsdorf, D. J., Pike, J. W., Haussler, M. R., and O'Malley, B. W. (1987). Molecular cloning of complementary DNA encoding the avian receptor for vitamin D. *Science* **235**, 1214–1217.

McKee, M. D., and Murray, T. M. (1985). Binding of intact parathyroid hormone to chicken renal plasma membranes: Evidence for a second binding site with carboxyl-terminal specificity. *Endocrinology (Baltimore)* **117**, 1930–1939.

McSheehy, P. M. J., and Chambers, T. J. (1986). Osteoblastic cells mediate osteoclastic responsiveness to parathyroid hormone. *Endocrinology (Baltimore)* **118**, 824–828.

Milhaud, G., Perault-Staub, A. M., and Staub, J. F. (1972). Diurnal variations in plasma calcium and calcitonin concentration functions in the rat. *J. Physiol. (London)* **222**, 559–567.

Miller, B., and Norman, A. W. (1979). Studies on the metabolism of calciferol. XIV. Evidence of a circadian rhythm in the activity of the 25-hydroxyvitamin D_3-1-hydroxylase. *Biochem. Biophys. Res. Commun.* **88**, 730–734.

Miller, S. C., and Kenny, A. D. (1985). Activation of avian medullary bone osteoclasts by oxidized synthetic parathyroid hormone (1–34). *Proc. Soc. Exp. Biol. Med.* **179**, 38–43.

Miller, S. C., Bowman, B. M., and Myers, R. L. (1984). Morphological and ultrastructural aspects of the activation of avian medullary bone osteoclasts by parathyroid hormone. *Anat. Rec.* **208**, 223–231.

Minvielle, S., Cressent, M., Lasmoles, F., Jullienne, A., Milhaud, G., and Moukhtar, M. S. (1986). Isolation and partial characterization of the calcitonin gene in lower vertebrate. Predicted structure of avian calcitonin gene-related peptide. *FEBS Lett.* **203**, 7–10.

Miyaura, C., Segawa, A., Nagasawa, H., Abe, E., and Suda, T. (1986). Effects of retinoic acid on the activation and fusion of mouse alveolar macrophages induced by $1\alpha,25$-dihydroxy vitamin D_3. *J. Bone Miner. Res.* **1**, 359–368.

Montecuccoli, G., Bar, A., Cohen, A., and Hurwitz, S. (1977). The role of 25-hydroxycholecalciferol-1-hydroxylase in the response of calcium absorption to reproductive activity in birds. *Comp. Biochem. Physiol. A* **57A**, 335–339.

Moore-Ede, M. C. (1986). Physiology of the circadian timing system: Predictive versus reactive homeostasis. *Am. J. Physiol.* **250**, R735–R762.

Navickis, R. J., Katzenellenbogen, B. S., and Nalbandov, A. V. (1979). Effect of sex steroid hormones and vitamin D_3 on calcium-binding proteins in the chick shell gland. *Biol. Reprod.* **21**, 1153–1162.

Nemere, I., Theofan, G., and Norman, A. W. (1987). 1,25-Dihydroxyvitamin D_3 regulates tubulin expression in chick intestine. *Biochem. Biophys. Res. Commun.* **148**, 1270–1276.

Nemeth, E. F., and Scarpa, A. (1986). Cytosolic Ca^{2+} and the regulation of secretion in parathyroid cells. *FEBS Lett.* **203**, 15–19.

Nemeth, E. F., and Scarpa, A. (1987). Rapid mobilization of cellular Ca^{2+} in bovine parathyroid cells evoked by extracellular divalent cations. *J. Biol. Chem.* **262**, 5188–5196.

Neuman, M., Neuman, W. F., and Lane, K. (1979). Formation and serum disappearance of fragments of parathyroid hormone in the infused dog. *Calcif. Tissue Int.* **28**, 70–81.

Niall, H., Keutmann, H., Sauer, R., Hogan, M., Dawson, B., Aurbach, G. D., and Potts, J. T., Jr. (1970). The amino acid sequence of bovine parathyroid hormone. I. *Hoppe-Seyler's Z. Physiol. Chem.* **351**, 1586–1588.

Nicholson, G. C., Livesey, S. A., Mosley, J. M., and Martin, T. J. (1986). Action of calcitonin, parathyroid hormone, and prostaglandin E_2 on cAMP formation in chicken and rat osteoclasts. *J. Cell. Biochem.* **31**, 229–241.

Nicholson, G. C., Moseley, J. M., Sexton, P. M., and Martin, T. J. (1987). Chicken osteoclasts do not possess calcitonin receptors. *J. Bone Miner. Res.* **2**, 53–60.

Nicolayesen, R., Eeg-Larsen, R. N., and Malm, O. J. (1953). Physiology of calcium metabolism. *Physiol. Rev.* **33**, 424–444.

Nieto, A., Noya, F., and R-Candela, J. L. (1973). Isolation and properties of two calcitonins from chicken ultimobranchial gland. *Biochim. Biophys. Acta* **322**, 383–391.

Nijweide, P. J., Burger, E. H., and Feyen, J. H. M. (1986). Cells of bone: Proliferation, differentiation, and hormonal regulation. *Physiol. Rev.* **66**, 855–886.

Nissenson, R. A., and Arnaud, C. D. (1979). Properties of the parathyroid hormone receptor-adenylate cyclase system in chicken renal plasma membranes. *J. Biol. Chem.* **254**, 1469–1475.

Norman, A. W., Roth, J., and Orci, L. (1982). The vitamin D endocrine system: Steroid metabolism, hormone receptors, and biological responses (calcium-binding proteins). *Endocr. Rev.* **3**, 331–366.

Norman, A. W. (1987). Studies on the vitamin D endocrine system in the avian. *J. Nutr.* **117**, 797–807.

Norman, A. W., Myrtle, J. F., Midgett, R. J., Nowicki, H. G., Williams, V., and Popjak, G. (1971). 1,25-Dihydroxycholecalciferol: Identification of the proposed active form of vitamin D_3 in the intestine. *Science* **173**, 51–54.

Nys, Y., N'guyen, T. M., and Garabedian, M. (1984). Involvement of 1,25-dihydroxycholecalciferol in the short- and long-term increase in intestinal calcium absorption in laying hens: Stimulation by gonadal hormones is partly independent of 1,25-dihydroxycholecalciferol. *Comp. Biochem. Physiol. A* **53A**, 54–59.

Omdahl, J. L., and DeLuca, H. F. (1973). Regulation of vitamin D metabolism and function. *Physiol. Rev.* **53**, 327–372.

Omdahl, J. L., Hunsaker, L. A., Evan, A. P., and Torrez, P. (1980). *In vitro* regulation of kidney 25-hydroxyvitamin D_3-hydroxylase enzyme activities by vitamin D_3 metabolites. *J. Biol. Chem.* **225**, 7460–7466.

Ornoy, A., Goodwin, D., Noff, D., and Edelstein, S. (1978). 24,25-Dihydroxyvitamin D is a metabolite of vitamin D essential for bone formation. *Nature (London)* **276**, 517–519.

Pang, P. K. T., Zhang, R. H., and Yang, M. C. M. (1984). Hypotensive action of parathyroid hormone in chicken. *J. Exp. Zool.* **232**, 691–696.

Parfitt, A. M. (1987). Bone and plasma calcium homeostasis, *Bone* **8**, Suppl. 1, S1–S8.

Pearson, T. W., and Goldner, A. M. (1973). Calcium transport across avian uterus. I. Effect of electrolyte substitution. *Am. J. Physiol.* **225**, 1508–1512.

Pike, J. W., Gooze, L. L., and Haussler, M. R. (1980). Biochemical evidence for 1,25-dihydroxyvitamin D receptor macromolecules in parathyroid, pancreatic, pituitary and placental tissues. *Life Sci.* **26**, 407–414.

Pines, M., and Hurwitz, S. (1988). The effect of parathyroid hormone and atrial natriuretic peptide on cyclic nucleotides production and proliferation of avian epiphyseal growth plate chondroprogenitor cells. *Endocrinology (Baltimore)* **123**, 360–305.

Pines, M., Polin, D., and Hurwitz, S. (1983). Urinary cyclic AMP excretion in birds: Dependence on parathyroid hormone activity. *Gen. Comp. Endocrinol.* **49**, 90–96.

Pines, M., Bar, A., and Hurwitz, S. (1984). Isolation and purification of avian parathyroid hormone using high performance liquid chromatography, and some of its properties. *Gen. Comp. Endocrinol.* **53**, 224–231.

Proscal, D. A., Okamura, W. H., and Norman, A. W. (1975). Structural requirements for the interaction of $1\alpha,25(OH)_2$-vitamin D_3 with its chick intestinal receptor system. *J. Biol. Chem.* **250**, 8382–8388.

Raisz, L. G. (1963). Stimulation of bone resorption by parathyroid hormone in tissue culture. *Nature (London)* **197**, 1015–1016.

Rappaport, M. S., and Stern, P. (1986). Parathyroid hormone and calcitonin modify mosital phospholipid metabolism in fetal rat limb bones. *J. Bone Miner. Res.* **1**, 173–179.

Rasmussen, H., Fontain, O., Max, E. E., and Goodman, D. B. P. (1979). The effect of 1-hydroxyvitamin D_3-administration on calcium transport in chick intestine brush border vesicles. *J. Biol. Chem.* **254**, 2993–2999.

Ribovich, M. L., and DeLuca, H. F. (1976). Intestinal calcium transport: Parathyroid hormone and adaptation to dietary calcium. *Arch. Biochem. Biophys.* **175**, 256–261.

Rodan, G. A., and Rodan, S. B. (1983). Expression of the osteoblastic genotype. *Bone Miner. Res.* **2**, 244–285.

Rodan, S. B., and Rodan, G. A. (1974). The effect of parathyroid hormone and thyrocalcitonin on the accumulation of cyclic adenosine $3',5'$-monophosphate in freshly isolated bone cells. *J. Biol. Chem.* **249**, 3068–3074.

Rosenberg, J., Pines, M., and Hurwitz, S. (1987). Stimulation of chick adrenal stereogenesis by avian parathyroid hormone. *J. Endocrinol.* **116**, 91–95.

Rosenberg, R., Hurwitz, S., and Bar, A. (1986). Regulation of kidney calcium-binding protein in the bird (*Gallus domesticus*). *Comp. Biochem. Physiol. A* **83A**, 277–281.

Rosenblatt, M. (1982). Structure–activity relations in the calcium-regulating peptide hormones. *In* "Endocrinology of Calcium Metabolism" (J. A. Parsons, ed.), pp. 103–141. Raven Press, New York.

Russell, J., and Sherwood, L. M. (1989). Nucleotide sequence of the DNA complementary to avian (chicken) pre-proparathyroid hormone mRNA and the deduced sequence of the hormone precursor. *Mol. Endocrinol.* **3**, 325.

Sauer, R. T., Niall, H. D., Hogan, M. L., Keutmann, H. T., O'Riordan, J. L. H., and Potts, J. T., Jr. (1974). The amino acid sequence of porcine parathyroid hormone. *Biochemistry* **13**, 1994–1999.

Sauveur, B., and Mongin, P. (1974). Effect of time-limited calcium meal upon food and calcium ingestion and egg quality. *Br. Poult. Sci.* **15**, 305–313.

Sauveur, B., and Mongin, P. (1983). Plasma inorganic phosphorus concentration during eggshell formation. II. Inverse relationships with intestinal calcium content and eggshell weight. *Reprod. Nutr. Dev.* **23**, 755–764.

Schachter, D., Dowdle, E. B., and Schenker, H. (1960). Active transport of calcium by the small intestine of the rat. *Am. J. Physiol.* **200**, 263–268.

Schneider, N., Teitelbaum, A. P., and Neuman, W. F. (1980). Tissue deposition and metabolism of ^{125}I-labeled synthetic amino-terminal parathyroid hormone bPTH (1–34). *Calcif. Tissue Int.* **30**, 147–150.

Seino, Y., Yamaoka, K., Ishida, M., Yabuuchi, H., and Ichikawa M. (1982). Biochemical characterization of $1,25(OH)_2D_3$ receptors in chick embryonal duodenal cytosol. *Calcif. Tissue Int.* **34,** 265–269.

Simkiss, K. (1961). Calcium metabolism and avian reproduction. *Biol. Rev. Cambridge Philos. Soc.* **36,** 321–367.

Spanos, E., Barrett, D., MacIntyre, I., Pike, J. W., Safilian, E. F., and Haussler, M. R. (1978). Effect of growth hormone on vitamin D metabolism. *Nature (London)* **273,** 246.

Spanos, E., Brown, D. J., Stevenson, J. C., and MacIntyre, I. (1981). Stimulation of 1,25-dihydroxycholecalciferol production by prolactin and related peptides in intact renal preparations *in vitro. Biochim. Biophys. Acta* **672,** 7–15.

Staub, J. F., Tracqui, P., Brezillon, P., Milhaud, G., and Perault-Staub, A. M. (1988). Calcium metabolism in the rat: A temporal self-organized model. *Am. J. Physiol.* **254,** R134–R149.

Steenbock, H., Kletzien, S. W. F., and Halpin, J. G. (1932). The reaction of the chicken to irradiated ergosterol or irradiated yeast as contrasted with the natural vitamin D of fish liver oils. *J. Biol. Chem.* **97,** 249–264.

Stern, P. H. (1980). The D vitamins and bone. *Pharmacol. Rev.* **32,** 47–80.

Takahashi, N., Abe, E., Tanabe, R., and Suda, T. (1980). A high-affinity cytosol binding protein for $1\alpha,25$ dihydroxyvitamin D_3 in the uterus of Japanese quail. *Biochem. J.* **190,** 513–518.

Talmage, R. V., Roycroft, J. H., and Anderson, J. J. B. (1975). Morphological and physiological considerations in a new concept of calcium transport in bone. *Am. J. Anat.* **129,** 467–476.

Tam, C. S., Heersche, J. N. M., Murray, T. M., and Parsons, J. A. (1982). Parathyroid hormone stimulates the bone apposition rate independently of its resorptive action: Differential effects of intermittent and continuous administration. *Endocrinology (Baltimore)* **110,** 506–512.

Tanaka, Y., Castillo, L., and DeLuca, H. F. (1976). Control of renal vitamin D hydroxylases in birds by sex hormones. *Proc. Natl. Acad. Sci. U.S.A.* **731,** 2701.

Tata, J. R., and Smith, D. F. (1979). Vitellogenesis: A versatile model for hormonal regulation of gene expression. *Recent Prog. Horm. Res.* **35,** 47–90.

Tauber, S. D. (1967). The ultimobranchial origin of thyrocalcitronin. *Proc. Natl. Acad. Sci. U.S.A.* **58,** 1684–1687.

Theofan, G., King, M. W., Hall, A. K., and Norman, A. W. (1987). Expression of calbindin-D_{28k} mRNA as a function of altered serum calcium and phosphorus levels in vitamin D-replete chick intestine. *Mol. Cell. Endocrinol.* **54,** 135–140.

Turner, R. T., and Schraer, H. (1977). Estrogen-induced sequential changes in avian bone metabolism. *Calcif. Tissue Res.* **24,** 157–160.

Wasserman, R. H. (1963). Vitamin D and the absorption of calcium and strontium *in vivo. In* "The Transfer of Calcium and Strontium across Biological Membranes" (R. H. Wasserman, ed.), pp. 197–228. Academic Press, New York.

Wasserman, R. H., and Combs, G. F. (1978). Relation of vitamin D-dependent intestinal calcium-binding protein to calcium absorption during the ovulatory cycle in Japanese quail. *Proc. Soc. Exp. Biol. Med.* **159,** 286–287.

Wasserman, R. H., and Corradino, R. A. (1973). Vitamin D, calcium, and protein synthesis. *Vitam. Horm. (N.Y.)* **31,** 43–103.

Wasserman, R. H., and Fullmer, C. S. (1983). Calcium transport proteins, calcium absorption, and vitamin D. *Annu. Rev. Physiol.* **45,** 375–390.

Wasserman, R. H., and Taylor, A. N. (1966). Vitamin D -induced calcium-binding protein in chick intestinal mucosa. *Science* **152,** 791–793.

Wecksler, W. R., and Norman, A. W. (1980). Biochemical properties of 1α,25-dihydroxy-vitamin D receptors. *J. Steroid Biochem.* **13,** 977–989.

Wideman, R. F., Jr. (1987). Renal regulation of avian calcium and phosphorus metabolism. *J. Nutr.* **117,** 808–815.

Wideman, R. F., Jr., and Braun, E. J. (1981). Stimulation of avian renal phosphate secretion by parathyroid hormone. *Am. J. Physiol.* **241,** F263–F272.

Wideman, R. F., Jr., and Youtz, S.L. (1985). Comparison of avian renal responses to bovine parathyroid extract, synthetic bovine (1–34) parathyroid hormone, and synthetic human (1–34) parathyroid hormone. *Gen. Comp. Endocrinol.* **57,** 480–490.

Wilson, P. W., and Lawson, D. E. M. (1977). 1,25-Dihydroxyvitamin D stimulation of specific membrane proteins in chick intestine. *Biochim. Biophys. Acta* **497,** 805–811.

Wilson, P. W., and Lawson, D. E. M. (1978). Incorporation of [³H] leucine into an actin-like protein in response to 1,25-dihydroxycholecalciferol in chick intestinal brush borders. *Biochem. J.* **173,** 627–631.

Wilson, P. W., Harding, M., and Lawson, D. E. M. (1985). Putative amino acid sequence of chick calcium-binding protein deduced from a complementary DNA sequence. *Nucleic Acids Res.* **13,** 8867–8880.

Wilson, P. W., Rogers, J., Harding, M., Pohl, V., Pattyn, G., and Lawson, D. E. M. (1988). Structure of chick chromosomal genes for calbindin and calretinin. *J. Mol. Biol.* **200,** 615–625.

Wilson, T. H., and Wiseman, G. (1954). The use of sacs of everted small intestine for the study of transference of substances from the mucosal to the serosal surface. *J. Physiol. (London)* **123,** 116–125.

Windeck, R., Brown, E. M., Gardner, D. G., and Aurbach, G. D. (1978). Effect of gastrointestinal hormones on isolated bovine parathyroid cells. *Endocrinology (Baltimore)* **103,** 2020–2026.

Wrobel, J., and Nagel, G. (1979). Diurnal rhythm in active calcium transport in rat intestine. *Experientia* **35,** 1581–1582.

Zull, J. E., Czarnowska-Misztal, F., and DeLuca, H. F. (1956). On the relationship between vitamin D and actinomycin-sensitive processes. *Proc. Natl. Acad. Sci. U.S.A.* **55,** 177–184.

Pyrroloquinoline Quinone: A Novel Cofactor

JOHANNIS A. DUINE AND JACOB A. JONGEJAN

Department of Microbiology and Enzymology
Delft University of Technology
2628 BC Delft, The Netherlands

I. COFACTOR RESEARCH

A. SIGNIFICANCE

About half of the enzymes known today contain or require the addition of a cofactor for activity (see International Union of Biochemistry, 1984). It is curious that despite the obvious importance of these compounds, which form an integral part of the enzyme, current enzymology concentrates mainly on the apoenzymes, e.g., the protein part of the enzymes, as is apparent from the massive attention paid to topics such as protein structure and protein engineering. Although continuing research on individual cofactors is regularly discussed (for instance, in symposia devoted to flavins and flavoproteins and the

223

biochemistry of vitamin B_6), equivalent topics for cofactor research in general are lacking. As a consequence, no general strategies have been developed for the analysis of cofactors in enzymes, while opinions about their distribution are based on vague notions derived from typical examples discussed in textbooks.

B. INSIGHT INTO DISTRIBUTION

The cofactors regarded as the most important ones with respect to the number of enzymes dependent on them were discovered long ago. For instance, the structure of the well-known cofactor FMN was elucidated in 1935 (Theorell, 1935). Subsequently, several oxidoreductases were found to contain flavins (either FMN or FAD), compounds indispensible for the transfer of reduction equivalents derived from substrates to either the respiratory chain or directly to O_2. Textbooks discussing the composition of the respiratory chain invariably show a scheme in which flavoprotein dehydrogenases [NAD(P) independent] are coupled to the respiratory chain at the level of ubiquinones, indicated as Q in Fig. 1. Also, other enzyme classes are typified by examples for which the identity of the cofactor has been well established. This and the fact that data about the real distribution are not given have probably led to the generally prevailing opinion that the basic concepts of this field of enzymology have been formulated, and further research is needed only to verify the details.

To obtain real insight into the distribution of cofactors is not easy. The system used for classification of enzymes is based on the reaction catalyzed, not on the cofactor involved. Consequently many enzymes have been recognized through codification in the system, but the nature of their cofactors is still unknown. Table I, compiled from *Enzyme Nomenclature Recommendations* (International Union of Bio-

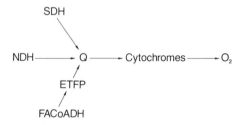

FIG. 1. Scheme of the mitochondrial electron transport chain indicating the coupling of some flavoproteins. SDH, Succinate dehydrogenase; NDH, NADH dehydrogenase; ETFP, electron transfer flavoprotein; FACoADH, fatty acyl-coenzyme A dehydrogenase.

TABLE I

COFACTOR DISTRIBUTION IN SOME SUBCLASSES OF OXIDOREDUCTASES AND LYASES

Subclass	Cofactors (present/addition required; %)				
	NAD(P)	Flavin	Other organic cofactor	Metal ion	Not indicated
Dehydrogenases/reductases [NAD(P)-dependent (350)][a]	100[b]	3	1		
Dehydrogenases/reductases [NAD(P)-independent (127)]	2	39	10	11	38
Oxidases (76)		38	8	13	41
Monooxygenases (79)	41	33	19	15	33
Dioxygenases (46)		4	2	67	27
Hydratases/dehydratases (77)	4	4	13 (10% PLP)	4	79

[a] Total number of enzymes considered is given in parentheses.

[b] As a percentage of the total number of enzymes in that subclass. Some enzymes contain/require more than one cofactor.

chemistry, 1984) and from the *European Journal of Biochemistry* (1986), reveals the remarkably high number of enzymes to which this applies and the randomness of the distribution among some subclasses.

Conclusions derived from such compilations are the following. The action of a cofactor is not restricted to a certain class or subclass. Conversely, cofactor diversity exists to a varying extent among the classes and subclasses. Although some subclasses seem homogeneous with respect to the type of cofactor, some enzymes have a second cofactor, but it is not clear whether this has been checked for all enzymes in that subclass. Although some subclasses show a high incidence of "not indicated" cofactors, on mechanistic grounds it is clear that a nonproteinaceous compound should be present. Perhaps a lack of knowledge of these facts has led to the neglect of cofactor identification. Research on this aspect of enzymology might indeed turn up something new.

C. NOVEL COFACTORS

Extensive research on the biochemistry of methanogens (bacteria able to produce CH_4, a subgroup of the archaebacteria), has revealed several novel cofactors: coenzyme M (Taylor and Wolfe, 1974), factor F_{420} (a 5-deazaflavin derivative) (Eirich *et al.*, 1978), factor F_{430} (a unique nickel tetrapyrrole compound) (Pfaltz *et al.*, 1982), methanopterin (van Beelen *et al.*, 1984), methanofuran (Leigh *et al.*, 1984), and a phosphorylated mercaptan (Noll *et al.*, 1986). The function of these compounds is, however, restricted to this specialized group of organisms [factor F420 is somewhat exceptional since it also plays a role in photoreactivating enzyme (Eker *et al.*, 1980) and in a reductase involved in the biosynthesis of chlortetracycline (McCormick and Morton, 1982)].

A compound with a wider distribution is the molybdopterin cofactor (Kramer *et al.*, 1987) [the slightly deviating compound found in bacterial molybdoproteins is called bactopterin (Meyer *et al.*, 1986)] present in several oxidoreductases from mammalian as well as microbial origin. However, just as for most of the compounds isolated from methanogens, the novelty of the structure is debatable, since it is merely a variation on a familiar theme.

Another group of specialized bacteria, the methylotrophs (dissimilating C_1 compounds such as methane, methanol, and methylamine), has also revealed a novel cofactor, namely, pyrroloquinoline quinone (PQQ), the topic of this review. As will be shown here, PQQ is rather exceptional since it occurs not only in several different bacterial dehydrogenases (quinoproteins) but has been overlooked in the study of many well-known enzymes involved in the biosynthesis or conversion of mammalian bioregulators. For that reason, this novel field of enzymology can be expected to have an impact on certain fields of pharmacology as well. In view of the rapid developments during the past few years, it seems highly relevant to review the current status of the cofactor and to discuss the possible role of PQQ or PQQ-like compounds as vitamins and their biosynthesis. Earlier reviews have appeared on the role of PQQ in microbial oxidations (Duine *et al.*, 1986) and on the enzymology of microbial quinoproteins (Duine and Frank, 1981; Duine *et al.*, 1987a). Specific enzymological topics, dealing with the recently discovered mammalian quinoproteins, are reviewed elsewhere (Duine and Jongejan, 1989).

D. The Discovery of PQQ

Upon screening the literature, it now appears that early hints that PQQ might exist can be traced back about 40 years. At that time several research groups working on glucose oxidation by gramnegative bacteria discovered that the enzyme fraction responsible for this activity was not an oxidase but a dehydrogenase, an activity independent of NAD(P) but detectable with an artificial electron acceptor. Such a finding might suggest that the enzyme is a flavoprotein, but certain properties were against such a supposition (see, for instance, Wood and Schwerdt, 1953). (It should be mentioned, though, that the arguments used by the authors to reject the idea of a flavoprotein were not correct.) Continuing work on this topic in the 1960s by Hauge and co-workers clearly demonstrated that this enzyme, indicated as glucose dehydrogenase (although the substrate specificity is so broad that a more appropriate name would be aldose dehydrogenase), possessed an unfamiliar cofactor (Hauge, 1964). Unfortunately, this excellent work on the cofactor was neither continued nor picked up by others, and the compound remained forgotten until 1979, when similarity to a cofactor from a quite different enzyme became apparent from the work by Imanaga's group (Imanaga *et al.*, 1979) and by us (Duine *et al.*, 1979).

In the mid-1950s interest developed in single-cell proteins and, related to this topic, in the physiology of methylotrophic bacteria. It appeared that not only were the pathways for C_1 compound dissimilation exceptional (compared to the familiar pathways), but so was the enzyme catalyzing methanol oxidation. The latter appeared to be a dye-linked dehydrogenase (EC 1.1.99.8), but the low-molecular-weight compound obtained in the supernatant after denaturing the enzyme was definitely not a flavin. From its fluorescence properties, it was proposed to be a pterin derivative (Anthony and Zatman, 1967). This idea was gained support in following years when it was claimed by Forrest and co-workers that the compound was neopterin cyclic phosphate (Urushibara *et al.*, 1971) and, later on, a lumazine derivative (Sperl *et al.*, 1974).

When research on methanol dehydrogenase was undertaken by our group, we originally believed that the concept of a pterinlike compound was correct. A curious property of the purified enzyme, however, was that methanol addition did not change the absorption spectrum of the preparation. Thus, the possibility was considered that the chromophore of the enzyme, presumed to be the pterin, was not directly involved in the reaction mechanism but that a (paramagnetic) transition metal ion could be the actual cofactor. One of the techniques used to research this possibility was electron spin resonance (ESR). ESR detected no paramagnetic metal ions but, unexpectedly, an organic free radical with properties dissimilar to those of flavin or pterin radicals was found (Duine *et al.*, 1978). On the other hand, the properties were compatible with those of o-quinones. After detachment of the radical species from the protein, the hyperfine structure ESR spectrum could be measured. This revealed three hydrogens and two nitrogens and provided evidence that the fluorescing compound was indeed the cofactor (Westerling *et al.*, 1979). Since we discovered that methylotrophic bacteria excrete substantial amounts of the factor into their media, the latter provided an adequate supply of material (Duine and Frank, 1980) so that the structure could be elucidated with common techniques such as nuclear magnetic resonance (NMR) and mass spectrometry (MS) (Duine *et al.*, 1980). Meanwhile, the structure had been found for a derivative of the cofactor, extracted from methylotrophic bacteria with acetone. From this, a structure was proposed for the cofactor, in agreement with ours, and the compound was called methoxatin (Salisbury *et al.*, 1979). Since we had already discovered that the cofactor exists in other bacterial enzymes (Duine *et al.*, 1979; de Beer *et al.*, 1980) and that the o-quinone moiety is the active site of the molecule, the semisystematic name pyrroloquinoline quinone was proposed (Duine *et al.*, 1980), with the structure as indicated in Fig. 2. The name can be abbreviated to PQQ, while biologically relevant redox forms can be identified using PQQH·(the semiquinone form) and $PQQH_2$ (the quinol form) (Fig. 2). In analogy with flavoproteins, hemoproteins, and the like, PQQ-containing enzymes are called quinoproteins.

After the initial survey had indicated that several bacterial enzymes

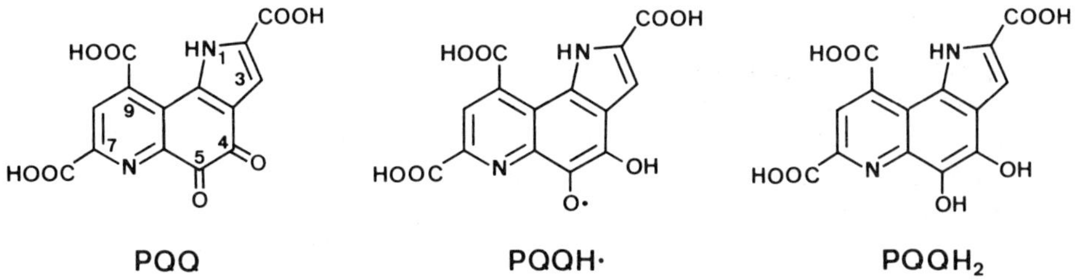

FIG. 2. Structures of PQQ, PQQH·, and PQQH$_2$.

were quinoproteins and that PQQ was widespread among bacteria, the next question could be posed: namely, whether the evolutionary history of the cofactor was dead-ended or not. One of the bacterial quinoproteins already discovered was methylamine dehydrogenase (EC 1.4.99.3), the first example indicating that PQQ exists in covalently bound form (de Beer *et al.*, 1980). This enzyme (Vellieux *et al.*, 1986) is remarkably similar to copper-containing amine oxidases (EC 1.4.3.6) found in plants and animals. Apart from copper, these enzymes were reported to have a covalently bound organic cofactor with a reactive carbonyl group. Mainly for that reason, they had been claimed to be pyridoxal-containing enzymes (International Union of Biochemistry, 1984), notwithstanding the fact that several spectroscopic as well as mechanistic features reported in the literature were incompatible with such an idea. From this discrepancy and the overall similarity with methylamine dehydrogenase, we reasoned that PQQ could be a good candidate for the second cofactor in the amine oxidases, indicating that investigation of these enzymes might shed light on the evolutionary success of PQQ. However, how could we cope with the problem of the covalency? Straightforward hydrolysis of the protein did not seem feasible, since chemical studies had already revealed the reactivity of PQQ toward nucleophilic compounds such as amino acids (Dekker *et al.*, 1982), leading to a variety of adducts which degrade into several unidentifiable compounds. The solution to this problem appeared to be derivatization of the cofactor *in situ* with a hydrazine, forming an adduct stable enough to survive enzymatic proteolysis, enabling comparison of the adduct with a model compound (Lobenstein-Verbeek *et al.*, 1984). This approach has been successfully applied to several members of this group of enzymes, showing that the cofactor is not pyridoxal phosphate but covalently bound PQQ. From this, it can be concluded that PQQ has made the jump from prokaryotes to eukaryotes, being functional in microbes as well as in humans.

So far, no systematic study has been reported on the distribution of

PQQ in enzymes or in organisms. The finding of PQQ as a cofactor in copper-containing amine oxidases and strong indications that both cofactors interact with one another (Jongejan et al., 1987) bring us to the question of whether such an interplay could be a common feature. Upon screening the literature for metalloproteins, it becomes clear that the assumption of a metal ion as a single cofactor is untenable, at least in some cases. Application of the "hydrazine method" indeed revealed that covalently bound PQQ is the second cofactor in dopamine β-hydroxylase (EC 1.14.17.1) (van der Meer et al., 1988) and in soybean lipoxygenase-1 (EC 1.13.11.12) (van der Meer and Duine, 1988). Since these enzymes have been studied for more than 40 years without revealing the presence of PQQ, this cofactor may have been overlooked in other enzymes as well. Indications that support this view can indeed be found in the literature, so that it may eventually turn out that PQQ is ubiquitous in nature and a versatile cofactor with respect to the reactions catalyzed. At any rate, this problem already has drawn the attention of several research groups, and the first International Symposium on PQQ and Quinoproteins was held in September 1988 in Delft.

In reviewing the history of PQQ, some remarkable facts are apparent which may have relevance for cofactor identification in general. First, after the initial evidence for a novel cofactor had been revealed, it took a long time before its structure was elucidated. Second, as is apparent from the recently discovered mammalian metalloquinoproteins, efforts to screen these enzymes for other nonproteinaceous compounds or to elucidate the structures of products formed by inhibition were seldom made (despite the fact that sometimes spectroscopic or mechanistic data were hardly explainable from the assumption of a single metal ion). Therefore, the history of PQQ may be exemplary so that, contrary to general feeling, cofactor identification is not a dead pursuit, and surprises may still await the alert investigator.

II. Properties

A. Structures of Naturally Occurring Forms

1. *PQQ and Its Adducts*

Absorption, fluorescence, and NMR spectroscopy of aqueous PQQ solutions show two interconverting species. The explanation is that an equilibrium exists between unhydrated and hydrated PQQ (PQQ–

H_2O) (Fig. 3). This is due to the reactivity of the C-5 carbonyl group toward nucleophiles, leading to the hydrate, adduct formation with amino groups, thiol groups, etc. (Fig. 3). These adducts could also exist in quinoproteins, providing an explanation for the variety of absorption spectra aberrant from those of free PQQ and PQQ–H_2O. On the other hand, model studies (M. A. G. van Kleef, J. A. Jongejan, and J. A. Duine, unpublished observations) show that adducts of PQQ and amino acids are not stable but decompose with formation of the corresponding amine, CO_2, and a reduced form of PQQ, which becomes reoxidized under aerobic conditions so that a cyclic process takes place with catalytic amounts of PQQ. A recently reported assay (Flueckiger *et al.*, 1988) is based on reoxidation with nitroblue tetrazolium. Depending on the type of amino acid used, however, a dead-end yellow product, the so-called oxazole (Fig. 4), is formed slowly or rapidly. This product is devoid of activity, as demonstrated by the concomitant loss of activity (measured with a biological assay) upon incubation of PQQ with mixtures of amino acids under aerobic conditions. Chelating agents, bivalent and trivalent metal ions, and NH_3 strongly influence these processes. Intermediates will be stabilized by some metal ions [it should be realized that several constituents of the cycle are excellent chelators for ions, such as Cu(II) and Fe(III)]. Although no systematic studies have been made on the occurrence of oxazoles in the natural environment, it is expected that free PQQ will exist only under rather clean conditions, such as in the culture fluid of methylotrophic or acetic aid bacteria, grown on a mineral medium with alcohols as a carbon and energy source.

2. *Protein-Bound Forms*

Apart from adduct formation, PQQ can be found derivatized in other ways. For instance, all mammalian quinoproteins (and some bacterial quinoprotein dehydrogenases) investigated so far contain PQQ in

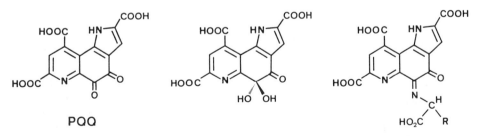

PQQ

FIG. 3. Covalently hydrated PQQ and an amino acid adduct of PQQ.

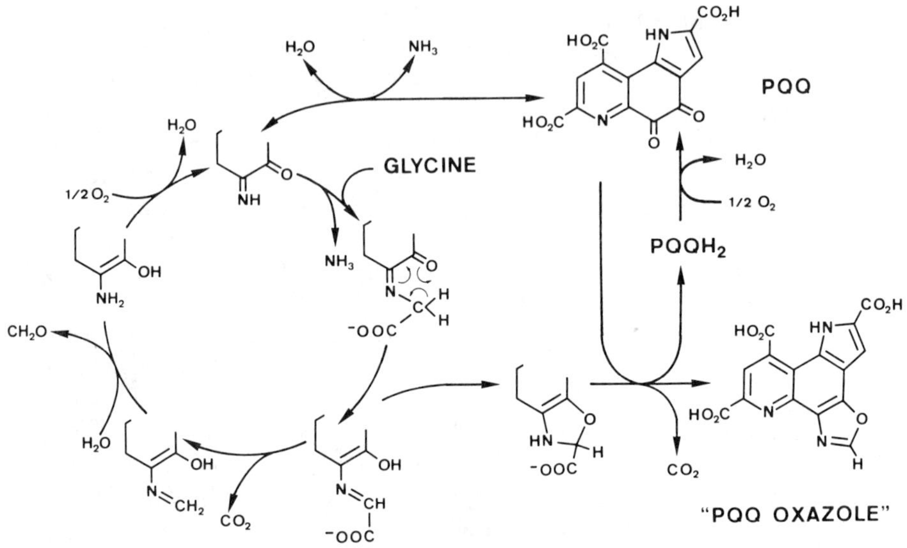

FIG. 4. Reaction cycle for PQQ and amino acids, showing the decarboxylation process as well as oxazole formation.

covalently bound form. Since the cofactor becomes detached upon incubation with proteolytic enzymes (pronase), PQQ might well be anchored to the protein by an amide or an ester bond via its carboxylic acid group(s). Studies of a peptide obtained after limited digestion of porcine kidney diamine oxidase with trypsin indicated that there is a link between an unknown amino acid residue (indicated X), converted into norleucine by hydrolysis, and one of the carboxylic acid groups of PQQ (perhaps in view of its acidity, the COOH group at the C-2 position) (Fig. 5). Norleucine is not a natural amino acid and hence is not a candidate site for attachment of PQQ. The unknown amino acid might be lysine, forming an amide bond with PQQ via its ε-amino group and degrading into norleucine during hydrolysis. Comparison of a synthetic compound, consisting of PQQ coupled with an amide bond via one of its carboxylic acid groups to the ε-amino group of lysine, with the product from the peptide has shown indeed that they are identical (van der Meer *et al.*, 1989b). Since not all proteases are able to cleave the bond, partial hydrolysis of mammalian quinoproteins might lead to production in nature of PQQ in a form released by trypsin (Fig. 5).

A recent surprising discovery is an enzyme-bound form of the cofactor which is indicated as pro-PQQ. From studies on the three-

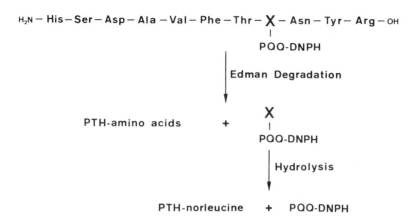

H_2N − His − Ser − Asp − Ala − Val − Phe − Thr − X − Asn − Tyr − Arg − OH

PQQ-DNPH

Edman Degradation

PTH-amino acids   +   X

PQQ-DNPH

Hydrolysis

PTH-norleucine   +   PQQ-DNPH

FIG. 5. Structure of the PQQ-containing peptide from hog kidney diamine oxidase. DNPH, 2,4-Dinitrophenylhydrazine.

dimensional structure elucidation of methylamine dehydrogenase, it appeared that the cofactor may consist of the indole structure of PQQ, connected to a glutamic acid residue attached at two positions to the protein chain of the small subunit in this enzyme (F. M. D. Vellieux, F. Huitema, H. Groendijk, K. H. Kalk, J. Frank, J. A. Jongejan, J. A. Duine, J. Drenth, and W. G. J. Hol, unpublished observations). Since application of the hydrazine method to this enzyme produces an adduct which is completely identical to the model compound prepared from authentic PQQ and the hydrazine, it appears that during cofactor derivatization cyclization to PQQ may occur. The implication is that all enzymes in which the hydrazine method has indicated the presence of covalently bound PQQ (e.g., all enzymes from eukaryotes) should be reexamined to see whether the cofactor is PQQ or pro-PQQ.

3. Redox Forms

Being a redox cofactor, PQQ should also occur in reduced form. Two natural forms have so far been discovered: $PQQH_2$ and PQQH· (Fig. 2). Since $PQQH_2$ becomes very rapidly oxidized above pH 4 and PQQH· is stable only at very high pH under anaerobic conditions (Duine *et al.*, 1981), it can be assumed that these forms do not exist under (aerobic) physiological conditions in free form. However, PQQH· and $PQQH_2$ are very stable in quinoprotein dehydrogenases, obviously because they are stabilized by the protein environment and shielded from O_2 attack.

TABLE II
ABSORPTION COEFFICIENTS AND MAXIMA OF PQQ REDOX FORMS AND IN QUINOPROTEINS

Substance	Absorption maximum (nm)	Molar absorption coefficient $(M^{-1}\ cm^{-1})$	References
PQQ	249	22,500	Duine et al. (1987a)
	325	10,200	
	475	800	
PQQH·	460	3200	Faraggi et al. (1986)
PQQH$_2$	302	30,500	Duine et al. (1987a)
Methanol dehydrogenase	345	13,700	Duine et al. (1987a)
Glucose dehydrogenase	349	9700	Duine et al. (1987a)
Methylamine dehydrogenase	440	10,600	Duine et al. (1987a)
Methylamine oxidase	480	1900	Duine et al. (1987a)

B. SPECTROSCOPIC DATA

Absorption, fluorescence, NMR, and MS spectra have been discussed previously (Duine et al., 1986). A recapitulation of the essentials is presented below.

Spectra are complex, representing contributions from two components, PQQ and PQQ–H$_2$O. Spectra of PQQ recorded at high temperature or in organic solvents are very similar to those of unhydrated PQQ, whereas spectra at low temperature or PQQ complexed with metal ions closely resemble those of PQQ–H$_2$O [see Dekker et al. (1982) for the genuine spectra of the two species, calculated by mathematical procedures]. Fluorescence spectra are relatively simple since only PQQ–H$_2$O shows fluorescence; unhydrated PQQ does not. Table II shows some absorption maxima and molar absorption coefficients of PQQ, its adducts, and its reduced forms. For comparison, the values are also given for some quinoproteins. As appears from Table II, striking differences exist among the proteins and with the redox forms of the cofactor, so that it is clear that identification of an enzyme as a quinoprotein cannot be based solely on its absorption spectrum.

Electron spin resonance (ESR) and electron nuclear double resonance (ENDOR) spectroscopy of PQQH· in free and enzyme-bound forms have been discussed (Duine et al., 1987a).

C. CHEMICAL REACTIVITY AND SYNTHESIS

The most prevailing property of PQQ is the reactivity of its C-5 carbonyl group toward nucleophiles, leading to adducts. The redox behavior, as far as two-electron processes are concerned, probably forms an extension of this property since, once the adduct is formed, doublet migration can occur. In this respect, PQQ is comparable to pyridoxal phosphate. However, a significant difference is the ability of PQQ to participate in one-electron transfer processes. The combination of these two properties may be crucial to the functioning of PQQ as a cofactor in dehydrogenases: two-electron transition in the PQQ substrate adduct constitutes the substrate oxidation step (although a double one-electron step mechanism cannot be excluded at the moment), followed by one-electron transfer to the natural one-electron acceptors (copper–proteins, cytochromes) functioning in the respirato-

TABLE III
SYNTHETIC ROUTES FOR PQQ, PQQ
DERIVATIVES, AND PQQ ANALOGS

Compound[a]	Biological activity[b] (%)	Reference[c]
PQQ	100	1–5
7-Decarboxy-PQQ	15[d]	8, 9
9-Decarboxy-PQQ	0[d]	7, 8
7,9-Didecarboxy-PQQ	0[d]	6, 9
PQ	0	3
4-Hydroxy-PQ	0	4
5-Hydroxy-PQ	0	1
N-1-Alky-PQQ	0.5–3	9, 10
C-3-Alkyl-PQQ	1–10	10
C-8-Alkyl-PQQ	5	10
C-3-Nitro-PQQ		2
PQQ–DNPH adduct		11
PQQ–PH adduct		12

[a] The numbering is as indicated in Fig. 2. P, 4,5-Dehydro-4,5-desoxy-PQQ; PQQ-PH adduct, the C-5 hydrazone of PQQ and phenylhydrazine; PQQ-DNPH adduct, the C-5 hydrazone of PQQ and 2,4-dinitrophenylhydrazine.

[b] Biological activity was measured (J. A. Jongejan, B. W. Groen and J. A. Duine, unpublished observations) using the quinohenoprotein alcohol dehydrogenase apoenzyme (Groen et al., 1986).

[c] References: (1) Corey and Tramontano, 1981; (2) Gainor and Weinreb, 1982; (3) Hendrickson and de Vries, 1984; (4) MacKenzie et al., 1986; (5) Buechi et al., 1985; (6) Sleath et al., 1985; (7) Noar et al., 1985; (8) Noar and Bruice, 1987; (9) Itoh et al., 1987; (10) Jongejan et al., 1988; (11) van Koningsveld et al., 1985; (12) van der Meer et al., 1987.

[d] Data are from Shinagawa et al. (1986).

ry chain. Details on derivatization, degradation, etc., are given in an earlier review (Duine *et al.*, 1987a).

PQQ can be produced either by microbial fermentation or by chemical synthesis. Apart from factors such as economy and purity, the latter method is crucial for the preparation of certain intermediates or analogs of PQQ. A survey of the analogs described to date is given in Table III. Of the six routes developed so far, one of the most attractive is that of Corey and Tramontano (1981), especially since it has been improved substantially and modified to prepare specifically labeled PQQ and derivatives (Jongejan *et al.*, 1988).

D. ANALYSIS

1. *Problems in Detection and Quantification*

As discussed before, the natural occurrence of free PQQ will be the exception rather than the rule. Only spent culture media of bacterial PQQ producers free of nucleophiles or extracts from purified quinoproteins (those with PQQ in noncovalently bound form) will contain underivatized PQQ. For those samples, a number of chromatographic methods or biological assays are available, as indicated in Sections II,D,2 and II,D,3. Reaction of PQQ with certain nucleophilic amino acids, as noted above, leads to (among others) oxazole formation, the amount and rate of formation depending on many factors. Although decomposition of the oxazoles into PQQ has been achieved under acid conditions (M. A. G. van Kleef and J. A. Duine, unpublished observations), problems arise with tryptophan. For all these reasons, detection of PQQ in such biological materials with methods developed for free PQQ is not feasible. Preliminary experiments (R. A. van der Meer and J. A. Duine, unpublished observations) in which quinoproteins under strongly acidic conditions are refluxed with a large surplus of hexanol indicate that reaction with amino acids can be prevented, since the hexanol adduct formed is extracted into the organic layer (the strong acid detaches PQQ from the protein and decomposes any oxazole). If it appears that all adducts of PQQ can be converted into the hexanol adduct or at least to a single compound, this novel method may eventually turn out to be the method of choice for analysis of PQQ and its derivatives in complex biological systems. The procedure has been successfully applied to dopa decarboxylase (Groen *et al.*, 1988) and glutamic acid decarboxylase (van der Meer *et al.*, 1989a).

Analysis of PQQ in laboratories in which milligram amounts of the compound are used may be plagued by contamination problems. PQQ easily adheres to the glassware, while chromatographic columns that have been loaded with an appreciable amount of PQQ may bleed for a long time. This problem is especially pertinent if biological assays are used, since such methods are so sensitive that special precautions must be taken. These include treatment of culture media and buffers with anion exchanger and decomposition of adhering PQQ by heating the glassware to very high temperatures (van Kleef *et al.*, 1987).

In order to detect and quantify PQQ in covalently bound form, development of a special procedure, the so-called hydrazine method (Section II,D,4), is required. Since no specific method has been found to detach PQQ from a protein, one must avoid in some way its conversion into unidentifiable compounds during protein hydrolysis. We reasoned that derivatization of the cofactor *in situ* might circumvent this problem and allow comparison of the adduct with the model compound. Screening of a number of candidates revealed that 2,4-dinitrophenylhydrazine (DNPH) reacted with PQQ to a product surviving hydrolytic conditions. Since the reaction of DNPH with the diethylmethyltriester of PQQ gave crystals suitable for X-ray diffraction analysis (van Koningsveld *et al.*, 1985), its structure could be elucidated (the 2,4-dinitrophenylhydrazone of PQQ-triester at the C-5 position). Hydrolysis of this compound gave the same product as that obtained from PQQ and DNPH, so that the structure was obviously the C-5 hydrazone of PQQ and DNPH. Despite its bulky groups, DNPH reacted with bovine serum amine oxidase so that the feasibility of the method could be proved (Lobenstein-Verbeek *et al.*, 1984).

At that time, however, for unknown reasons, the yield was rather low. Moreover, not all enzymes suspected to be quinoproteins reacted with DNPH. Therefore, the method was further elaborated (see Section II,D,4). As will be shown, the reliability and precision of this method have been established in several instances.

2. *Chromatographic Methods*

PQQ behaves as a relatively strong acid, allowing adequate removal of the cofactor from spent culture media of PQQ-producing bacteria by anion exchanger. However, desorption is not easy, requiring high salt concentrations plus alcohols. Otherwise, significant tailing and severe losses are encountered. It follows then that anion exchangers are unsuited for the analyses of small amounts of PQQ, although they are quite suited for concentration and purification purposes (Duine and Frank, 1980).

Gel filtration has been used in screening a large number of biological materials for PQQ (Ameyama *et al.*, 1985a). Since the material used (Sephadex G-25) is of low resolving power with respect to size of the compounds concerned, one can expect contamination with other compounds. Moreover, the method frequently used to detect PQQ in the eluates was fluorescence spectroscopy. Here again, the discriminating power is not high enough, since hydrolyzed nonquinoproteins show fluorescence spectra very similar to that of PQQ (van Kleef *et al.*, 1987) (apart from the high improbability that free PQQ occurs in these samples, as has already been pointed out).

So far, the most suitable and frequently used chromatographic procedure appears to be high-performance liquid chromatography (HPLC) on a reversed-phase column, as originally described by Duine and Frank (1980). Applying a low pH, the polarity can be decreased sufficiently to induce adsorption and subsequent elution on raising the methanol content of the eluent. The reactivity of PQQ also introduces problems here. Presumably, water and/or methanol react (reversibly) at the C-5 group to give adducts, leading to a broad peak, thus lowering the sensitivity and selectivity of the system. Fortunately, the same reactivity can also be used to advantage: To assess the identity of a peak as belonging to PQQ, the sample is treated with acetone or butyraldehyde, giving a rather stable adduct. Comparison of the chromatograms before and after derivatization reveals loss of the PQQ peak and the appearance of the novel (sharp) adduct peak (Duine and Frank, 1980). To improve the chromatographic system for PQQ as such, ion pairing seems the method of choice, as it gives a much sharper peak (Duine *et al.*, 1983).

In view of its rather high molar absorption coefficient at 249 nm (Table II), ultraviolet (UV) monitoring of the HPLC eluate is well suited for detection and quantification purposes. If the samples contain interfering UV-absorbing substances, more selective monitoring is required. Fluorescence detection can be helpful in these cases. To increase selectivity even further, derivatization of PQQ to a highly fluorescing compound has been utilized (Duine *et al.*, 1983). Incubation with 2 M NaOH at 100°C in a sealed ampule has also been used for this purpose (Lobenstein-Verbeek *et al.*, 1984). It should be recognized, however, that it is uncertain whether these procedures are quantitative or whether they detect preexisting adducts. The same applies to a novel approach (Suzuki *et al.*, 1989) consisting of gas chromatography of derivatized PQQ.

3. Biological Assays

a. Apoquinoproteins. Without realizing it, Hauge (1964) was the first who developed a biological assay for PQQ. After purifying the soluble form of glucose dehydrogenase (EC 1.1.99.17) from *Acinetobacter calcoaceticus* LMD 79.41 (at that time indicated as *Bacterium anitratum*), slightly denaturing conditions and dialysis almost completely abolished activity, which could be restored by addition of then unknown PQQ in the form of boiled enzyme extract. Similar results were reported by Niederpruem and Doudoroff (1965), who found that from *Rhodopseudomonas spheroides* grown under anaerobic conditions, a cell-free extract could be prepared which showed glucose dehydrogenase activity only after addition of the same compound, now known to be PQQ. Thus, when it was found that glucose dehydrogenase is a quinoprotein, the apoenzyme was prepared more or less analogously to the description by Hauge, affording a biological assay system for PQQ (Duine *et al.*, 1979). Although this test has been used by others (Kilty *et al.*, 1982), a serious drawback in our hands was the irreproducibility of the procedure to prepare apoenzyme. The problem can be circumvented by preparing apoenzyme from the membrane-bound form of glucose dehydrogenase of *Pseudomonas aeruginosa* [in contrast to the soluble enzyme form, PQQ of this enzyme can be easily removed by dialysis against an ethylenediaminetetraacetic acid (EDTA)-containing buffer (Duine *et al.*, 1983)] or by using a mutant from *Pseudomonas florescens,* unable to provide its apoglucose dehydrogenase with PQQ (Ameyama *et al.*, 1981). A somewhat unattractive aspect, however, is the fact that purification of these enzymes is very difficult to achieve, so that, in practice, cell-free extracts are used. This may lead to nonspecific adsorption of PQQ, a danger which could also apply to the use of cytoplasmic membranes of *Escherichia coli.* In the latter case, use is made of the property of this bacterium (Hommes *et al.*, 1984) to synthesize constitutively the apoenzyme but not the holoenzyme [although synthesis of free PQQ by this organism has been claimed (Ameyama *et al.*, 1984b), all of the strains checked by us (van Kleef *et al.*, 1987) failed to do this]. A similar situation exists in *Pseudomonas testosteroni.* The quinohemoprotein alcohol dehydrogenase is always found in its apo form but never in its holo form (Groen *et al.*, 1986). Since the apoenzyme can be easily purified and is stable, one can develop a very sensitive test which is routinely used in our laboratory. A list of naturally occurring or prepared apoenzymes and reported application in biological assays is given in Table IV.

   b. Whole Bacteria. After it appeared that *Acinetobacter lwoffi* synthesizes glucose dehydrogenase only in its apoform (van Schie *et al.*, 1984), several gram-negative bacteria were found to possess this curious property (Table IV). Since these dehydrogenases are most probably situated in the periplasmic space, transport of PQQ from outside

TABLE IV

BACTERIA PRODUCING APOQUINOPROTEINS AND BIOLOGICAL ASSAYS

Organism	Apoenzyme[a]	Assay[a]
Acinetobacter lwoffi	Glucose dehydrogenase (1)[b]	
Escherichia coli	Glucose dehydrogenase (2)[b]	3–5
Pseudomonas testosteroni	Alcohol dehydrogenase (6)[b]	6
Agrobacterium and *Rhizobium* species	Glucose dehydrogenase (7)[b]	
Flavobacterium and *Proteus* species	Glucose dehydrogenase (8)[b]	
Salmonella typhimurium	Glucose dehydrogenase (9)[b]	
Acinetobacter calcoaceticus	Glucose dehydrogenase[c]	10–12
Pseudomonas aeruginosa	Glucose dehydrogenase[c]	13
Pseudomonas fluorescens	Glucose dehydrogenase[c]	14

[a] References: (1) van Schie *et al.*, 1984; (2) Hommes *et al.*, 1984; (3) Ameyama *et al.*, 1985d; (4) Geiger and Goerisch, 1987; (5) van Kleef *et al.*, 1987; (6) Groen *et al.*, 1986; (7) van Schie *et al.*, 1987; (8) Ameyama *et al.*, 1985c; (9) P. Postma, personal communication; (10) Hauge, 1964; (11) Duine *et al.*, 1979; (12) Kilty *et al.*, 1982; (13) Duine *et al.*, 1983; (14) Ameyama *et al.*, 1981.

[b] Natural apoenzyme.

[c] Apoenzyme prepared from a holoenzyme.

across the cytoplasmic membrane is not necessary, so that, in principle, reconstitution can be easily achieved. Very rapid and effective reconstitution has indeed been reported so that this also forms an attractive assay system (although the same objection can be made as for the unpurified apoenzymes with respect to adventitious adsorption). The effective recombination and the stability of the enzyme in the organism (as opposed to enzyme in the *in vitro* assay), assure the achievement of a very high amplification factor and the analysis of tiny amounts of PQQ or of large samples of low concentration (van Kleef *et al.*, 1987).

4. *The Hydrazine Method*

As mentioned in Section II,D,1, the search for quinoproteins in mammalian organisms required a technique for detection and quantification of PQQ in enzymes in which it is covalently bound. In the first instance, a concern was the low yield in which adduct could be isolated from hydrazine-inhibited enzyme. Apart from the drawback that quantitative determinations were not possible, it also laid a heavy burden on the credibility of the technique, as possible contamination with PQQ could not be excluded from a stoichiometric amount of cofactor found with respect to the enzyme present. After some insight was obtained into the conditions for proteolysis and into hydrazone formation, it became clear that initially an almost complete conversion to a product, indicated as the azo compound (Fig. 6), occurs under the usual conditions of hydrazine inhibition of amine oxidases. The azo compound in the enzyme can be converted (in a slow process) into the corresponding hydrazone under high oxygen tensions (van der Meer *et al.*, 1987). Another drawback was the fact that DNPH does not react with all quinoproteins. Since other hydrazines tend to reduce PQQ under conditions initially used for preparing model compounds, these reagents could not be used. When we realized that inhibition with hydrazines can lead either to hydrazone or to azo compounds, we were able to prepare similar adducts from various hydrazines using the apropriate conditions (Table V).

Derivatization with DNPH has also been used by others (Moog *et al.*, 1986; Williamson *et al.*, 1986; Knowles *et al.*, 1987). Unfortunately, the conditions essential for azo compound or hydrazone formation were neglected or not realized, and adducts were not isolated but investigated *in situ* with Raman spectroscopy. From the scarce data given for preparing the model compound, the adduct in the enzyme, and some

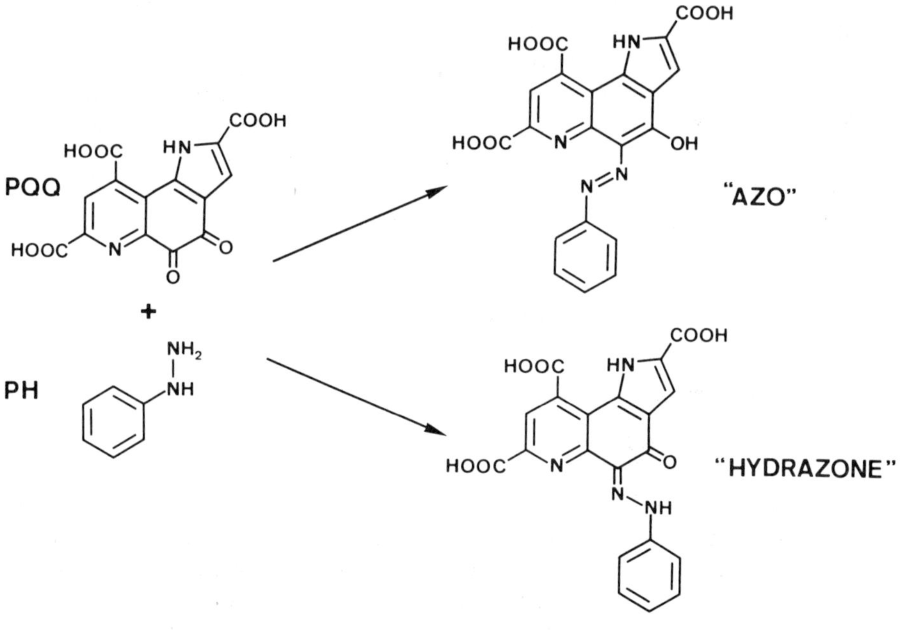

FIG. 6. The azo adduct and the hydrazone of PQQ and phenylhydrazine (PH).

TABLE V

HYDRAZONES AND AZO ADDUCTS OF PQQ[a]

Adduct	Absorption maximum (nm)	Absorption coefficient (M^{-1} cm^{-1})	Reference
PQQ-DNPH	335, 445	31, 400	Duine et al. (1987b)
PQQ-azo-DNPH	454		Duine et al. (1987b)
PQQ-PH	335		van der Meer et al. (1987)
PQQ-azo-PH	365, 440		van der Meer et al. (1987)
PQQ-azo-MH	383		van Iersel et al. (1986)

[a] PQQ-DNPH, The C-5 hydrazone of PQQ and 2,4-dinitrophenylhydrazine; PQQ-azo-DNPH, the azo adduct of PQQ and 2,4-dinitrophenylhydrazine; PQQ-PH, the C-5 hydrazone of PQQ and phenylhydrazine; PQQ-azo-PH, the azo adduct of PQQ and phenylhydrazine; PQQ-azo-MH, the azo adduct of PQQ and methylhydrazine.

absorption spectra, it appears that *in vivo* azo compound was compared with the model hydrazone. Despite the fact that the Raman spectra were clearly different (the difference attributed by the authors to the influence of the protein environment in the case of the adduct), it was nevertheless concluded that these results proved the existence of PQQ in these enzymes. Although Raman spectroscopy can be used as one of the spectroscopic techniques for comparison purposes (provided that the correct comparisons are made), estimation of the exact number of PQQs in an enzyme requires the complete detachment of the adduct so that it can be analyzed by quantitative methods, and slight differences in structure, if any, can be revealed from comparisons of absorption spectra and chromatographic behavior.

III. Distribution in Organisms and Enzymes

A. Distribution in Organisms

So far, no reliable, systematic search has been reported for PQQ in biological materials. The reasons for this are related to the problems of analysis (Section II,D,1): Only free PQQ can be quantified with high sensitivity; mammalian organisms contain quinoproteins with PQQ in covalently bound form, and although several of these purified enzymes have been successfully analyzed with the hydrazine method, it is by no means certain that this method will be applicable in all cases. With microorganisms growing on complex culture media or mammals or plants synthesizing PQQ, one may assume that nucleophilic compounds in the environment will convert PQQ into nondetectable compounds. Hence, all studies to date on the distribution of PQQ have depended on the identification of quinoproteins.

1. *Bacteria*

Structural elucidation, noted above, was performed with material extracted from methylotrophic bacteria. All gram-negative methylotrophic bacteria investigated so far contain quinoprotein methanol dehydrogenase. Moreover, the gram-positive methylotroph, *Nocardia* species 239, also produces PQQ in its culture medium and contains a quinoprotein, probably involved in methanol oxidation, while the acetogenic anaerobe, *Clostridium thermoautotrophicum,* is claimed to contain PQQ-dependent methanol dehydrogenase (Winters-Ivey and Ljungdahl, 1989). Quinoprotein glucose dehydrogenase is widely distributed among bacteria growing aerobically. Moreover, it appears that an anaerobe such as *Zymomonas mobilis* also contains this enzyme (M. Strohdeicher, personal communication). Bacteria growing on alkanes or alcohols frequently contain a quinoprotein alcohol dehydrogenase, such as quinoprotein ethanol dehydrogenase of *Pseudomonas aeruginosa* and quinohemoprotein ethanol dehydrogenase of *Pseudomonas testosteroni.* Other types are polyethylene glycol dehydrogenase, polyvinylalcohol dehydrogenase, and glycerol dehydrogenase of *Gluconobacter industrius.*

Also widespread is the capability of dissimilating quinate via an NAD(P)-independent quinate dehydrogenase, an enzyme which was shown to be a quinoprotein in several bacterial species. In addition, quinoproteins have been detected in bacteria where PQQ is found covalently bound: methylamine dehydrogenase and methylamine oxidase (the latter is a copper–quinoprotein). Eukaryotic cells contain copper–quinoprotein amine oxidases able to oxidize compounds such as spermine and spermidine, which play a role in the regulation of cell division. These or similar compounds are also found in prokaryotes, but the corresponding enzymes acting on them have not been described. If these enzymes exist and also represent quinoproteins, PQQ would be omnipresent among bacteria. In any event, the many species in which quinoproteins have been detected indicate that the cofactor is widespread among bacteria. Table VI shows some enzymes discussed in earlier reviews (Duine *et al.,* 1986, 1987a) as well as some novel examples. Criteria to incorporate enzymes in this table were that the identification of PQQ as a cofactor was established by checking that the quantity of PQQ was stoichiometric to the enzyme, by attaining

TABLE VI
ESTABLISHED QUINOPROTEINS

Organism	Enzyme[a]
Bacteria	
Methylotrophic bacteria	Methanol dehydrogenase
Pseudomonas aeruginosa	Ethanol dehydrogenase
Pseudomonas testosteroni	Ethanol dehydrogenase (quinohemoprotein)
Many bacteria	Glucose dehydrogenase
Some methylotrophic bacteria	Methylamine dehydrogenase
Arthrobacter P1	Methylamine oxidase (1)
Several bacteria	Quinate dehydrogenase (2)
Gluconobacter industrius	Glycerol dehydrogenase
Flavobacterium sp.	Polyethylene glycol dehydrogenase
Pseudomonas sp.	Polyvinyl alcohol dehydrogenase
Yeasts, fungi	
Several yeasts	Amine oxidase[b]
Several fungi	Amine oxidase[b]
Several fungi	Galactose oxidase (3)
Plants	
Pea (*Pisum sativum*)	Amine oxidase (4)
Soybean	Lipoxygenase-1 (5)
Animals	
Cow	Serum amine oxidase
Cow	Dopamine β-hydroxylase (6)
Pig	Kidney diamine oxidase (7)
Human	Placental lysyl oxidase (8)

[a] Most of the enzymes have been mentioned already in other reviews (Duine *et al.*, 1986, 1987a). For the others, the following references apply: (1) van Iersel *et al.*, 1986; (2) van Kleef and Duine, 1988a; (3) R. A. van der Meer, J. A. Jongejan, and J. A. Duine, unpublished observations; (4) Glatz *et al.*, 1987; (5) van der Meer and Duine, 1988; (6) van der Meer *et al.*, 1988; (7) van der Meer *et al.*, 1986; (8) van der Meer and Duine, 1986.

[b] These enzymes are very similar to the mammalian amine oxidases.

reconstitution with PQQ of the apoenzyme produced by PQQ⁻ mutants, or by strong analogy with well-established quinoproteins.

2. *Yeasts and Fungi*

Copper-containing amine oxidases have been detected in many yeasts and fungi. Since these enzymes are very similar to the mammalian amine oxidases, they are most probably also copper–quinoproteins. Several fungal species produce galactose oxidase (EC 1.1.3.9), an enzyme which was formerly considered to be a simple copper–protein. Besides the metal ion, we recently discovered that this enzyme also contains covalently bound PQQ as a cofactor (R. A. van der Meer and J. A. Duine, unpublished results).

3. *Plants*

Several plants contain copper-containing amine oxidases, further indicating the wide distribution of PQQ. Indeed, it is found in amine oxidase from peas (*Pisum sativum*). Many plant species contain lipoxygenase, an enzyme which appears now to be an iron–quinoprotein in the case of soybean lipoxygenase-1. In addition, plants should be able to convert quinate, and if it is assumed that this takes place via the already mentioned quinoprotein quinate dehydrogenase, the distribution of PQQ among plants becomes even wider.

4. *Animals*

A number of mammalian quinoprotein enzymes have now been detected, such as plasma amine oxidases, diamine oxidase, lysyl oxidase, and dopamine β-hydroxylase. In addition, mammalian lipoxygenases are very similar to soybean lipoxygenase-1 (both being iron–proteins), and since this contains PQQ, mammalian lipoxygenases may also be iron–quinoproteins. An enzyme has been detected with α-amidation activity which is very similar to dopamine β-hydroxylase, containing copper and requiring ascorbic acid for activity (Eipper *et al.*, 1983). Therefore, this might also be a quinoprotein. PQQ is widespread, if not omnipresent, among these organisms.

B. Established Quinoproteins

Quinoproteins appear to be distributed among several types of oxidoreductases. In addition, they are claimed to be part of nitrilase (Nagasawa and Yamada, 1987), an enzyme belonging to the class of hydrolases. Moreover, it appears that PQQ has been overlooked in many metalloprotein enzymes and might be found in other well-established groups of enzymes with an already established cofactor. Some subclasses are discussed below.

1. *Dehydrogenases*

Until recently, NAD(P)-independent dehydrogenases were generally considered to be flavoproteins. In bacteria, a number of enzymes belonging to this subclass appear now to be quinoproteins. Several of these enzymes, found in gram-negative bacteria, have been found in the periplasm, a property which might be relevant in explaining their role in the bioenergetics of this group of organisms. A review on this topic in relation to incomplete microbial oxidations has been reported elsewhere (Duine *et al.*, 1986). So far, no representatives of this subclass have been found in eukaryotic cells.

2. *Oxidases*

Copper-containing amine oxidases have been known for a long time but, as it appears now, they have been incorrectly classified with respect to the nature of their organic cofactor. Except methylamine oxidase, an enzyme in the gram-positive bacterium *Arthrobacter* P1, all quinoprotein amine oxidases have been detected in eukaryotes, especially in mammalian organisms. Since many of them fulfill important physiological functions, an extensive line of research exists related to this aspect. Therefore, the finding that PQQ, but not pyridoxal, is the cofactor will have important consequences on the view of the role of vitamin B_6 and on the development of drugs directed against these enzymes. The enzymes will be briefly described below.

a. Plasma or Serum Amine Oxidase. The confusion with respect to nomenclature of amine oxidases is particularly striking for this enzyme, since it is also known under the names benzylamine oxidase, spermine oxidase, and semicarbazide sensitive amine oxidase, among others. The variety in names is illustrative of the lack of knowledge on the genuine physiological substrate and thus the role of the enzymes. The distinction with flavoprotein amine oxidases (EC 1.4.3.4) is not always clear, although it is generally agreed that the copper-containing class only converts primary amines and not secondary or tertiary amines. The reason for the lack of knowledge is that most of the work has been performed with unpurified extracts and both classes have overlapping substrates (with respect to the primary amines) and inhibitor specificities [in spite of the fact that the lathyrogenic compound aminoacetonitrile is a specific inhibitor for the copper-containing class (Riceberg *et al.*, 1975), application of this compound to distinguish between the classes is seldom utilized].

It will be clear that this confusion has seriously hampered studies aimed at elucidating the specific role of this class of enzymes. Since the polyamines spermine and spermidine (or their products formed by the amine oxidase) are regarded as compounds involved in the regulation of cell proliferation, selective inhibitors for these enzymes might reveal their precise function in this process.

Another uncertainty exists with respect to the localization of the enzyme. As apparent from the name, the enzyme is detected in the blood but since a similar or identical enzyme is found in the arterial walls, the occurrence in the circulation might be an artifact. A similar situation is found during pregnancy: high levels are found in the serum and a similar or an identical form is found in the placenta.

b. Lysyl Oxidase. This enzyme oxidizes lysyl residues in the precursors of collagen and elastin, so that cross-linking can occur between the aldehyde group formed and an unmodified lysine residue. It has been solubilized from placental material, cartilage, and arterial walls. Although it has been claimed that the enzyme from chicken cartilage contains pyridoxal phosphate (Bird and Levene, 1982), evidence for this is indirect and the enzyme from human placenta is clearly a quinoprotein (van der Meer and Duine, 1986).

c. Diamine Oxidase. Another name for this enzyme is histaminase, indicating a role which it might have in mammals. The enzyme is found in the kidneys and the gut. For the latter tissue, it has been proposed that the function of the enzyme is to keep histamine at a sufficiently low level.

3. Hydroxylases (Monooxygenases)

Dopamine β-hydroxylase (EC 1.14.17.1) is the only quinoprotein hydroxylase detected so far. It is found in the chromaffin granules of the adrenal medulla as well as in the andrenergic nervous system, and it converts dopamine into the neurotransmitter noradrenaline. In the reaction, one oxygen atom of O_2 is attached to the benzylic carbon of dopamine; the other is reduced to H_2O with ascorbic acid. Until recently, the enzyme was indicated as a colorless copper–protein. Although the enzyme has been studied for decades, the mechanistic properties could be accommodated, with difficulty, by copper as the only cofactor. Inhibition with hydrazines had been reported and the product is assumed to be a modified amino acid residue without performing structural determinations. Application of the hydrazine method showed that PQQ is present, and its possible role as a cofactor has been discussed (van der Meer *et al.*, 1988).

4. Dioxygenases

Many iron-containing enzymes catalyze insertion of dioxygen into substrate. With insertion at a C–H bond, distribution of the two oxygen atoms can take place over two sites or at one site, the latter leading to a hydroperoxide product. Soybean lipoxygenase (EC 1.13.11.12), a representative from the latter group, is a nonheme iron protein which dioxygenates lipids with *cis,cis*-pentadiene structures. It has been extensively studied with respect to spectroscopic as well as mechanistic properties, leading to the conclusion that it is a unique iron protein. From the finding that it contains one covalently bound PQQ per enzyme molecule, a complex has been proposed in which PQQ forms ligands for the Fe ion. The electron relay system formed explains well the anomalous properties of the Fe ion and the steps in the catalytic cycle (van der Meer *et al.*, 1988). Several of the products of mammalian lipoxygenases are potent physiological effectors involved in vasoconstriction, blood clotting, hypersensitivity, and inflammation.

Several pyridoxal phosphate-containing enzymes among amino acid decarboxylases and amino transferases show atypical behavior—that is, upon removal of this cofactor, the apoenzyme still contains a nonproteinaceous chromophore frequently indicated as a vitamin B_6-like compound. Investigation of a representative of this group, L-aromatic amino acid (dopa) decarboxylase from pig kidney, revealed that the second cofactor is covalently bound PQQ (Groen *et al.*, 1988). A mechanism in which an interplay of the two cofactors is suggested has already been proposed (Duine and Jongejan, 1989). Meanwhile, it has also been found that glutamic acid decarboxylase from *E. coli* contains PQQ (van der Meer *et al.*, 1989a), indicating that an organism can harbor covalently bound PQQ, although it does not produce the free form of the cofactor (Hommes *et al.*, 1984). Therefore, pyridoxoquinoproteins might be common enzymes in prokaryotic as well as eukaryotic organisms.

IV. BIOSYNTHESIS

As mentioned already, PQQ has an unfamiliar structure. Although kynurenic acid, xanthurenic acid, and pseudanes partially resemble PQQ, it is difficult to see how these compounds could act as precursors for PQQ. On the other hand, one might readily imagine pairs of amino acids such as phenylalanine or tyrosine and glutamic acid, glutamine, or its corresponding keto acids as precursors. Knowledge about PQQ production and the availability of PQQ$^-$ mutants are indispensible factors in the elucidation of the biosynthesis route. These aspects are, therefore, also dealt with in the following sections.

A. PRODUCTION BY BACTERIA

A rich source of PQQ is the culture fluid of methylotrophic bacteria, with concentrations in the micromolar range. Similar levels are attained by *Acinetobacter* or *Pseudomonas* species growing on alcohols or alkanes (Table VII). Excretion of PQQ is clearly related to the synthesis of quinoprotein alcohol dehydrogenases and not per se to the presence of a special substrate acting as an inducer. For instance, *Acinetobacter calcoaceticus,* a bacterium able to produce PQQ but which converts ethanol via NAD- and NADP-dependent alcohol dehydrogenases, produces levels with ethanol comparable to those observed with acetate as a carbon and energy source. On the other hand, *Pseudomonas* species produce a large amount of PQQ with ethanol as growth substrate (they contain quinoprotein alcohol dehydrogenase) (Table VII). The view is also strengthened by the observation that *A. calcoaceticus* produces higher levels when growing on quinate, a substrate which is degraded via a quinoprotein quinate dehydrogenase (van Kleef and Duine, 1988). Thus, production rates of PQQ and quinoprotein seem more or less in tune with one another, the type of quinoprotein being important for the levels of PQQ attained (it should be noted that the values indicated in Table VII refer to batch cultures, and much higher values can be obtained in fed batch cultures). Although PQQ is generally overproduced (with respect to the amount of quinoprotein), at certain growth conditions it is underproduced so that part of the quinoprotein is found in its apo form. PQQ production by other microbes or by higher organisms has never been reported. This

TABLE VII
PQQ PRODUCTION BY BACTERIA[a]

Organism	Growth substrate	Type of quinoprotein synthesized	PQQ in the culture medium (nM)
Acinetobacter calcoaceticus	Ethanol	(GDH)	ND[b]
A. calcoaceticus	Quinate	QDH (GDH)	200
Pseudomonas aeruginosa	Ethanol	EDH (GDH)	3000
P. aeruginosa	Glucose	GDH	ND[b]
Hyphomicrobium X	Methanol	MDH	6000
Thiobacillus versutus	Methylamine	MADH	6000
Arthrobacter P1	Methylamine	MeAO	ND[b]

[a] GDH, Glucose dehydrogenase; QDH, quinate dehydrogenase; EDH, ethanol dehydrogenase; MDH, methanol dehydrogenase; MADH, methylamine dehydrogenase; MeAO, methylamine oxidase. Quinoproteins in parentheses are synthesized by the organism but are not necessary for dissimilation of the growth substrate. Data are from a recent compilation (van Kleef and Duine, 1989).

[b] ND, Nondetectable (i.e., the concentration is below 5 nM).

may be due to the inability of these organisms to synthesize free PQQ or to the conversion of PQQ into an as yet unknown compound due to the complex environment in these cases (see Section II,D,1). Commercially PQQ is currently produced via microbial fermentation with methylotrophs (Mitsubishi Gas Chemical Company and Ube Industries, both in Japan) and by chemical synthesis (Fluka, Switzerland).

B. PQQ-Deficient Mutants

Several mutants have been isolated from *A. calcoaceticus* that cannot produce quinoprotein glucose dehydrogenase activity, but this activity can be reconstituted upon addition of PQQ. Genetic studies showed that the mutants could be subdivided into four complementation groups. The genes have been cloned, sequenced, and brought to expression in *E. coli* and *A. lwoffi* (Goosen *et al.*, 1987). Although many mutants have been described for methylotrophic bacteria, in only one instance was a mutant for methanol dehydrogenase activity obtained that could be reconstituted by PQQ supplementation (Biville *et al.*, 1988) [however, several other PQQ⁻ mutants of *Methylobacterium organophilum* have been obtained, and these can be subdivided into five genetic complementation groups (F. Gasser, personal communication)]. The finding that the natural PQQ⁻ mutants (e.g., *E. coli*, *A. lwoffi*) are able to produce PQQ after introduction of these four genes from *A. calcoaceticus* indicates that the biosynthetic route must be relatively simple (but see the evidence for covalently bound PQQ biosynthesis in Section III,B,5, which could imply that the four genes are only necessary for production of the free form of the cofactor and the genes for covalently bound PQQ are still unknown). Studies on deletion mutants of *A. calcoaceticus* and *Pseudomonas aureofaciens* have provided evidence that one of the genes for PQQ biosynthesis and a gene for anthranilate hydroxylase are in close proximity (van Kleef and Duine, 1988c).

C. Precursors and Intermediates

Studies with methylotrophic bacteria growing on ^{13}C-labeled methanol and unlabeled amino acids have provided evidence that glutamate and tyrosine are precursors for PQQ biosynthesis. These results were independently obtained by the group of Unkefer (Houck *et al.*, 1988), using *Methylobacterium* AM1 and of Duine (van Kleef and Duine, 1988b), using *Hyphomicrobium* X. Although both groups used

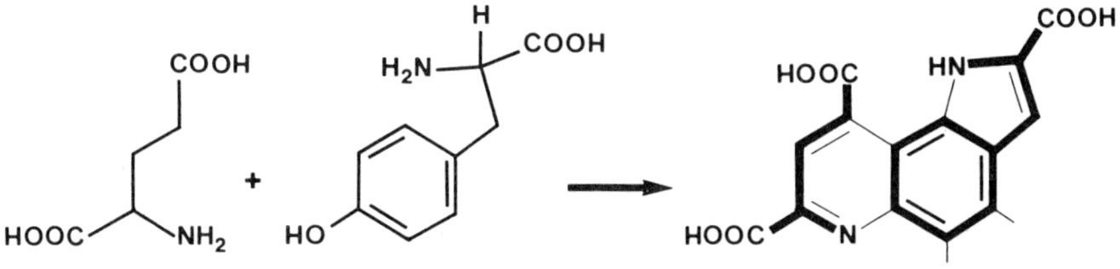

FIG. 7. Tyrosine and glutamic acid as precursors for PQQ biosynthesis.

^{13}C-NMR to trace biosynthesis, the experimental set-ups were independent, providing strong evidence for the synthetic scheme depicted in Fig. 7.

Since the *A. calcoaceticus* PQQ⁻ mutants could be genetically grouped into four classes, this opened up possibilities to probe for intermediates with cross-feeding studies (van Kleef and Duine, 1988c). Results were negative with normal cells, permeabilized cells, and cells growing under stress to induce quinoprotein production. Analysis of the culture media of very efficient PQQ producers (e.g., *Methylobacterium organophilum, Pseudomonas aureofaciens*), comparing PQQ⁻ mutants and wild-type strains, did not reveal differences. Supplementation of growth media with the amino acids concerned did not increase the yield of PQQ or lead to detectable intermediates of the biosynthetic route. The lack of detectable intermediates can be explained in several ways. However, since only four genes have been discovered for biosynthesis and one of the genes is so small that it will not code for an enzyme (Goosen *et al.*, 1987), an attractive explanation could be that biosynthesis proceeds on a peptide matrix by cyclization of tyrosine and glutamic acid, desaturation, and hydroxylation, all without free intermediates. For enzymes containing covalently bound PQQ, the cofactor might be processed on the peptide chain itself; for noncovalently bound PQQ, a special matrix/carrier protein could exist from which the completed PQQ is removed by scission of amide bonds. A model for such a process is depcited in Fig. 8. Finally, it should be mentioned in this context that processing of an amino acid residue in a protein chain to cofactor has already been proposed for another carbonyl group containing cofactor, the pyruvoyl prosthetic group (Recsei and Snell, 1984). An even more interesting example is the tyrosyl free radical cofactor, recently detected in a number of enzymes (Prince, 1988). This cofactor could be the evolutionary precursor of pro-PQQ, eventually leading to the "amino acid cofactor" PQQ.

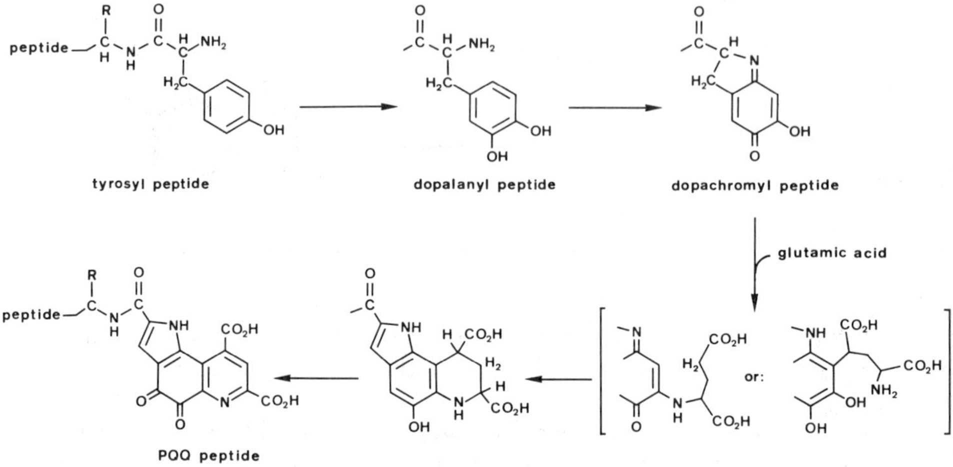

FIG. 8. Proposed model for the assemblage of PQQ on a matrix peptide.

V. BIOLOGICAL ROLE

A. THE EFFECT OF PQQ ADDITION

1. Growth Factor for Microbia

Several bacteria produce apoquinoprotein dehydrogenases during growth on a carbon and energy source not requiring the participation of the dehydrogenase concerned (Table IV). Culturing these organisms on substrates related to this quinoprotein yields one of two possibilities. One type of bacteria grows only in medium supplemented with PQQ. Another type shows suboptimal growth; PQQ supplementation is not absolutely necessary but improves growth significantly. In the latter instance, either the organism has an escape in the form of an enzyme catalyzing the same reaction as the quinoprotein but with a different cofactor [for example, *Pseudomonas testosteroni* growing on ethanol produces quinohemoprotein alcohol dehydrogenase apoenzyme as well as NAD-dependent alcohol dehydrogenase, while PQQ supplementation improves growth rates enormously (Groen *et al.*, 1986)] or the quinoprotein forms an element in an auxiliary energy-providing system (for example, many *A. calcoaceticus* strains do not grow on glucose or gluconate but possess the quinoprotein glucose dehydrogenase which converts glucose into gluconolactone and generates useful energy for transport processes, adenosine triphosphate production, etc.). It would seem that PQQ is not vital for these bacteria, but is a growth factor only when a quinoprotein is a key enzyme in the dissimilation route. This conclusion may be premature, however, since quinoproteins with covalently bound PQQ are essential for mammalian organisms. If it is assumed that similar enzymes occur in bacteria and syntheses of covalently and noncovalently PQQ occur independently, it may eventually turn out that PQQ is also essential for bacteria, and is synthesized (in covalently bound form) even in the natural PQQ^- mutants (see Section III,B,5).

Also, bacteria producing holoquinoproteins show reduction in growth lag time upon PQQ addition, e.g., *Acetobacter* and *Gluconobacter* (Ameyama *et al.*, 1984a). Since apoquinoprotein and PQQ synthesis can proceed in an uncoordinated manner (van Schie *et al.*, 1984), the stimulation could result from imbalance in the synthesis so that insufficient quantities of holoquinoproteins are available [another possibility could be the removal of PQQ from holoquinoprotein during manipulations, in accordance with the fact that the effect is only observable after the cells are rinsed several times (Ameyama *et al.*, 1985b)]. This effect was also claimed for *Saccharomyces cereviseae*, but this is difficult to explain, since no quinoprotein dehydrogenases have been reported for this organism. This finding has not yet been confirmed.

2. A Role as Vitamin?

The occurrence of PQQ in so many mammalian enzymes raises the question of whether these organisms are able to synthesize this compound themselves or whether they require an outside source (for instance, from the intestines where the source might be ingested food or overproduction by the microbial flora). In principle, the first possibility could be tested, were there mutants producing insufficient amounts of PQQ. In view of the involvement of several quinoproteins in the regulation of important physiological processes (e.g., dopamine β-hydroxylase, lysyl oxidase, lipoxygenase), however, inadequate provision of PQQ might impair viability of offspring, making this approach impracticable. On the other hand, were such a disorder to yield only lower levels of PQQ, the result might not be fatal and PQQ supplementation could relieve certain defects related to underproduction (the same effect could be achieved under conditions of suboptimal PQQ supply from external sources).

Inadequate amounts of PQQ could also develop upon administration of carbonyl group-reactive drugs or upon unwitting ingestion of like substances (e.g., lathyrogens). Until now, such effects have been attributed to a reduction in concentrations of vitamin B_6 or to blocking of enzymes requiring this compound. It should be recognized, however, that the same phenomena could apply to PQQ and quinoproteins. Claims that certain disorders are related to vitamin B_6 shortage might be challenged. Such evidence is generally based on improvement (artificially induced by the carbonyl group-reactive compounds) upon administration of vitamin B_6. Another explanation, however, might be that vitamin B_6 acts as a scavenger for the carbonyl group-reactive agent, thus shifting the equilibrium so that inhibited quinoproteins become deblocked. It could even be possible that PQQ administration would have the same effect. In any event, an intimate relationship between PQQ and vitamin B_6 may exist based on their reactive carbonyl groups. Hence, the role of vitamin B_6 may require reexamination. Construction of inhibitors specifically aimed at one of the cofactors, as well as comparative studies, will be necessary to elucidate each specific function. Finally, it should be noted that several compounds not only react with cofactors bearing reactive carbonyl groups, but also with other cofactors (e.g., hydrazines also block certain flavoproteins and hemoproteins). In principle, such effects could be counteracted by PQQ and vitamin B_6, implying a complex interrelationship among drugs, cofactors, and enzymes.

To prove that PQQ is a vitamin, one must also consider availability and assemblage into quinoprotein. The existence of free PQQ in complex mammalian tissues and blood seems out of the question. Transport via specific carriers or existence of "oxazolases" at appropriate loci could circumvent the problem of degradation or derivatization, but such possibilities are speculative. All mammalian quinoproteins contain PQQ in covalently bound form, and preliminary studies in bacteria indicate that PQQ may be biosynthesized on the enzyme itself (directly from the building blocks by ring closure, desaturation, and hydroxylation steps). If the latter view were correct, PQQ would not be a vitamin, since its administration would not lead to incorporation into quinoproteins. On the other hand, indirect effects due to its reactive carbonyl group cannot be excluded. A proposal has already been made (Hanauske-Abel *et al.*, 1987) that PQQ is a modulator of connective tissue formation based on the fact that it is the cofactor of lysyl oxidase and that it is a strong inhibitor of another enzyme in the route, proline hydroxylase. Nutritional studies could shed light on this. It is interesting that vinegar contains significant amounts of PQQ (Duine *et al.*, 1985) (ethanol-growing *Acetobacter* strains excrete PQQ into their culture medium and the industrial production of vinegar is carried out with a relatively clean mineral medium).

So far, PQQ supplementation in plant and animal systems has not shown significant effects. On the other hand, recent reports claim efects on rats (Matsumoto *et al.*, 1989) and *Lilium* pollen (Xiong *et al.*, 1988). In the light of the foregoing, one must distinguish indirect from direct effects in order to attribute to PQQ a possible role as a vitamin.

B. The Significance of Quinoproteins

1. *In Microorganisms*

So far, no unique property has been revealed for quinoproteins in microorganisms, since quinoprotein dehydrogenases find their counterparts in flavoprotein- and NAD-linked dehydrogenases (Duine, 1988). In fact, some microbia contain the whole set of enzymes catalyzing the same reaction but using different cofactors. Perhaps quinoprotein dehydrogenases become important only under certain circumstances. Special features of a particular catalyst may fit it to the task, e.g., the unique properties of PQQ may impose special catalytic characteristics (turnover number, affinity for the substrate, stability under certain conditions of pH, etc.) on quinoproteins, characteristics not conferred by other cofactors. Such properties might govern localization of dehydrogenases (periplasm, cytoplasm) or the nature of the component in the respiratory chain to which the electrons derived from the substrate are transferred. This could affect, in turn, energetics required or available for transport and ATP yield. From the fragmentary data available at the moment, one cannot define such unique features of quinoproteins (Duine, 1988). Comparative studies among enzymes catalyzing the same reaction but using different cofactors are necessary to achieve that goal. Related to these structure–function aspects is the question concerning the evolutionary significance of quinoproteins. Since PQQ is not unique to microorganisms, it may be a relic which has survived because it somehow escaped natural selection pressure. On the other hand, this has no bearing on the significance of quinoproteins in mammalian organisms.

2. *In Mammalian Organisms*

Lysyl oxidase plays a crucial role in the synthesis of elastin and collagen. The other mammalian quinoproteins are involved in important physiological processes of regulation. A list of bioregulators (as-

TABLE VIII

QUINOPROTEINS IN THE CONVERSION/BIOSYNTHESIS OF MAMMALIAN BIOREGULATORS

Enzyme	Bioregulator
Plasma amine oxidase	Spermine, spermidine
Diamine oxidase	Histamine
Dopamine β-hydroxylase	Noradrenaline
Lipoxygenase	Lipoxins, leukotrienes, prostaglandins, thromboxanes
Dopa decarboxylase	Dopamine
α-Amidating enzyme (acting on glycine-extended peptides)	Many bioactive peptides operating in neural and endocrine tissue (e.g., corticotropin, growth hormone, oxytocin, vasopressin, gastrin, melanocyte-stimulating hormone)

sumed to be) synthesized or converted by quinoprotein enzymes is given in Table VIII. Obviously, quinoproteins play a key role in mammals utilizing this type of regulation because as far as is known, there are no alternate pathways via enzymes catalyzing the same reactions with other cofactors (except the quinoprotein amine oxidases, which show a certain overlap in substrate specificity with their flavoprotein counterparts).

VI. IMPLICATIONS AND PERSPECTIVES

1. Although PQQ is an essential cofactor for several key enzymes in physiological processes in mammals, it has not yet been proved to be a vitamin.

2. Development of inhibitors specifically directed to PQQ might reveal not only the role of PQQ and quinoproteins, but also that of vitamin B_6 and enzymes depending on it (and vice versa). This could also be afforded by developing inhibitors specifically blocking the biosynthesis of PQQ or feeding animals a PQQ-free diet.

3. Analytical procedures should be developed to determine PQQ and its derivatives unambiguously in biological materials. This will provide answers to questions related to biosynthesis and vitamin function.

4. The recent discovery of PQQ suggests that there are still other unknown cofactors yet to be found. Systematic procedures for cofactor identification will stimulate progress on cofactor enzymology.

5. The fact that PQQ has been detected in many well-known metal-

loenzymes implies that it may also have been overlooked in enzymes already believed to or known to utilize recognized cofactors.

6. The finding of PQQ implies evolutionary variation not only in the apoprotein of an enzyme but also in its cofactor.

ACKNOWLEDGMENTS

We thank Hoffmann La Roche, Basel, Switzerland, for generous financial support of part of our research and our colleagues for providing us their unpublished results.

REFERENCES

Ameyama, M., Matsushita, K., Ohno, Y., Shinagawa, E., and Adachi, O. (1981). Existence of a novel prosthetic group, PQQ, in membrane-bound, electron transport chain-linked, primary dehydrogenase of oxidative bacteria. *FEBS Lett.* **130,** 179–183.

Ameyama, M., Shinagawa, E., Matsushita, K., and Adachi, O. (1984a). Growth stimulation of microorganisms by pyrroloquinoline quinone. *Agric. Biol. Chem.* **48,** 2909–2911.

Ameyama, M., Shinagawa, E., Matsushita, K., and Adachi, O. (1984b). Growth stimulating substance for microorganisms produced by *Escherichia coli* causing the reduction of the lag phase in microbial growth and identity of the substance with pyrroloquinoline quinone. *Agric. Biol. Chem.* **48,** 3099–3107.

Ameyama, M., Shinagawa, E., Matsushita, K., and Adachi, O. (1985a). Growth stimulating activity for microorganisms in naturally occurring substances and partial characterization of the substance for the activity as pyrroloquinoline quinone. *Agric. Biol. Chem.* **49,** 699–709.

Ameyama, M., Shinagawa, E., Matsushita, K., and Adachi, O. (1985b). How many times should the inoculum be rinsed before inoculation in the assay for growth stimulating activity of pyrroloquinoline quinone? *Agric. Biol. Chem.* **49,** 853–854.

Ameyama, M., Nonobe, M., Hayashi, M., Shinagawa, E., Matsushita, K., and Adachi, O. (1985c). Mode of binding of pyrroloquinoline quinone to apo-glucose dehydrogenase. *Agric. Biol. Chem.* **49,** 1227–1231.

Ameyama, M., Nonobe, M., Shinagawa, E., Matsushita, K., and Adachi, O. (1985d). Method of enzymatic determination of pyrroloquinoline quinone. *Anal. Biochem.* **151,** 263–267.

Anthony, C., and Zatman, L. J. (1967). The microbial oxidation of methanol. The prosthetic group of the alcohol dehydrogenase of *Pseudomonas* spec. M27: A new oxidoreductase prosthetic group. *Biochem. J.* **104,** 960–969.

Bird, T. A., and Levene, C. I. (1982). Lysyl oxidase: Evidence that pyridoxal phosphate is a cofactor. *Biochem. Biophys. Res. Commun.* **108,** 1172–1180.

Biville, F., Mazodier, P., Gasser, F., van Kleef, M. A. G., and Duine, J. A. (1988). Physiological properties of a pyrroloquinoline quinone mutant of *Methylobacterium organophilum*. *FEMS Microbiol. Lett.* **52,** 53–58.

Buechi, G., Botkin, J. H., Lee, G. C. M., and Yakushijin, K. (1985). A synthesis of methoxatin. *J. Am. Chem. Soc.* **107,** 5555–5556.

Corey, E. J., and Tramontano, A. (1981). Total synthesis of the quinonoid alcohol dehydrogenase coenzyme of methylotrophic bacteria. *J. Am. Chem. Soc.* **103,** 5599–5600.

de Beer, R., Duine, J. A., Frank, J., and Large, P. J. (1980). The prosthetic group of methylamine dehydrogenase from *Pseudomonas* AM1. *Biochim. Biophys. Acta* **622,** 370–374.

Dekker, R. H., Duine, J. A., Frank, J., Verwiel, P. E. J., and Westerling, J. (1982). Covalent addition of H_2O, enzyme substrates and activators to pyrroloquinoline quinone, the coenzyme of quinoproteins. *Eur. J. Biochem.* **125**, 69–73.

Duine, J. A. (1988). Unity and diversity in biological redox catalysis: Comparative enzymology of some microbial oxidoreductases showing variation in cofactor identity. *In* "The Roots of Modern Biochemistry" (Kleinkauf, von Dohren, and Jaenicke, eds.), pp. 671–682. de Gruyter, Berlin and New York.

Duine, J. A., and Frank, J. (1980). The prosthetic group of methanol dehydrogenase. Purification and some properties. *Biochem. J.* **187**, 213–219.

Duine, J. A., and Frank, J. (1981). Quinoproteins: A novel class of dehydrogenases. *Trends Biochem. Sci.* **6**, 278–280.

Duine, J. A., and Jongejan, J. A. (1989). Quinoprotein enzymes. *Annu. Rev. Biochem.* **58**, 403–426.

Duine, J. A., Frank, J., and Westerling, J. (1978). Purification and properties of methanol dehydrogenase from *Hyphomicrobium* X. *Biochim. Biophys. Acta* **524**, 277–287.

Duine, J. A., Frank, J., and van Zeeland, J. K. (1979). Glucose dehydrogenase from *Acinetobacter calcoaceticus:* A quinoprotein. *FEBS Lett.* **108**, 443–446.

Duine, J. A., Frank, J., and Verwiel, P. E. J. (1980). Structure and activity of the prosthetic group of methanol dehydrogenase. *Eur. J. Biochem.* **108**, 187–192.

Duine, J. A., Frank, J., and Verwiel, P. E. J. (1981). Characterization of the second prosthetic group in methanol dehydrogenase from *Hyphomicrobium* X. *Eur. J. Biochem.* **118**, 395–399.

Duine, J. A., Frank, J., and Jongejan, J. A. (1983). Detection and determination of pyrroloquinoline quinone, the coenzyme of quinoproteins. *Anal. Biochem.* **133**, 239–243.

Duine, J. A., Frank, J., and Jongejan, J. A. (1985). The coenzyme PQQ and quinoproteins, a novel class of oxidoreductases. *In* "Proceedings of the 16th FEBS Congress, Part A" (Yu. Ovchinikov, ed.), pp. 79–88. VNU Science Press, Utrecht, The Netherlands.

Duine, J. A., Frank, J., and Jongejan, J. A. (1986). PQQ and quinoprotein enzymes in microbial oxidations. *FEMS Microbiol. Rev.* **32**, 165–178.

Duine, J. A., Frank, J., and Jongejan, J. A. (1987a). Enzymology of quinoproteins. *Adv. Enzymol.* **59**, 169–212.

Duine, J. A., Jongejan, J. A., and van der Meer, R. A. (1987b). Copper-containing amine oxidases (EC 1.4.3.6) have covalently-bound PQQ and not PLP as organic cofactor. *In* "Biochemistry of Vitamin B6" (T. Korpela and P. Christen, eds.), pp. 243–252. Birkhaeuser, Basel.

Eipper, B. A., Mains, R. E., and Glembotski, C. C. (1983). Identification in pituitary tissue of a peptide α-amidation activity that acts on glycine-extended peptides and requires molecular oxygen, copper, and ascorbic acid. *Proc. Natl. Acad. Sci. U.S.A.* **80**, 5144–5148.

Eirich, L. D., Vogels, G. D., and Wolfe, R. S. (1978). Proposed structure for coenzyme F420 from Methanobacterium. *Biochemistry* **17**, 4583–4593.

Eker, A. P. M., Dekker, R. H., and Berends, W. (1980). Photoreactivating enzyme from *Streptomyces griseus*. *Photochem. Photobiol.* **33**, 65–72.

Faraggi, M., Chandrakesar, R., McWhirter, R. B., and Klapper, M. H. (1986). The methoxatin semiquinone. A pulse radiolysis study. *Biochem. Biophys. Res. Commun.* **139**, 955–960.

Flueckiger, R., Woodtli, T., and Gallop, P. M. (1988). The interaction of aminogroups with pyrroloquinoline quinone as detected by the reduction of nitroblue tetrazolium. *Biochem. Biophys. Res. Commun.* **153**, 353–358.

Gainor, J. A., and Weinreb, S. M. (1982). Synthesis of the bacterial coenzyme methoxatin. *J. Org. Chem.* **47**, 2833–2837.

Geiger, O., and Goerisch, H. (1987). Enzymatic determination of pyrroloquinoline quinone using crude membranes from *Escherichia coli. Anal. Biochem.* **164**, 418–423.

Glatz, Z., Kovar, J., Macholan, L., and Pec, P. (1987). Pea (*Pisum sativum*) diamine oxidase contains pyrroloquinoline quinone as a cofactor. *Biochem. J.* **242**, 603–606.

Goosen, N., Vermaas, D. A. M., and van de Putte, P. (1987). Cloning of the genes involved in synthesis of coenzyme pyrroloquinoline quinone from *Acinetobacter calcoaceticus. J. Bacteriol.* **169**, 303–307.

Groen, B. W., van Kleef, M. A. G., and Duine, J. A. (1986). Quinohaemoprotein alcohol dehydrogenase apoenzyme from *Pseudomonas testosteroni. Biochem. J.* **234**, 611–615.

Hanauske-Abel, H. M., Tschank, G., Guenzler, V., Baader, E., and Gallop, P. (1987). Pyrroloquinoline quinone and molecules mimicking its functional domains. Modulators of connective tissue formation? *FEBS Lett.* **214**, 236–243.

Hauge, J. G. (1964). Glucose dehydrogenase of *Bacterium anitratum:* An enzyme with a novel prosthetic group. *J. Biol. Chem.* **239**, 3630–3639.

Hendrickson, J. B. and de Vries, J. G. (1984). Total synthesis of the novel coenzyme methoxatin. *J. Org. Chem.* **50**, 1688–1695.

Hommes, R. W. J., Postma, P. W., Neijssel, O. M., Tempest, D. W., Dokter, P., and Duine, J. A. (1984). Evidence of a quinoprotein glucose dehydrogenase apoenzyme in several strains of *Escherichia coli. FEMS Microbiol. Lett.* **24**, 329–333.

Houck, D. R., Hanners, J. L., and Unkefer, C. J. (1988). PQQ: Biosynthetic studies in *Methylobacterium* AM1 using specific ^{13}C-labeling and NMR. *J. Am. Chem. Soc.* **110**, 6920–6921.

Imanaga, Y., Hirano-Sawatake, Y., Arito-Hashimoto, Y., Itou-Shibouta, Y., and Katoh-Semba, R. (1979). Glucose dehydrogenase from *Pseudomonas fluorescens. Proc. Jpn. Acad.* **558**, 264–269.

International Union of Biochemistry (1984). "Enzyme Nomenclature." Academic Press, Orlando, Florida.

Itoh, S., Kato, J., Inoue, T., Kitamura, M., and Oshiro, Y. (1987). Synthesis of pyrroloquinoline quinone derivatives: Model compounds of a novel coenzyme PQQ (methoxatin). *Synthesis* **12**, 163–168.

Jongejan, J. A., van der Meer, R. A., van Zuylen, G. A., and Duine, J. A. (1987). Spectrophotometric studies on pyrroloquinoline quinone–Cu(II) complexes as possible models for copper–quinoprotein amine oxidases. *Recl. Trav. Chim. Pays-Bas* **106**, 365.

Jongejan, J. A., Bezemer, R. P., and Duine, J. A. (1988). Synthesis of [13]C- and [2]H-labelled PQQ. *Tetrahedron Lett.* **29**, 3709–3712.

Kilty, C. G., Maruyama, K., and Forrest, H. S. (1982). Reconstitution of glucose dehydrogenase using synthetic methoxatin. *Arch. Biochem. Biophys.* **218**, 623–625.

Knowles, P. F., Pandeya, K. B., Rius, F. X., Spencer, C. M., Moog, R. S., McGuirl, M. A., and Dooley, D. M. (1987). The organic cofactor in plasma amine oxidase: Evidence for pyrroloquinoline quinone and against pyridoxal phosphate. *Biochem. J.* **241**, 603–608.

Kramer, S. P., Johnson, J. L., Ribeiro, A. A., Millington, D. S., and Rajagopolan, K. V. (1987). The structure of the molybdenum cofactor. Characterization of di-(carboxamidomethyl)molybdopterin from sulfite oxidase and xanthine oxidase. *J. Biol. Chem.* **262,** 16357–16363.

Leigh, J. A., Rinehart, K. L., and Wolfe, R. S. (1984). Proposed structure for coenzyme F420 from Methanobacterium. *J. Am. Chem. Soc.* **106,** 3636–3640.

Lobenstein-Verbeek, C. L., Jongejan, J. A., Frank, J., and Duine, J. A. (1984). Bovine serum amine oxidase: A mammalian enzyme having covalently-bound PQQ as prosthetic group. *FEBS Lett.* **170,** 305–309.

MacKenzie, A. R., Moody, C. J., and Rees, C. W. (1986). Synthesis of the bacterial coenzyme methoxatin. *Tetrahedron* **42,** 3259–3268.

Matsumoto, T., Hori, A., Hayakawa, H., Ogiso, S., Hayakawa, N., Nimura, Y., Takahashi, I., and Shionoya, S. (1989). Effects of exogenous PQQ on mortality rate and some biochemical parameters during endotoxin shock in rats. *In* "Proceedings of the First International Symposium on PQQ and Quinoproteins" (J. A. Duine and J. A. Jongejan, eds.), pp. 162–164. Kluwer Academic, Dordrecht, The Netherlands.

McCormick, J. R. D., and Morton, G. O. (1982). Identity of cosynthetic factor 1 of *Streptomyces aureofaciens* and fragment FO of Methanobacterium species. *J. Am. Chem. Soc.* **104,** 4014–4015.

Meyer, O., Jacobitz, S., and Krueger, B. (1986). Biochemistry and physiology of aerobic carbon monoxide-utilizing bacteria. *FEMS Microbiol. Rev.* **39,** 161–179.

Moog, R. S., McGuirl, M. A., Cote, C. E., and Dooley, D. M. (1986). Evidence for methoxatin (pyrroloquinoline quinone) as the cofactor in bovine plasma amine oxidase from resonance Raman spectroscopy. *Proc. Natl. Acad. Sci. U.S.A.* **83,** 8435–8439.

Nagasawa, T., and Yamada, H. (1987). Nitrile hydratase is a quinoprotein. A possible new function of pyrroloquinoline quinone: Activation of H_2O in an enzymatic hydration reaction. *Biochem. Biophys. Res. Commun.* **147,** 701–709.

Niederpruem, D. J., and Doudoroff, M. (1965). Cofactor-dependent aldose dehydrogenase of *Rhodopseudomonas spheroides*. *J. Bacteriol.* **89,** 697–705.

Noar, J. B., and Bruice, T. C. (1987). Decarboxylated methoxatin analogues. Synthesis of 7- and 9-decarboxymethoxatin. *J. Org. Chem.* **52,** 1942–1945.

Noar, J. B., Rodriguez, E. J., and Bruice, T. C. (1985). Synthesis of 9-decarboxymethoxatin. Metal complexation of methoxatin as a possible requirement for its biological activity. *J. Am. Chem. Soc.* **107,** 7198–7201.

Noll, K. M., Rinehart, K. L., Tanner, R. S., and Wolfe, R. S. (1986). Structure of component B (7-mercaptoheptanoylthreonine phosphate) of the methylcoenzyme M methylreductase system of *Methanobacterium autotrophicum*. *Proc. Natl. Acad. Sci. U.S.A.* **83,** 4238–4242.

Pfaltz, A., Jaun, B., Fassler, A., Eschenmoser, A., Jaenchen, R., Gilles, H. H., Diekert, G., and Thauer, R. K. (1982). Zur Kenntniss des Faktors F430 aus methanogenen Bacterien: Struktur des porphinoiden Ligand Systems. *Helv. Chim. Acta* **65,** 828–865.

Prince, R. C. (1988). Tyrosyl radicals. *Trends Biochem. Sci.* **13,** 286–288.

Recsei, P. A., and Snell, E. E. (1984). Pyruvoyl enzymes. *Annu. Rev. Biochem.* **53,** 357–387.

Riceberg, L. J., Simon, H., Vunakis, H. V., and Abeles, R. H. (1975). Effects of aminoacetonitrile, an amine oxidase inhibitor, on mescaline metabolism in the rabbit. *Biochem. Pharmacol.* **24,** 119–125.

Salisbury, S. A., Forrest, H. S., Cruse, W. B. T., and Kennard, O. (1979). A novel coenzyme from bacterial primary alcohol dehydrogenases. *Nature (London)* **280,** 843–844.

Shinagawa, E., Matsushita, K., Nonobe, M., Adachi, O., Ameyama, M., and Oshiro, Y. (1986). The 9-carboxyl group of pyrroloquinoline quinone, a novel prosthetic group, is essential in the formation of holoenzyme of D-glucose dehydrogenase. *Biochem. Biophys. Res. Commun.* **139,** 1279–1284.

Sleath, P. R., Noar, J. B., Eberlein, G. A., and Bruice, T. C. (1985). Synthesis of 7,9-didecarboxymethoxatin (4,5-dihydro-4,5-dioxo-1*H*-pyrrolo[2,3-*f*]quinoline-2-carboxylic acid) and comparison of its chemical properties with those of methoxatin and analogous *o*-quinones. Model studies directed toward the action of PQQ requiring bacterial oxidoreductases and mammalian plasma amine oxidase. *J. Am. Chem. Soc.* **107,** 3328–3338.

Sperl, G. T., Forrest, H. S., and Gibson, D. T. (1974). Substrate specificity of the purified primary alcohol dehydrogenase from methanol oxidizing bacteria. *J. Bacteriol.* **118,** 541–550.

Suzuki, O., Seno, H., Kumazawa, T., and Urakami, T. (1989). Gas chromatography of PQQ. In "Proceedings of the First International Symposium on PQQ and Quinoproteins" (J. A. Duine and J. A. Jongejan, eds.), pp. 123–130. Kluwer Academic, Dordrecht, The Netherlands.

Taylor, C. D., and Wolfe, R. S. (1974). Structure and methylation of coenzyme M (HSCH$_2$CH$_2$SO$_3$). *J. Biol. Chem.* **249,** 4879–4885.

Theorell, H. (1935). Reindarstellung der Wirkungsgruppe der gelben Ferment. *Biochem. Z.* **275,** 344–349.

Urushibara, T., Forrest, H. S., Hoare, D. S., and Patel, R. N. (1971). Pteridines produced by *Methylococcus capsulatus.* Isolation and identification of neopterin 2′,3′-phosphate. *Biochem. J.* **125,** 141–146.

van Beelen, P., Stasser, A. P. M., Bosch, J. W. G., Vogels, G. D., Guyt, W., and Haasnoot, C. A. G. (1984). Elucidation of the structure of methanopterin, a coenzyme from *Methanobacterium autotrophicum,* using two-dimensional nuclear-magnetic-resonance techniques. *Eur. J. Biochem.* **138,** 563–571.

van der Meer, R. A., and Duine, J. A. (1986). Covalently-bound pyrroloquinoline quinone is the organic prosthetic group in human placental lysyloxidase. *Biochem. J.* **239,** 789–791.

van der Meer, R. A., and Duine, J. A. (1988). Pyrroloquinoline quinone (PQQ) is the organic cofactor in soybean lipoxygenase-1. *FEBS Lett.* **235,** 194–200.

van der Meer, R. A., Jongejan, J. A., Frank, J., and Duine, J. A. (1986). Hydrazone formation of 2,4-dinitrophenylhydrazine with PQQ in porcine kidney diamine oxidase. *FEBS Lett.* **206,** 211–214.

van der Meer, R. A., Jongejan, J. A., and Duine, J. A. (1987). Phenylhydrazine as probe for cofactor identification in amine oxidoreductases. Evidence for PQQ as the cofactor in methylamine dehydrogenase. *FEBS Lett.* **221,** 299–304.

van der Meer, R. A., Jongejan, J. A., and Duine, J. A. (1988). Dopamine β-hydroxylase from bovine medulla contains covalently-bound pyrroloquinoline quinone. *FEBS Lett.* **231,** 303–307.

van der Meer, R. A., Groen, B. W., and Duine, J. A. (1989a). On the biosynthesis of free and covalently bound PQQ. Glutamic acid decarboxylase from *Escherichia coli* is a pyridoxo-quinoprotein. *FEBS Lett.* **246,** 109–112.

van der Meer, R. A., van Wassenaar, P. D., van Brouwershaven, J. H., and Duine, J. A. (1989b). Primary structure of a pyrroloquinoline quinone (PQQ) containing peptide isolated from procine kidney diamine oxidase. *Biochem. Biophys. Res. Commun.* **159,** 726–733.

van Iersel, J., van der Meer, R. A., and Duine, J. A. (1986). Methylamine oxidase from

Arthrobacter P1: A bacterial copper–quinoprotein amine oxidase. *Eur. J. Biochem.* **161**, 415–419.

van Kleef, M. A. G., and Duine, J. A. (1988a). Bacterial NAD(P)-independent quinate dehydrogenase is a quinoprotein. *Arch. Microbiol.* **150**, 32–36.

van Kleef, M. A. G., and Duine, J. A. (1988b). L-tyrosine is the precursor of PQQ biosynthesis in *Hyphomicrobium* X. *FEBS Lett.* **237**, 91–97.

van Kleef, M. A. G., and Duine, J. A. (1988c). A search for intermediates in the bacterial biosynthesis of PQQ. *BioFactors* **1**, 297–302.

van Kleef, M. A. G., and Duine, J. A. (1989). Factors relevant in bacterial pyrroloquinoline quinone production. *Appl. Environ. Microbiol.* **55**, in press.

van Kleef, M. A. G., Dokter, P., Mulder, A. C., and Duine, J. A. (1987). Detection of PQQ. *Anal. Biochem.* **162**, 143–149.

van Koningsveld, H., Jansen, J. C., Jongejan, J. A., Frank, J., and Duine, J. A. (1985). Structure of the 2,4-dinitrophenylhydrazine adduct of pyrroloquinoline quinone (PQQ) dimethyl ethyl triester, C24H18N6011. *Acta Crystallogr., Sect. C* **C41**, 92–95.

van Schie, B. J., van Dijken, J. P., and Kuenen, J. G. (1984). Non-coordinated synthesis of glucose dehydrogenase and its prosthetic group PQQ in Acinetobacter and Pseudomonas species. *FEMS Microbiol. Lett.* **24**, 133–138.

van Schie, B. J., de Mooy, O. H., Linton, J. D., van Dijken, J. P., and Kuenen, J. G. (1987). PQQ-dependent production of gluconic acid by Acinetobacter, Agrobacterium and Rhizobium species. *J. Gen. Microbiol.* **133**, 867–875.

Vellieux, F. M. D., Frank, J., Swarte, M. B. A., Groenendijk, H., Duine, J. A., Drenth, J., and Hol, W. G. J. (1986). Purification, crystallization and preliminary X-ray investigation of quinoprotein methylamine dehydrogenase from *Thiobacillus versutus*. *Eur. J. Biochem.* **154**, 383–386.

Westerling, J., Frank, J., and Duine, J. A. (1979). The prosthetic group of methanol dehydrogenase from *Hyphomicrobium* X: Electron spin evidence for a quinone structure. *Biochem. Biophys. Res. Commun.* **87**, 719–724.

Williamson, P. R., Moog, R. S., Dooley, D. M., and Kagan, H. M. (1986). Evidence for pyrroloquinoline quinone as the carbonyl cofactor in lysyl oxidase by absorption and resonance Raman spectroscopy. *J. Biol. Chem.* **261**, 16302–16305.

Winters-Ivey, D. K., and Ljungdahl, L. G. (1989). PQQ-dependent methanol dehydrogenase from *Clostridium thermoautotrophicum*. *In* "Proceedings of the First International Symposium on PQQ and Quinoproteins" (J. A. Duine and J. A. Jongejan, eds.), pp. 35–39. Kluwer Academic, Dordrecht, The Netherlands.

Wood, W. A., and Schwerdt, R. F. (1953). Carbohydrate oxidation by *Pseudomonas fluorescens*. I. The mechanism of glucose and gluconate oxidation. *J. Biol. Chem.* **201**, 501–511.

Xiong, L. B., Sekiya, J., and Shimose, N. (1988). Stimulation of Lillium pollen germination by pyrroloquinoline quinone. *Agric. Biol. Chem.* **52**, 1065–1066.

Folylpolyglutamate Synthesis and Role in the Regulation of One-Carbon Metabolism

BARRY SHANE

Department of Nutritional Sciences
University of California
Berkeley, California 94720

I. Introduction

Folate coenzymes act as acceptors or donors of one-carbon units in a variety of reactions involved in amino acid and nucleotide metabolism in mammalian tissues (MacKenzie, 1984). These reactions, known as one-carbon metabolism, were initially studied using pteroylmonoglutamates as substrates. It has been known for many years that tissue folates exist primarily as polyglutamate derivatives with the glutamate moieties linked via γ-carboxyl peptide bonds (Fig. 1). These derivatives were thought to be storage forms of the vitamin. The devel-

263

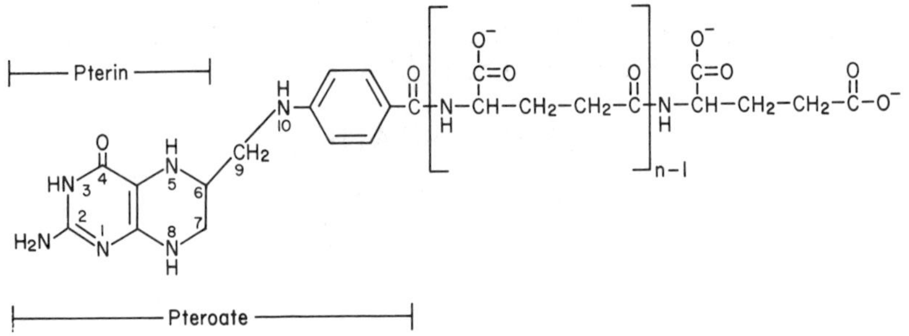

FIG. 1. Structure of tetrahydropteroylpoly-γ-glutamate (H₄PteGlu$_n$).

opment of methods for the chemical synthesis of folylpolyglutamates and for the identification of intracellular folate derivatives over the last 15 years (reviewed by Krumdieck *et al.*, 1983) has allowed detailed studies on the physiological role of these compounds.

It is now apparent that intracellular metabolism of folates to polyglutamate derivatives plays an important role in the regulation of folate homeostasis and is absolutely required for the normal functioning of the metabolic cycles of one-carbon metabolism. Rather than acting as storage forms of the vitamin, folylpolyglutamates are the physiological substrates for the enzymes of one-carbon metabolism, they are potential regulators of different cycles of one-carbon metabolism, and they are required for normal cellular retention of folates. The physiological roles of folylpolyglutamates have been the subject of several reviews (Kisliuk, 1981; McGuire and Bertino, 1981; Cichowicz *et al.*, 1981; McGuire and Coward, 1984).

The physiological importance of folylpolyglutamate synthesis was first clearly demonstrated in cultured Chinese hamster ovary (CHO) cell mutants (AUX B1) which require exogenous glycine, thymidine, and a purine for growth (McBurney and Whitmore, 1974a,b). Although folate transport appeared normal, the mutant cells contained low intracellular folate levels, all of which appeared to be pteroylmonoglutamate. Later studies confirmed that the mutant phenotype was due to a lack of detectable folylpolyglutamate synthetase activity (Taylor and Hanna, 1977) and that AUX B1 cells contain pteroylmonoglutamates, while pteroylpolyglutamates, primarily hexa- and heptaglutamates, comprise over 95% of intracellular folates in wild-type CHO cells (Foo and Shane, 1982). Normalizing intracellular folate levels in AUX B1 cells, by increasing the medium folate content, does not eliminate the mutant phenotype, indicating that the phenotype is due to a lack of folylpolyglutamates rather than low intracellular folate levels. The observation that the proportion of folylpolyglutamates did not decrease in mammalian cells cultured in medium containing suboptimal folate concentrations also suggested that the polyglutamates are not storage forms of the vitamin (Moran *et al.*, 1976). The current review focuses on the mechanisms by which folylpolyglutamates are synthesized in mammalian cells and discusses how regulation of folylpolyglutamate synthesis by physiological and nutritional factors can modulate intracellular folate levels and the types of folylpolyglutamates in tissues. The potential effects of such modulations on the regulation of one-carbon metabolism and recent studies on the role of folylpolyglutamates are also discussed.

II. FOLATE AND ONE-CARBON METABOLISM

Folic acid (pteroylmonoglutamate, PteGlu) consists of a 2-amino-4-hydroxypteridine (pterin) moiety linked via a methylene group at the C-6 position to a p-aminobenzoylglutamate moiety. Folate metabolism involves the reduction of the pyrazine ring of the pterin moiety to the coenzymatically active tetrahydro form (Fig. 1), the elongation of the glutamate chain by the addition of glutamate residues in γ-peptide linkage, and the acquisition and oxidation or reduction of one-carbon units at the N-5 and/or N-10 positions.

The various metabolic cycles of one-carbon metabolism in the cytoplasm and mitochondria of mammalian tissues are shown in Figs. 2 and 3. Folate coenzymes act as cosubstrates in these reactions. Consequently, folate metabolism and its regulation are interwoven with the regulation of the synthesis of products of one-carbon metabolism, and factors that regulate any one cycle of one-carbon metabolism would be expected to influence folate availability for the other cycles of one-carbon metabolism. Before discussing the synthesis and the role of folylpolyglutamates in one-carbon metabolism, a brief review on the organization of these metabolic cycles is presented.

A. CYTOPLASMIC PATHWAYS

1. *Amino Acid Metabolism*

a. Serine–Glycine Interconversion. Serine hydroxymethyltransferase, a pyridoxal phosphate containing enzyme, catalyzes the reversible transfer of formaldehyde from serine to $H_4PteGlu_n$[1] to generate 5,10-methylene-$H_4PteGlu_n$ and glycine (Fig. 2, reaction 3), as follows:

---

[1]$H_4PteGlu_n$, 5,6,7,8-Tetrahydropteroylpoly-γ-glutamate, n indicating the number of L-glutamate moieties.

$$\text{serine} + H_4PteGlu_n \rightleftharpoons \text{glycine} + 5,10\text{-methylene-}H_4PteGlu_n$$

Although $H_4PteGlu_n$ is not absolutely required for the serine-to-glycine conversion, $H_4PteGlu_n$ increases the reaction rate by several orders of magnitude and changes the kinetic mechanism (Schirch, 1984) from ordered to random. Mammalian cells contain two isozymes of the hydroxymethyltransferase, one cytosolic and one mitochondrial (Schirch and Peterson, 1980). The cytosolic enzyme appears to be the predominant species in liver (Schirch and Peterson, 1980; Matthews *et al.*, 1982), although a predominant distribution in mitochondria has been reported for cultured cells (Chasin *et al.*, 1974). Serine hydroxymethyltransferase is an abundant protein in the cytoplasm and the C-3 of serine is the major source of one-carbon units for folate metabolism. The 5,10-methylene-$H_4PteGlu_n$ formed in this reaction plays a central role in one-carbon metabolism, as its one-carbon moiety can be directed into the three cytoplasmic one-carbon cycles of methionine, *de novo* purine, and thymidylate synthesis.

b. Methionine Cycle. A major cycle of one-carbon utilization involves the reduction of 5,10-methylene-$H_4PteGlu_n$ to 5-methyl-$H_4PteGlu_n$ (Fig. 2, reaction 10) followed by the transfer of the methyl group to homocysteine to form methionine and to regenerate $H_4PteGlu_n$ (Fig. 2, reaction 11; Matthews, 1984).

5,10-Methylene-$H_4PteGlu_n$ reduction is catalyzed by the flavoprotein methylene tetrahydrofolate reductase as follows:[2]

$$5,10\text{-methylene-}H_4PteGlu_n + NADPH + H^+ \rightarrow 5\text{-methyl-}H_4PteGlu_n + NADP^+$$

The reaction is irreversible under *in vitro* and *in vivo* conditions (Green *et al.*, 1988) and is the committed step in methionine synthesis. Mammalian tissues contain low levels of the reductase protein (Daubner and Matthews, 1982).

Methionine synthase catalyzes the transfer of the methyl group from 5-methyl-$H_4PteGlu_n$ to homocysteine, as follows:

$$5\text{-methyl-}H_4PteGlu_n + \text{homocysteine} \rightarrow H_4PteGlu_n + \text{methionine}$$

Although methionine is an essential amino acid, the methionine synthase reaction plays a major role in methyl group metabolism, as it allows the reutilization of the homocysteine backbone as a carrier of methyl groups derived primarily from the three carbon of serine. The

---

[2]NADPH, The reduced form of nicotinamide–adenine–dinucleotide phosphate (NADP); ATP, adenosine triphosphate; ADP, adenosine diphosphate; dUMP, deoxyuridine monophosphate; dTMP, thymidine monophosphate; NADH, the reduced form of nicotinamide–adenine dinucleotide (NAD).

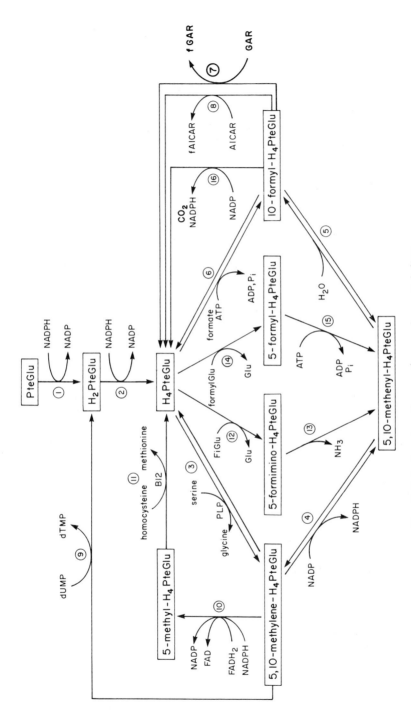

FIG. 2. Cytoplasmic pathways of one-carbon metabolism.

enzyme contains tightly bound cobalamin and the reaction proceeds via a methylcobalamin intermediate (Taylor and Weissbach, 1973). Utley *et al.* (1985) have reported the only purification of the synthase to homogeneity from any mammalian tissue. Their 1000-fold purified human placental enzyme contains three dissimilar subunits. Placenta may be a particularly rich source of the enzyme, as other studies have suggested that the synthase is a low-abundance protein (Matthews *et al.*, 1987).

The methionine synthase reaction is the sole reaction whereby the methyl group of 5-methyl-$H_4PteGlu_n$ can be metabolized in mammalian cells. Under conditions of vitamin B_{12} deprivation, loss of holoenzyme results in the trapping of folate in the 5-methyl-$H_4PteGlu_n$ form (Shane and Stokstad, 1985). The enzyme is also inactivated by nitrous oxide. Inactivation requires enzyme turnover and proceeds through a free-radical mechanism (Frasca *et al.*, 1986). Methionine is a weak inhibitor of mammalian methionine synthase. The major site of regulation of the methionine cycle is via adenosylmethionine inhibition of methylenetetrahydrofolate reductase. Adenosylmethionine is a potent allosteric inhibitor of the reductase (Kutzbach and Stokstad, 1971; Jencks and Matthews, 1987). At normal physiological levels of adenosylmethionine, much of the reductase activity would be expected to be repressed.

c. Histidine Catabolism. The C-2 position of the imidazole ring of histidine provides one-carbon units at the oxidation level of formate for one-carbon metabolism (Shane and Stokstad, 1984). Formiminoglutamate formiminotransferase catalyzes the transfer of a formimino group from formiminoglutamate, an intermediate in the histidine catabolism pathway, to $H_4PteGlu_n$ (Fig. 2, reaction 12), as follows:

$$\text{formiminoglutamate} + H_4PteGlu_n \rightarrow \text{5-formimino-}H_4PteGlu_n + \text{glutamate}$$

The formimino moiety cannot be utilized as such in one-carbon metabolism and has to be converted to 5,10-methenyl-$H_4PteGlu_n$ in a formiminotetrahydrofolate cyclodeaminase-catalyzed reaction (Fig. 2, reaction 13):

$$\text{5-formimino-}H_4PteGlu_n + H^+ \rightarrow [\text{5,10-methenyl-}H_4PteGlu_n]^+ + NH_3$$

In mammalian tissues, formiminotransferase and cyclodeaminase activities reside on a single bifunctional protein (Drury *et al.*, 1975). Under conditions of folate deficiency, formiminoglutamate catabolism is impaired and is excreted in elevated amounts in urine.

Formiminotransferase also catalyzes, at a slow rate, the conversion of formylglutamate to glutamate (Fig. 2, reaction 14; MacKenzie, 1984), and this reaction is unlikely to be physiologically significant. Any 5-formyl-H_4PteGlu$_n$ formed is converted to 5,10-methenyl-H_4PteGlu$_n$ by methenyltetrahydrofolate synthetase (Fig. 2, reaction 15; Hopkins and Schirch, 1984)[2]:

$$5\text{-formyl-}H_4\text{PteGlu}_n + \text{MgATP} \rightarrow [5,10\text{-methenyl-}H_4\text{PteGlu}_n]^+ + \text{MgADP} + P_i$$

5-Formyl-H_4PteGlu$_n$ is often found in tissue extracts but is believed to arise primarily from 10-formyl-H_4PteGlu$_n$ during tissue extraction. 5-Formyl-H_4PteGlu is used clinically and experimentally as a source of reduced folate, due to its greater stability than other reduced folates.

2. Thymidylate Cycle

Folates are not involved in the *de novo* synthesis of pyrimidines. However, folate is required for the synthesis of thymidylate (Fig. 2, reaction 9). Thymidylate synthase catalyzes the transfer of formaldehyde from folate to the 5-position of deoxyuridylate, as follows[2]:

$$5,10\text{-methylene-}H_4\text{PteGlu}_n + \text{dUMP} \rightarrow H_2\text{PteGlu}_n + \text{dTMP}$$

The pyrazine ring of H_4PteGlu$_n$ provides the reducing component for the reduction of the transferred one-carbon moiety to the level of methanol, and H_4PteGlu$_n$ is oxidized to H_2PteGlu$_n$ in the process.

H_2PteGlu$_n$ is inactive as a coenzyme and has to be reduced back to H_4PteGlu$_n$ in a reaction catalyzed by dihydrofolate reductase (Fig. 2, reaction 2):

$$H_4\text{PteGlu}_n + \text{NADPH} + H^+ \rightarrow H_4\text{PteGlu}_n + \text{NADP}^+$$

Dihydrofolate reductase also catalyzes the reduction of PteGlu$_n$ to H_2PteGlu$_n$ (Fig. 2, reaction 1). PteGlu is not normally found in unsupplemented foods and is unlikely to occur in tissues, although some could arise from nonenzymatic oxidation of reduced folates. The major role of dihydrofolate reductase is the reduction of H_2PteGlu$_n$ formed during thymidylate synthesis.

The level of thymidylate synthase in mammalian tissues is related to replication rates. Expression of the synthase and dihydrofolate reductase is highest during the S phase of the cell cycle (Navalgund *et al.*, 1980; Farnham and Schimke, 1985). A multienzyme complex containing thymidylate synthase, dihydrofolate reductase, DNA polymerase, thymidine kinase, deoxycytidine monophosphate kinase, nucleoside diphosphate kinase, and ribonucleotide reductase has been described (Reddy and Pardee, 1980, 1982). This complex, termed a replitase, forms during the S phase of the cell cycle, during which the individual cytosolic activities become associated with the nuclear fraction of the cell. The complex, which contains all of the enzymes required for the synthesis of deoxynucleoside triphosphates, appears to channel ribonucleotides directly to replication forks. Ayusawa *et al.* (1983) have restored normal growth rates to thymidylate synthase-negative mouse cells by transfection with human thymidylate synthase cDNA. Although the transfectants grew normally, they had abnormally high levels of the human enzyme, which did not cosediment with the replitase complex. It appears that human thymidylate synthase will not form protein–protein interactions with the mouse proteins of the replitase complex and, under these conditions, normal production of thymidylate for DNA synthesis requires very high levels of thymidylate synthase. Similar complexes have been reported in T4 phage (Chiu *et al.*, 1982; Allen *et al.*, 1983).

3. *Purine Cycle*

a. C_1 Synthase. One-carbon moieties at the oxidation level of formate are utilized in *de novo* purine biosynthesis. They can arise by the oxidation of 5,10-methylene-$H_4PteGlu_n$, which is catalyzed reversibly by methylenetetrahydrofolate dehydrogenase and methenyltetrahydrofolate cyclohydrolase (Fig. 1, reactions 4 and 5):

$$\text{5,10-methylene-}H_4PteGlu_n + NADP^+ \rightleftharpoons \text{[5,10-methenyl-}H_4PteGlu_n]^+ + NADPH$$

$$\text{[5,10-methenyl-}H_4PteGlu_n]^+ + H_2O \rightleftharpoons \text{10-formyl-}H_4PteGlu_n + H^+$$

Alternatively, 10-formyl-$H_4PteGlu_n$ can be obtained by the direct formylation of $H_4PteGlu_n$ (Fig. 2, reaction 6), catalyzed by formyltetrahydrofolate synthetase:

$$\text{formate} + MgATP + H_4PteGlu_n \rightarrow \text{10-formyl-}H_4PteGlu_n + MgADP + P_i$$

The dehydrogenase, cyclohydrolase, and synthetase are associated on a single trifunctional protein in mammalian tissues (Paukert *et al.*, 1976; Tan *et al.*, 1977) which has been given the name C_1 synthase. The synthase consists of two separate domains, each containing a folate-binding site. One domain contains the dehydrogenase and cyclohydrolase activities and the other, the synthetase activity (Tan and MacKenzie, 1977; Cohen and MacKenzie, 1978; Villar *et al.*, 1985).

A separate 5,10-methylenetetrahydrofolate dehydrogenase–cyclohydrolase which uses NAD^+ rather than $NADP^+$ as the acceptor has recently been described (Mejia and MacKenzie, 1985). This activity has only been found in embryonic, undifferentiated, or transformed tissues and cells. One suggested role for this enzyme is to increase the one-carbon flux into purine biosynthesis and away from other one-carbon cycles, such as methionine synthesis.

   b. Purine Synthesis Enzymes. The C-8 and C-2 positions of the purine ring are derived from 10-formyl-H_4PteGlu$_n$ in reactions catalyzed by glycinamide ribonucleotide (GAR) transformylase and 5-amino-4-imidazolecarboxamide ribonucleotide (AICAR) transformylase (Fig. 2, reactions 7 and 8; Smith *et al.,* 1981):

$$10\text{-formyl-}H_4\text{PteGlu}_n + \text{GAR} \rightarrow H_4\text{PteGlu}_n + \text{formyl-GAR}$$

$$10\text{-formyl-}H_4\text{PteGlu}_n + \text{AICAR} \rightarrow H_4\text{PteGlu}_n + \text{formyl-AICAR}$$

   Mammalian purine enzymes have not been well characterized, although GAR transformylase has recently been purified to near-homogeneity from several transformed mouse cell lines (Caperelli, 1985; Daubner and Benkovic, 1985). Considerably more information is available on purine enzymes isolated from uricotelic sources. The chicken liver GAR transformylase is the second activity of a trifunctional protein which also possesses glycinamide ribonucleotide synthetase and aminoimidazole ribonucleotide synthase activities (Daubner *et al.,* 1985). A similar trifunctional protein has also been identified in *Drosophila* (Henikoff *et al.,* 1986). The chicken liver AICAR transformylase is a bifunctional protein also possessing inosine monophosphate cyclohydrolase activity (Mueller and Benkovic, 1981). Two other enzymes in the *de novo* purine pathway, aminoimidazole ribonucleotide carboxylase and aminoimidazolesuccinocarboxamide synthetase, also appear to be part of a bifunctional protein (Patey and Shaw, 1973). GAR and AICAR transformylases copurify from chicken liver in association with C_1 synthase and serine hydroxymethyltransferase under mild purification conditions, and the C_1 synthase copurifies with the transformylases from GAR and AICAR affinity columns (Rowe *et al.,* 1978; Caperelli *et al.,* 1980; Smith *et al.,* 1980), suggesting a multienzyme complex for directing one-carbon units into purine synthesis. The individual activities, however, are easily separated without loss of activity (Benkovic, 1984). Evidence for complexes in uricotelic animals does not necessarily indicate complexes in mammalian tissues. However, Allegra *et al.* (1985a) have reported that serine hydroxymethyltransferase remains associated with AICAR transformylase during partial purification of the transformylase from a human breast cancer cell line.

4. Disposal of One-Carbon Units

   One-carbon moieties are oxidized to CO_2 in a reaction catalyzed by 10-formyltetrahydrofolate dehydrogenase (Fig. 2, reaction 16):

$$\text{10-formyl-}H_4\text{PteGlu}_n + \text{NADP}^+ + H_2O \rightarrow H_4\text{PteGlu}_n + CO_2 + \text{NADPH} + H^+$$

This reaction is believed to be a mechanism for the disposal of excess one-carbon units (Krebs *et al.*, 1976; Scrutton and Beis, 1979). The purified enzyme also catalyzes the hydrolysis of 10-formyl-H_4PteGlu$_n$ to H_4PteGlu$_n$ and formate (Kutzbach and Stokstad, 1968; Scrutton and Beis, 1979) at 20–30% of the oxidative rate. Recent studies suggest that the dehydrogenase and hydrolase activities can occur simultaneously and that the dehydrogenase–hydrolase is a bifunctional protein (Rios-Orlandi *et al.*, 1986). The physiological significance of the hydrolase activity is not clear, although it does represent an additional mechanism for regenerating unsubstituted H_4PteGlu$_n$ under conditions in which utilization of substituted folate for biosynthetic purposes is impaired.

B. Mitochondrial Pathways

1. *Choline Catabolism*

Choline is oxidized in mitochondria to betaine. Liver contains a betaine methyltransferase, which catalyzes the transfer of one of the methyl groups of betaine to homocysteine to generate methionine and dimethylglycine (Skiba *et al.*, 1982). The enzyme does not contain bound cobalamin and does not use a folate coenzyme as a substrate. It is present in high concentrations in liver, but its physiological significance in terms of methionine and methyl group status is not clear.

Flavoproteins dimethylglycine dehydrogenase and sarcosine dehydrogenase catalyze the oxidative demethylation of dimethylglycine to sarcosine and sarcosine to glycine (Fig. 3, reactions 19 and 20), respec-

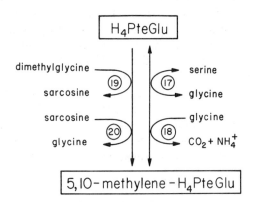

FIG. 3. Mitochondrial pathways of one-carbon metabolism.

tively, with the generation of formaldehyde. Wittwer and Wagner (1981) isolated two mitochondrial folate-binding proteins from rat liver and demonstrated their coidentity with dimethylglycine and sarcosine dehydrogenases. Both proteins contained $H_4PteGlu_5$, the major polyglutamate species in rat liver. Formaldehyde generated in these reactions is incorporated into 5,10-methylene-$H_4PteGlu_n$. Although $H_4PteGlu_n$ binds tightly to the dehydrogenases, product formation is unaffected in the absence of folate (Porter et al., 1985).

Cytoplasmic sarcosine, if transported into the mitochondria, is an additional potential source of one-carbon units for mitochondrial metabolism. Cytoplasmic sarcosine is formed by methylation of glycine by adenosylmethionine in a reaction catalyzed by glycine N-methyltransferase. The N-methyltransferase is a major cytoplasmic protein, accounting for about 1% of hepatic protein (Ogawa and Fujioka, 1982). Cook and Wagner (1984) characterized a major folate-binding protein of rat cytoplasm and demonstrated coidentity with the methyltransferase. The enzyme contained bound 5-methyl-$H_4PteGlu_5$, which is a potent inhibitor of enzyme activity (Wagner et al., 1985). It is suggested that the glycine N-methyltransferase reaction is a sink for removing excess methyl groups in the form of adenosylmethionine. Under conditions of low adenosylmethionine or methionine levels, 5-methyl-$H_4PteGlu_n$ synthesis is increased and the methyltransferase would be inhibited. High levels of methionine or methyl groups would decrease the level of 5-methyl-$H_4PteGlu_n$ and increase the activity of glycine methyltransferase. Excess methionine is toxic and results in elevated levels of sarcosine, some of which is excreted in urine (London et al., 1987). Part of the toxicity is due to a decrease in glycine levels (Sugiyama et al., 1987). Although sarcosine oxidation in the mitochondria would regenerate some of the glycine, it is interesting to note that a significant amount of glycine and methyl groups is directed into creatine synthesis in liver.

2. Serine and Glycine Metabolism

As discussed above, mitochondria contain a distinct serine hydroxymethyltransferase isozyme for the reversible interconversion of serine and glycine and the concomitant interconversion of $H_4PteGlu_n$ and 5,10-methylene-$H_4PteGlu_n$ (Fig. 3, reaction 17). The major pathway of glycine catabolism is via the glycine cleavage system (Kikuchi, 1973; Schirch, 1984), a reaction in which an additional one-carbon moiety is supplied to the folate pool (Fig. 3, reaction 18)[2]:

$$\text{glycine} + H_4PteGlu_n + NAD^+ \rightleftharpoons$$
$$\text{5,10-methylene-}H_4PteGlu_n + NADH + CO_2 + NH_4^+$$

The glycine cleavage system is a multienzyme complex with four components. P protein, which contains pyridoxal phosphate, catalyzes glycine decarboxylation and transfer of methylamine to lipoic acid on H protein. The lipoic acid is reduced and the carbon moiety from glycine is oxidized to the level of formaldehyde. T protein catalyzes the transfer of formaldehyde to $H_4PteGlu_n$, and the reduced lipoate on H protein is reoxidized by NAD^+ in a reaction catalyzed by L protein (Kikuchi, 1973; Okamura-Ikeda *et al.*, 1982, 1987; Fujiwara *et al.*, 1984). Although reversible, the glycine cleavage system does not appear to play a role in the synthesis of glycine, and kinetic data suggest that this would be unlikely (Okamura-Ikeda *et al.*, 1987). Coupling of the serine hydroxymethyltransferase and glycine cleavage systems does provide a mechanism for the synthesis of serine from glycine. One molecule of serine can arise by reversal of the hydroxymethyltransferase, with the 5,10-methylene-$H_4PteGlu_n$ required arising from oxidative decarboxylation of an additional molecule of glycine via the cleavage system. Alternatively, the additional one carbon could arise from choline degradation as described above.

3. *Role of Mitochondrial One-Carbon Metabolism*

Approximately 75% of CHO cell serine hydroxymethyltransferase is located in the mitochondria. CHO cell mutants of the *glyA* complementation group lack mitochondrial enzyme activity but have normal levels of cytoplasmic activity and require exogenous glycine for growth (Chasin *et al.*, 1974). The glycine cleavage system is normal in these cells. Studies with *glyA* revertants demonstrated a general correlation between intracellular glycine concentration and the level of mitochondrial hydroxymethyltransferase activity and suggested that mitochondrial glycine synthesis may be required for normal rates of protein synthesis (Pfendner and Pizer, 1980). Serine and glycine are rapidly transported across the mitochondrial membrane, while transport of reduced folate is undetectable or occurs at a very slow rate (Cybulski and Fisher, 1976, 1981). It is not clear why the glycine requirement cannot be met by the cytoplasmic hydroxymethyltransferase when it can be satisfied by exogenous glycine. It is possible that the cytoplasmic enzyme is associated with the enzymes of cytoplasmic one-carbon metabolism and the serine-to-glycine flux in the cytoplasm is regulated by the needs for one-carbon units for the various cycles of one-carbon metabolism. If this is the case, insufficient glycine may be generated in the cytoplasm to support normal rates of protein synthesis. Serine hydroxymethyltransferase concentrations are elevated in mitogen-stimulated lymphocytes, and it has been suggested that proliferating cells may selectively synthesize serine *de novo* for utilization in pathways of nucleotide biosynthesis (Eichler *et al.*, 1981). It is interesting to note that the levels of a large number of enzymes of one-carbon metabolism are elevated in mitogen-stimulated cells (Rowe *et al.*, 1979).

Mitochondria may contain additional folate-dependent enzymes. Protein synthesis in this organelle presumably requires formylmethionine for initiation, which presumably requires the presence of a methionyl-tRNA transformylase, although it should be noted that mammalian cells grow normally in the absence of folate, provided products of one-carbon metabolism are supplied. A separate mitochondrial C_1 synthase has been reported in yeast (Shannon and Rabinowitz, 1986). It has also been reported that the two activities of the presumed bifunctional 10-formyltetrahydrofolate dehydrogenase–hydrolase from rat liver can be resolved into separate cytoplasmic dehydrogenase and mitochondrial hydrolase activities (Case and Steele, 1987). It is possible that the mitochondrial hydrolase activity represents the formylase activity associated with the formyltetrahydrofolate synthetase domain of the trifunctional enzyme.

III. FOLYLPOLYGLUTAMATES IN MAMMALIAN CELLS AND TISSUES

The types of folates that predominate in different tissues and species have been extensively documented in several recent reviews (Krumdieck *et al.*, 1983; Cossins, 1984). Endogenous folates in mammalian tissues are almost entirely pteroylpolyglutamate derivatives, while pteroylmonoglutamates are the only forms in plasma and urine. In a single tissue, a distribution of glutamate chain lengths is usually observed, with a particular species predominating. Pentaglutamates are the predominant derivatives in rat liver, and chain lengths up to the heptaglutamate are found (Shane, 1982). Pig liver contains the tetra- to nonaglutamates, with hexaglutamate predominating (Cichowicz and Shane, 1987a), and hexaglutamate is the major form in mouse liver (Priest *et al.*, 1981). Hepatic folate concentrations are several hundredfold higher than in plasma, while pteroylmonoglutamate concentrations are similar to plasma concentrations (Thenen and Stokstad, 1973). Within a single species, the distribution of polyglutamate forms can differ between tissues (Brody *et al.*, 1976).

Folate distributions in mammalian tissues have also been determined by identifying labeled vitamin derivatives at various times, following the administration of a tracer dose of the vitamin. For example, the major labeled folate derivatives in rat liver found 24 hours after a dose of [^{3}H]PteGlu is the pentaglutamate, which is similar to the endogenous folate distribution (Brody *et al.*, 1979). Significant labeling of the hexa- and heptaglutamate pools in this tissue is not found until much longer times after the dose is given (Leslie and Baugh, 1974). Consequently, distributions obtained after a single labeled dose of the vitamin do not reflect the endogenous steady-state distribution of folate derivatives. At early time periods after a labeled folate dose, short-chain-length folates are found, suggesting that extension of the polyglutamate chain occurs by the stepwise addition of glutamate moieties (Brody *et al.*, 1979).

Steady-state distributions of labeled folates in cultured cells can be obtained by culturing cells for many generations in media containing labeled folate. Human fibroblasts contain folates of chain length up to the decaglutamate, with heptaglutamates predominating (Foo *et al.*, 1982). Slightly shorter chain lengths, with the hexaglutamate as the major form, are found in CHO cells (Foo and Shane, 1982).

The subcellular distribution of folates has received limited study. Most of the cellular folate appears to be located in the cytoplasm, although a significant proportion is associated with the mitochondria (Brody *et al.*, 1975; McClain *et al.*, 1975; Shin *et al.*, 1976; Taylor and Hanna, 1982). Mitochondria contain folylpolyglutamates but it is not known whether these are of similar glutamate chain length to cytoplasmic folates. However, rat liver mitochondrial folate-binding proteins contain bound $H_4PteGlu_5$, which suggests a similar distribution to cytoplasmic folates.

IV. Role of Folylpolyglutamates

A. Enzyme Substrates and Inhibitors

As cellular folates are almost entirely folylpolyglutamates, they should be considered the normal substrates for the enzymes of one-carbon metabolism. In addition, as described above, a failure to synthesize folylpolyglutamates leads to an inability to retain cellular folates and to synthesize products of one-carbon metabolism in sufficient quantities to support growth. The advantages conferred on the folate molecule by the addition of the polyglutamate moiety have primarily been explored by assessing the substrate or inhibitory activity of folylpolyglutamates for purified enzymes of one-carbon metabolism (reviewed by Kisliuk, 1981; McGuire and Bertino, 1981; McGuire and Coward, 1984). This review emphasizes results obtained with mammalian enzymes. Most of the detailed studies in this area have used proteins purified from pig liver, a tissue that contains primarily pteroylhexaglutamates and a total intracellular folate concentration of about 30 μM. Results obtained from studies with the pig liver enzymes are summarized in Tables I and II. For many enzymes of one-carbon metabolism, the polyglutamate chain increases the affinity of the folate substrate or inhibitor for the enzyme and, in some cases, changes the kinetic mechanism.

1. Amino Acid Metabolism

a. Serine–Glycine Interconversion. 5-Methyl-H_4PteGlu$_n$ is an inhibitor of pig liver serine hydroxymethyltransferase. A decrease in free energy of binding of about 1 kcal/mol per residue is associated with the binding of the second and third glutamate moieties, and a smaller decrease (0.17 kcal/mol per residue) with binding of the fourth to seventh residues (Matthews et al., 1982). The binding energy is expressed partly by an increased affinity of glycine for the enzyme–folate complex and partly by an increased affinity of the inhibitor for the enzyme–glycine complex (Table II). The major changes in affinity occur with the di- and triglutamate derivatives. A similar phenomenon is seen with H_4PteGlu$_n$ substrates, with the major changes in binding energy occurring between the mono- and triglutamate derivatives (Matthews et al., 1982; Table I). However, with the folate substrate, the increased binding energy is expressed by an increased affinity of folate for the enzyme and for the enzyme–glycine binary complex, and the affinity of glycine for the enzyme–folate complex does not change. The increased binding energy is also reflected by a decrease in the K_m from 56 μM with the monoglutamate to 1.7 μM with the triglutamate, which is in the physiological range, with only a modest decrease in V_{max}. These data suggest that folates of glutamate chain length three and longer should be much more effective substrates of the hydroxymethyltransferase than the mono- and diglutamates. In addition, when pteroylmono- and polyglutamates are present in tissues, the enzyme should show a strong preference for utilization of the polyglutamate substrate.

The potent inhibition of the enzyme by 5-methyl-H_4PteGlu$_n$ (K_i 60 nM for the hexaglutamate for the enzyme–glycine binary complex) suggests a mechanism for regulating the flow of one-carbon units into the folate pool (Matthews et al., 1982). An increase in the level of 5-methyl-H_4PteGlu$_n$, glycine, or in the 5-methyl-H_4PteGlu$_n$/H_4PteGlu$_n$ ratio should cause increased inhibition of methyltransferase activity, the major route for one-carbon entry into the pool. 5-Methyl-H_4PteGlu$_n$

TABLE I

KINETIC CONSTANTS OF FOLYLPOLYGLUTAMATE SUBSTRATES FOR PIG LIVER ENZYMES[a]

Enzyme	Substrate	$n = 1$		$n = 2$		$n = 3$		$n = 4$		$n = 5$		$n = 6$		$n = 7$	
		K_m	V_{max}	K_m	V_{max}	K_m	V_{max}	K_m	V_{max}	K_m	V_{max}	K_m	V_{max}	K_m	V_{max}
Serine hydroxymethyltransferase	$H_4PteGlu_n$	5.2[b]		0.33		0.1								0.07	
		195[c]		7.2		3.1								2.8	
		56	1	3.9	0.6	1.7	0.6								
Thymidylate synthase	Methylene-$H_4PteGlu_n$	5.2	1	2.0	0.6	1.9	0.4	1.9	0.4	1.6	0.4	1.6	0.4	2.1	0.4
Methylene-THF reductase	Methylene-$H_4PteGlu_n$	7.1	1	5.2	1.8	1.7	1.7	0.62	1.7	0.26	0.6	1.10	0.7	0.51	0.7
Methionine synthase	Methyl-$H_4PteGlu_n$	6										0.05			
Formiminotransferase–cyclodeaminase	$H_4PteGlu_n$	48	1			27	0.4	0.7	0.5	0.7	0.6	0.6	0.5	0.7	0.7
	formimino-$H_4PteGlu_n$	149	1			21	0.4	2.9	0.2	2.0	0.12	1.2	0.11	2.1	0.13
C1 synthase:															
Methylene-THF dehydrogenase	Methylene-$H_4PteGlu_n$	4.8	1					4.2	1	2.4	1				
Formyl-THF synthetase	10-formyl-$H_4PteGlu_n$	25	1			7	0.8			3	1			3	0.8
Formyl-THF dehydrogenase–hydrolase	10-formyl-$H_4PteGlu_n$	89	1			2	1								
		7.5													
		21													

[a] All K_m and affinity values are μM. [Data are from Matthews and Baugh (1980), Matthew et al. (1982, 1987), Paquin et al. (1985), MacKenzie and Baugh (1980), Lu et al. (1984), Ross et al. (1984), and Rios-Orlandi et al. (1986)]. THF, tetrahydrofolate.
[b] Dissociation constant for enzyme–glycine complex.
[c] Dissociation constant for free enzyme.

TABLE II
FOLYLPOLYGLUTAMATES AS INHIBITORS OF PIG LIVER ENZYMES[a]

Enzyme	Inhibitor	Substrate	K_i (μM)						
			$n=1$	$n=2$	$n=3$	$n=4$	$n=5$	$n=6$	$n=7$
Serine hydroxymethyltransferase	Methyl-H$_4$PteGlu$_n$		3.8[b]	0.54	0.21	0.11	0.08	0.06	0.04
			22[c]	36	38	20	14	10	8
Thymidylate synthase	PteGlu$_n$	Methylene-H$_4$PteGlu	10	0.3	0.2	0.06	0.10	0.12	0.15
Methylene-THF reductase	H$_2$PteGlu$_n$	Methylene-H$_4$PteGlu	6.3	1.8	0.7	0.2	0.04	0.013	0.065
Formiminotransferase—	H$_4$PteGlu$_n$	—	14[c]		6	0.60	0.41	0.16	0.22
cyclodeaminase	PteGlu$_n$	Formimino-H$_4$PteGlu	70[d]		13		1.0		2.3
C$_1$ synthase:									
Methylene-THF dehydrogenase	PteGlu$_n$	Methylene-H$_4$PteGlu	55	58	70	57	16	16	18
Cyclohydrolase	PteGlu$_n$	Methenyl-H$_4$PteGlu	195[d]		60		18	18	18
Formyl-THF dehydrogenase—	H$_4$PteGlu$_n$	10-Formyl-H$_4$PteGlu	80[e]		37	31	24	10	17
hydrolase	H$_4$PteGlu$_n$		85[e]		49	40	25	19	23

[a] Data are from Matthews and Baugh (1980), Matthews et al. (1982, 1987), Paquin et al. (1985), MacKenzie and Baugh (1980), Lu et al. (1984), Ross et al. (1984), and Rios-Orlandi et al. (1986). THF, tetrahydrofolate.
[b] Dissociation constant for enzyme–glycine complex.
[c] Dissociation constant for free enzyme.
[d] Concentration required for 50% inhibition.
[e] Activity remaining in the presence of 0.3 μM inhibitor.

accumulates in tissues when the vitamin B_{12}-dependent methionine synthase is inhibited (Matthews, 1984; Shane and Stokstad, 1985). Under these conditions, all other metabolic cycles of one-carbon metabolism, including thymidylate synthesis, are depressed. Although part of this depression is due to a decrease in levels of folate coenzymes other than 5-methyl-H_4PteGlu$_n$, a decreased one-carbon flux into the folate pool may be a major contributing factor to this derangement of one-carbon metabolism (Matthews *et al.*, 1982).

   b. Methionine Cycle. Pig liver methylenetetrahydrofolate reductase, which catalyzes the physiologically irreversible and committed step in the methionine cycle, shows a very marked preference for folylpolyglutamate substrates and inhibitors (Tables I and II). H_2PteGlu is an inhibitor of the reductase (Matthews and Haywood, 1979). Extending the glutamate chain of H_2PteGlu$_n$ from the mono- to the hexaglutamate derivative produces a steady increase in affinity of the inhibitor equivalent to a free energy of binding of 0.75 kcal/mol for each additional glutamate moiety (Matthews and Baugh, 1980). The K_i is decreased from 6.5 μM to 13 nM. Addition of a further glutamate moiety (H_4PteGlu$_7$) decreases the affinity, with an increase in K_i to 65 nM. The reductase shows a striking preference for the folylpolyglutamate chain length that is endogenous to pig liver. A similar specificity is also observed with 5,10-methylene-H_4PteGlu$_n$ substrates (Matthews and Baugh, 1980; Table I), although decreases in K_m or increases in V_{max}/K_m with increasing chain length are not as large as the changes in affinity associated with H_2PteGlu$_n$ binding. V_{max} is slightly increased for the di- to tetraglutamate substrates and is slightly decreased for the longer glutamate derivatives. K_m(NADPH) is also increased, with folate substrates of chain length four and longer. Changes in inhibition patterns with the polyglutamate substrates are consistent with a change from a Ping-Pong to an sequential mechanism.

   As discussed above, methylenetetrahydrofolate reductase activity is regulated by methyl group status via allosteric inhibition by adenosylmethionine. The high affinity of H_2PteGlu$_6$ for the enzyme suggests an alternative regulatory feature of the methionine cycle. The concentration of 5,10-methylene-H_4PteGlu$_n$ in pig liver is not known, but, if similar to other species, is probably in the 1–5 μM range, which is considerably higher than the K_m for 5,10-methylene-H_4PteGlu$_6$ but similar to the K_m for the monoglutamate substrate. Under physiological conditions, the level of the polyglutamate substrate would be saturating. The H_2PteGlu$_n$ concentration is probably at least an order of magnitude lower. With 1 μM 5,10-methylene-H_4PteGlu$_6$ as substrate, the concentration of H_2PteGlu$_6$ required to inhibit activity 50% would be 0.13 μM, which is in the physiological range. With 1 μM pteroyl-monoglutamate substrate, 50% inhibition would require a nonphysio-logical 7 μM $H_2PteGlu$ (Matthews and Baugh, 1980). As tissue con-centrations of 5,10-methylene-$H_4PteGlu_6$ and $H_2PteGlu_6$ are higher than the K_m and K_i of these compounds for the reductase, the one-carbon flux through the reductase reaction should be regulated by the 5,10-methylene-$H_4PteGlu_n$: $H_2PteGlu_n$ ratio in the tissue. Increased thymidylate synthesis in growing cells elevates $H_2PteGlu_n$ levels and would be expected to decrease the one-carbon flux into methionine synthesis. This would be a mechanism to conserve one-carbon moieties for thymidylate and purine biosyntheses. In addition, the $H_2PteGlu_n$ pool is greatly expanded by antifolate-induced inhibition of dihydrofo-late reductase. The expected decrease in methionine synthesis under these conditions may be a factor in the cytotoxicity of these drugs.

Initial studies on the specificity of mammalian methionine synthase for polyglutamate substrates suggested only modest effects of poly-glutamate chain length on K_m and V_{max} of 5-methyl-$H_4PteGlu_n$ (Coward et al., 1975; Cheng et al., 1975). However, recent studies on the pig liver enzyme suggest a much higher degree of specificity for polyglutamate substrates (Matthews et al., 1987; Table I). Kinetic analyses with 5-methyl-$H_4PteGlu_6$ as the substrate suggested two classes of binding site with markedly different affinities, which may indicate negative cooperativity on substrate binding. Two K_m values were assigned for the hexaglutamate substrate, one of about 8 μM, which is similar to that found with the monoglutamate substrate, and one of 0.5 μM.

When a mixture of 5-[^{3}H]methyl-$H_4PteGlu_6$ and 5-[^{14}C]methyl-$H_4PteGlu$ was incubated with the synthase, [^{3}H]methionine was ini-tially generated at a linear rate, while there was a time lag in the appearance of [^{14}C]methionine which was equivalent to the nearly complete utilization of the hexaglutamate substrate (Matthews et al., 1987). This high degree of selectivity for the hexaglutamate substrate has important physiological implications. 5-Methyl-$H_4PteGlu$ is the major circulating form of folate and is the major form of folate taken up by tissues. Removal of the methyl group, via the methionine synthase reaction, is required before the entering folate can be utilized in other reactions of one-carbon metabolism or metabolized to folate derivatives that are retained by cells (Section VI,E). Methylfolates normally ac-count for a significant proportion of the folate one-carbon forms in the cell. These data suggest that incorporation of exogenous folate by tissues is repressed by physiological concentrations of 5-methyl-$H_4PteGlu$ polyglutamates. Conditions that result in reduction of the 5-

methyl-H_4PteGlu$_n$ pool, such as adenosylmethionine inhibition of methylenetetrahydrofolate reductase or folate depletion, should stimulate the accumulation of exogenous folate by tissues. Expansion of the 5-methyl-H_4PteGlu$_n$ pool, caused, for example, by vitamin B_{12} deficiency, would be expected to inhibit the accumulation of folate by tissues.

The significant proportion of methylfolates in cells suggests that the methionine synthase reaction is an important rate-limiting step in the metabolic cycles of one-carbon metabolism. The two enzymes in the methionine cycle are low-abundance proteins and are present at considerably lower concentrations, and specific activities in cell extracts, than some of the other enzymes involved in the metabolism of folate coenzymes. The labeled one carbon of 5-[^{14}C]methyl-H_4[^{3}H]PteGlu was metabolized rapidly by L1210 cells via methionine synthesis, while most of the tritium label remained associated with 5-methyl-H_4PteGlu (Nixon et $al.$, 1973), indicating that the synthase reaction, although rapid, was rate limiting for folate one-carbon interconversions. These studies used fairly high concentrations of labeled monoglutamate and, as discussed above, may not necessarily indicate steps that are rate limiting with polyglutamate substrates.

$c.$ $Histidine$ $Catabolism.$ The two activities associated with the bifunctional formiminoglutamate formiminotransferase–formiminotetrahydrofolate cyclodeaminase from pig liver show a preference for folate substrates and inhibitors typically found in pig liver (MacKenzie and Baugh, 1980; Paquin et $al.$, 1985; Tables I and II). The affinity of the substrate H_4PteGlu$_n$ for the formiminotransferase increases with increased glutamate chain length, reaches a maximum with the hexaglutamate, and drops off with the heptaglutamate derivative. The major changes in affinity occur as the glutamate chain is extended from the mono- to the tetraglutamate. The changes in affinity of the substrate are reflected by a large decrease in the K_m for H_4PteGlu$_n$, with only a modest decrease in V_{max} as the glutamate chain is extended. Again, the major change in K_m is associated with binding of the second, third, and fourth glutamate residues, and folates of glutamate chain length four or longer would all be effective substrates for the formiminotransferase (Table I). Under physiological conditions, saturating levels of the polyglutamate substrate would be present. Inhibition of cyclodeaminase by PteGlu$_n$ shows a similar effect, with the highest affinity displayed by the pentaglutamate (MacKenzie and Baugh, 1980; Table II). PteGlu$_6$ was not evaluated in this study. The K_m for 5-formimino-H_4PteGlu$_n$ also decreases rapidly with extension of the glutamate chain up to the tetraglutamate, but this is also accompanied by a significant drop in V_{max} (Paquin et $al.$, 1985;

Table I). Comparisons of V_{max}/K_m indicate a large increase in substrate effectiveness with increases in glutamate chain length up to the tetraglutamate but no significant increases in substrate effectiveness beyond the tetraglutamate. The advantages of folylpolyglutamate substrates in the channeling of intermediates with this bifunctional protein will be discussed in Section IV,B below.

2. Thymidylate Cycle

The enzymes of the thymidylate cycle show a very different specificity for folylpolyglutamates. Fetal pig liver thymidylate synthase is inhibited by $PteGlu_n$ (Lu et al., 1984; Table II). There is a large increase in affinity for this inhibitor between the mono- and diglutamate derivatives, but further increases in glutamate chain length cause only slight changes in affinity. Maximal affinity is observed with $PteGlu_4$ (K_i 60 nM). The large change in affinity between the mono- and diglutamate inhibitors (33-fold) is not reflected by an increased substrate effectiveness. The K_m for 5,10-methylene-H_4Pte-Glu_n decreases about 60% as the glutamate chain is increased from the mono- to diglutamate, and further extension has little additional effect. This is accompanied by a 40% decrease in V_{max} going from the mono- to diglutamate and a further 20% decrease with the triglutamate. Further extension of the glutamate chain does not affect V_{max} but does cause a modest increase in the K_m for deoxyuridylate (Lu et al., 1984; Table I). V_{max}/K_m values do not change significantly with pteroylmono- to heptaglutamate substrates, suggesting that the polyglutamate chain does not confer any advantage in this reaction. However, the increased affinity of folylpolyglutamates for this enzyme suggests that a polyglutamate substrate would be preferentially utilized under conditions in which both a mono- and a polyglutamate substrate were available for the synthase. Although this has not been tested with the pig liver enzyme, it has been shown that the Lactobacillus casei thymidylate synthase will preferentially use the hexaglutamate substrate over the monoglutamate when both substrates are present at equivalent V_{max}/K_m concentrations (Kisliuk et al., 1981). The kinetic mechanism of pig liver thymidylate synthase is ordered sequentially. Kinetic analyses with mono- and polyglutamate substrates and inhibitors suggest that the order of substrate addition and product release is reversed with polyglutamate substrates, due to the increased affinity of folate for the free enzyme, and consequently is not reflected by a decrease in K_m (Lu et al., 1984; Matthews et al., 1987). The K_m values for folate substrates for pig liver thymidylate synthase are in the physiological range. The flux through this reaction should be responsive to changes in the level of 5,10-methylene-H_4Pte-Glu$_n$ in this tissue.

Studies with other mammalian thymidylate synthases suggest similarities but also some differences from the pig liver studies. The K_m for 5,10-methylene-H_4PteGlu$_5$ with a human blast cell (2.2 μM; Dolnick and Cheng, 1978) and a human breast cancer cell line (0.6 μM; Allegra et al., 1985a) synthase is considerably lower than with the monoglutamate substrate (31 μM and 23 μM, respectively), while V_{max} is increased slightly. Methotrexate polyglutamates are potent inhibitors of human thymidylate synthase, with K_i values decreasing from 13 μM with the monoglutamate to 50 nM with the pentaglutamate, and most of the increased affinity occurs upon going from the mono- to the diglutamate (Allegra et al., 1985a). Similar K_i values are found when tested against mono- and pentaglutamate substrates. Methotrexate polyglutamates are noncompetitive inhibitors, while the monoglutamate is an uncompetitive inhibitor, which may reflect a change in the order of the kinetic mechanism.

Lactobacillus casei thymidylate synthase shows a similar specificity to the mammalian enzyme in that increased affinities for polyglutamate inhibitors (PteGlu$_n$ and H_2PteGlu$_n$) and decreases in K_m and V_{max} with polyglutamate substrates occur primarily among the mono-, di-, and triglutamate derivatives, but less dramatic changes in these parameters do occur beyond the triglutamate (Kisliuk et al., 1974, 1981). The marked increases in affinity with polyglutamate inhibitors, which were evaluated with 5,10-methylene-H_4PteGlu as the substrate, were not seen when affinities were assessed using substrates of the same glutamate chain length as the inhibitor under study (Matthews et al., 1987), which is consistent with the suggested change in kinetic mechanism.

Dihydrofolate reductase, the second enzyme in the thymidylate cycle, does not show any marked preference for folylpolyglutamate substrates or inhibitors (Coward et al., 1974). K_m values for H_2PteGlu$_n$ for a variety of mammalian dihydrofolate reductases are around 1–5 μM (McGuire and Bertino, 1981; Kisliuk, 1981; McGuire and Coward, 1984), and the flux through this reaction should be responsive to changes in folate substrate levels under physiological conditions.

3. Purine Cycle

a. C_1 Synthase. Pig liver methylenetetrahydrofolate dehydrogenase is inhibited by PteGlu$_n$. The K_i of the inhibitor for the folate substrate site is about 60 μM for mono- to tetraglutamates and drops to about 16 μM with penta-, hexa-, and heptaglutamates (Ross et al., 1984; Table II). The affinity of PteGlu$_n$ for the NADP$^+$ site on the enzyme is unaffected by glutamate chain length. The modest affinity of the inhibitor for the enzyme is enhanced by an interaction with the fifth glutamate residue of the chain. Initial studies with this enzyme suggested some decrease in K_m for penta- and hexaglutamates of 5,10-methylene-H_4PteGlu (MacKenzie and Baugh, 1980) which is consistent with the changes in affinity of the inhibitors. However, more recent studies indicate no significant changes in the K_m or V_{max} for the folate substrate, or in the K_m for NADP$^+$, with polyglutamate substrates (Ross *et al.*, 1984; Table I). The K_m for polyglutamate substrates is similar to the expected concentration of these folates in pig liver, and the metabolic flux through this reaction should be responsive to changes in folate substrate concentration *in vivo*.

Methenyltetrahydrofolate cyclohydrolase, the second activity of the bifunctional domain of the trifunctional protein, does show a preference for folylpolyglutamates. PteGlu$_n$ is also an inhibitor of this activity, and the affinity of the pentaglutamate is 10-fold higher than the monoglutamate (MacKenzie and Baugh, 1980; Table II).

Formyltetrahydrofolate synthetase activity is situated on a separate domain of the trifunctional protein. The pig liver enzyme shows a marked specificity for polyglutamate substrates, with the K_m for H_4PteGlu$_n$ dropping from 89 μM for the monoglutamate to a more physiological 2 μM for the triglutamate without any change in V_{max} (MacKenzie and Baugh, 1980; Table I). Interactions of folylpolyglutamates with the rabbit liver formyltetrahydrofolate synthetase have been studied by their effects on the denaturation temperature of the protein (Strong *et al.*, 1987). The data suggest a conformational change in the protein with the binding of the third glutamate of H_4PteGlu$_n$ and the β-phosphoryl of MgATP. The K_m for MgATP decreases from 130 to 40 μM and the K_m for formate from 2.5 mM to 4 μM when the H_4PteGlu$_n$ substrate is changed from the mono- to the pentaglutamate, and all of the decreases occur upon going from the mono- to the triglutamate (Strong *et al.*, 1987). The K_m for H_4PteGlu$_n$ is 15 μM with the monoglutamate and drops to well below 1 μM with polyglutamate substrates. The modest decrease in the K_m for MgATP is matched by a 6.5-fold decrease in V_{max} with the polyglutamate substrates. However, V_{max}/K_m is greatly increased for the folylpolyglutamate and formate substrates, which would make formate a much more effective contributor of one carbons to the folate pool. Despite the very low K_m for formate, mammalian tissues do not appear to contain saturating levels of formate, as the oxidation of formate to CO_2 by folate-dependent pathways is greatly increased in the rat after administration of a large dose of formate (Palese and Tephly, 1975).

The cyclohydrolase and formyltetrahydrofolate synthetase activities of the chicken liver C_1 synthase also show a preference for their triglutamate substrates when compared to monoglutamate (Wasserman *et al.*, 1983).

b. Purine Synthesis Enzymes. The specificity of mammalian GAR transformylase for folylpolyglutamate substrates has received little attention. The transformylase from a human breast cancer cell line shows only a modest decrease in K_m for 10-formyl-H_4PteGlu$_5$ compared to the monoglutamate substrate (3.2 μM versus 8.5 μM), which is in the physiological range for the folate substrate, and a modest increase in V_{max} (Allegra *et al.*, 1985c). However, the K_i of methotrexate, an inhibitor of enzyme activity, decreases from 80 μM for the monoglutamate to 2.5 μM for the pentaglutamate inhibitor when measured against the monoglutamate substrate. When 10-formyl-H_4PteGlu$_5$ is used as the substrate, a similar K_i is observed for methotrexate, but the K_i for the pentaglutamate is increased to 22 μM (Allegra *et al.*, 1985c). The different affinities of inhibitors when measured with the mono- and pentaglutamate substrates may result from a change in the kinetic mechanism with polyglutamate substrates.

Similarly, chicken liver AICAR transformylase shows a preference for polyglutamates of PteGlu as inhibitors of the enzyme, with K_i values decreasing up to the pentaglutamate (Chan and Baggott, 1982), and the inhibition patterns change with polyglutamate substrates. Only modest changes in K_m and V_{max}/K_m were observed between mono- and polyglutamate substrates. However, these studies used 5,10-methenyl-H_4PteGlu$_n$ as the substrate rather than 10-formyl-H_4PteGlu$_n$ (Chan and Baggott, 1982).

10-Formyl-H_4PteGlu$_5$ is a more effective substrate of human AICAR transformylase than the monoglutamate derivative (K_m 5.5 μM versus 44 μM), with a slightly enhanced V_{max} (Allegra *et al.*, 1985b). Methotrexate polyglutamates are potent inhibitors of the enzyme, when activity is measured with 10-formyl-H_4PteGlu as the substrate, and demonstrate a large increase in affinity with extension of the glutamate chain (Allegra *et al.*, 1985b; Chabner *et al.*, 1985). The second, third, and fourth glutamate residues each contribute about 1.5 kcal/mol, and the K_i falls from 140 μM with the monoglutamate to 56 nM with the tetraglutamate. The affinity of the pentaglutamate is similar to that of the tetraglutamate. The affinities of methotrexate polyglutamates are reduced when 10-formyl-H_4PteGlu$_5$ is the folate substrate. In this case, mono- and diglutamates have similar affinities (K_i 40 μM and 32 μM), and a large increase in affinity occurs with the triglutamate (K_i 2.3 μM) but no further increases occur with longer-chain-length derivatives. H_2PteGlu is a weak inhibitor of AICAR transformylase (K_i 63 μM) but

$H_2PteGlu_5$ is a potent inhibitor (K_i 43 nM). The affinity of the mono-glutamate is unchanged if measured with the pentaglutamate sub-strate, but that of $H_2PteGlu_5$ decreases (K_i 2.7 μM). Again, different affinities of inhibitors when mono- and pentaglutamate substrates are used may be due to a change in the kinetic mechanism with polygluta-mate substrates.

Antifolates such as methotrexate cause elevations in cellular H_2Pte-Glu_n levels. The accumulation of $H_2PteGlu_n$ is believed to be responsi-ble for the inhibition of purine synthesis that occurs with antifolate treatment (Baggott et al., 1986; Allegra et al., 1987).

The K_m of 10-formyl-$H_4PteGlu_n$ for the chicken liver AICAR trans-formylase greatly decreases between the mono- and triglutamate sub-strates (674 μM versus 1.7 μM, Baggott and Krumdieck, 1979; 84 μM versus 0.7 μM, Mueller and Benkovic, 1981), and this decrease is accom-panied by little or no change in V_{max}. Further extension of the gluta-mate chain of the substrate has only minor effects on these parameters.

4. Disposal of One-Carbon Units

The folylpolyglutamate substrate specificity of bifunctional for-myltetrahydrofolate dehydrogenase-hydrolase has not been reported. The K_m of the monoglutamate substrate, 10-formyl-$H_4PteGlu$, for the pig liver dehydrogenase is about 7 μM while the K_i of the product, $H_4PteGlu$, is about 1 μM. The K_m of 10-formyl-$H_4PteGlu$ for the hydro-lase activity is 42 μM (Kutzbach and Stokstad, 1968; Rios-Orlandi et al., 1986). Similar kinetic constants have been reported for the rat liver enzyme (Scrutton and Beis, 1979).

$H_4PteGlu_n$ are potent inhibitors of both activities (Rios-Orlandi et al., 1986; Table II). Affinities increase rapidly between the mono- and triglutamates and then more gradually up to the hexaglutamate. K_i values for $H_4PteGlu_n$ have not been determined. With 30 μM 10-formyl-$H_4PteGlu$ as the substrate, 0.3 μM $H_4PteGlu_6$ inhibits activity by 90%, demonstrating a very high affinity for the polyglutamate inhibitor (Table II). The high affinity of $H_4PteGlu_n$ for the protein is also reflected by the identification of the protein as a major intra-cellular folate-binding protein in rat and pig liver (Min et al., 1988).

The dehydrogenase reaction represents a mechanism for the disposal of excess one-carbon moieties (Krebs et al., 1976). The very high affinity of the product inhibitor $H_4PteGlu_6$ for the pig liver enzyme, and the presumed low K_m of the polyglutamate substrate, suggests that the metabolic flux through this reaction, and also the hydrolase reaction, is regulated by the 10-formyl-$H_4PteGlu_n$: $H_4PteGlu_n$ ratio rather than by the tissue concentration of 10-formyl-$H_4PteGlu_n$, as the concentrations of both of these folates are likely to be considerably in excess of their K_m and K_i values for the enzymes under physiological conditions. The physiological role of this protein would appear to be to regulate the proportion of folate present in the $H_4PteGlu_n$ form, presumably to make it available for other reactions of one-carbon metabolism, regardless of total folate levels in the tissue.

5. Mitochondrial Enzymes

The folylpolyglutamate substrate specificity of mitochondrial serine hydroxymethyltransferase has not been specifically addressed. The properties of the purified pig liver hydroxymethyltransferase used in the studies described above suggested that it was the cytoplasmic isozyme (Matthews et al., 1982). The high degree of homology between the cytoplasmic and mitochondrial isozymes suggests that the folylpolyglutamate substrate specificities of the enzymes are probably similar, but this remains to be investigated.

The folylpolyglutamate specificity of the glycine synthase complex has not been reported, and the activities of sarcosine and dimethylglycine dehydrogenases are unaffected by the presence or absence of a folate acceptor for formaldehyde. In fact, stoichiometric covalent binding of PteGlu to dimethylglycine dehydrogenase blocks binding of $H_4PteGlu_n$ but does not affect the rate of dehydrogenase activity in vitro (Wagner et al., 1984).

B. MULTIFUNCTIONAL COMPLEXES AND SUBSTRATE CHANNELING

Studies with isolated purified enzymes of one-carbon metabolism have suggested that the polyglutamate chain of the folate molecule plays an important role in modifying the substrate activity of folates and have also suggested potentially important regulatory features of folylpolyglutamates that would not be of physiological relevance if tissues contained only monoglutamates. However, kinetic analyses of individual enzyme activities do not address the potential role of folylpolyglutamates in multifunctional protein complexes. Many of the enzyme activities of one-carbon metabolism are associated on multifunctional proteins or possibly as multiprotein complexes.

1. Formiminotransferase–Cyclodeaminase

Pig liver formiminotransferase–cyclodeaminase is an octomeric protein arranged as a tetramer of dimers (MacKenzie et al., 1980; reviewed by Shane and Stokstad, 1984). Each monomer contains a formiminotransferase and a cyclodeaminase site, but there are only four

$H_4PteGlu_n$ binding sites per octomer (Paquin *et al.*, 1985). The protein can be cleaved by proteases to generate an active dimeric for-miminotransferase fragment lacking cyclohydrolase activity or can be modified to specifically inactivate formiminotransferase activity (Mac-Kenzie and Baugh, 1980).

Both enzyme activities show a strong preference for folylpolygluta-mate substrates of glutamate chain length four and above and pteroyl-hexaglutamate inhibitors have the highest affinity (Section IV,A,1,c). Although the K_m for $H_4PteGlu$ is unchanged with the protease-gener-ated formiminotransferase fragment, the increased substrate effec-tiveness of polyglutamates is completely lost, and the K_m values for polyglutamates increase to values higher than those with the mono-glutamate (MacKenzie *et al.*, 1980). The data suggest that the bifunc-tional protein contains one polyglutamate chain-binding site per pair of formiminotransferase–cyclodeaminase sites and that this site is re-moved by proteolysis.

Formiminotransferase–cyclodeaminase catalyzes two sequential metabolic reactions and the intermediate product, 5-formimino-$H_4PteGlu_n$, has no other metabolic function. The presence of both activities on a protein offers a potential kinetic advantage if the inter-mediate product is presented to the cyclodeaminase site without release from the protein. This phenomenon, called channeling, would increase the effective concentration of the substrate for the cyclodeaminase. This has been investigated by providing substrates for the formimino-transferase ($H_4PteGlu_n$) and by following the appearance of the inter-mediate and final products (5-formimino-$H_4PteGlu_n$ and 5,10-meth-enyl-$H_4PteGlu_n$). With mono-, di-, and triglutamate substrates, 5-formimino-$H_4PteGlu_n$ accumulates and there is a time lag in the ap-pearance of 5,10-methenyl-$H_4PteGlu_n$ (MacKenzie and Baugh, 1980; Paquin *et al.*, 1985). With tetra- to heptaglutamate substrates, no time lag is observed in the formation of the final product, demonstrating channeling. Some intermediate product is released with the tetra-, hexa-, and heptaglutamate substrates, but the amounts released are lower than the final product. With $H_4PteGlu_5$ as the substrate, essen-tially no intermediate product is released, demonstrating almost per-fect channeling with this chain length. To eliminate the possibility that the effects noted were due to the high affinity of 5-formimino-$H_4PteGlu_{4-7}$ for the cyclodeaminase, rather than channeling per se, the experiment was repeated using formiminotransferase-inactivated and cyclodeaminase-inactivated proteins, where both activities were present at the same concentration but were now on different proteins. The kinetics of appearance of products were unchanged with the monoglutamate substrate, but the channeling effect noted for polyglutamate substrates was lost and there was a time lag in the appearance of the final product. These data suggest that a single-site anchor for the polyglutamate tail on the protein aids in the transfer of the product of the formiminotransferase reaction to the active site of the cyclodeaminase. The triglutamate tail is not long enough to permit anchorage of the tail and pterin placement at the active sites while the pentaglutamate represents the optimal chain length. Slightly shorter or longer chain lengths allow channeling but also allow some dissociation of the intermediate product. The optimal chain length for channeling is different from that of the major folates in pig liver (hexaglutamate), but whether this has any regulatory significance is not clear.

2. C_1 Synthase

Channeling of folates has also been demonstrated for the methylenetetrahydrofolate dehydrogenase–methenyltetrahydrofolate cyclohydrolase domain of the C_1 synthase, while the formyltetrahydrofolate synthetase domain of this protein appears to be independent (Cohen and MacKenzie, 1978; MacKenzie and Baugh, 1980; Wasserman et al., 1983).

The dehydrogenase and cyclohydrolase share a common folate-binding site (Smith and MacKenzie, 1985). No time lag is observed in the appearance of 10-formyl-H_4PteGlu$_n$ when the pig liver and chicken liver proteins are incubated with 5,10-methylene-H_4PteGlu$_n$ (MacKenzie and Baugh, 1980; Wasserman et al., 1983), indicative of a channeling effect. Channeling with this complex differs from that observed with formiminotransferase–cyclodeaminase in that channeling occurs with the monoglutamate substrate as well as with polyglutamates, and the channeling is never complete, as some intermediate 5,10-methenyl-H_4PteGlu$_n$ product is always observed. Channeling of polyglutamates with the pig liver enzyme appears to be slightly more efficient than with the monoglutamate substrate (MacKenzie and Baugh, 1980). However, the interaction of the fifth glutamate moiety of folylpolyglutamates with the dehydrogenase (Ross et al., 1984) does not appear to influence the channeling process. The partitioning between the final and intermediate products with the chicken liver enzyme is higher with triglutamate (85 : 15) than with monoglutamate (46 : 54; Wasserman et al., 1983). Interestingly, exogenous 5,10-methenyl-H_4PteGlu$_n$ does not compete with the 5,10-methenyl-H_4PteGlu$_n$ formed in the dehydrogenase reaction as a substrate for the cyclohydrolase, suggesting that the intermediate product does not normally leave the protein. Channeling through the bifunctional domain of the C_1 synthase would avoid accumulation of 5,10-methenyl-H_4PteGlu$_n$, which has no known metabolic function. Incomplete channeling may not be too disadvantageous, as any 5,10-methenyl-H_4PteGlu$_n$ released would be converted nonenzymatically to 10-for-myl-H_4PteGlu$_n$ at physiological pH, although at a slower rate than the enzyme catalyzed reaction, provided the final product is not channeled directly to some other protein.

3. Other Complexes

Associations among C_1 synthase, serine hydroxymethyltransferase, and the enzymes of de novo purine biosynthesis have been suggested, but no studies have been carried out on the possible role of folylpoly-glutamates in the functioning of this putative complex. Similarly, the possible role of folylpolyglutamates in the functioning of the replitase complex, which contains thymidylate synthase and dihydrofolate reductase, remains to be explored.

C. INTRACELLULAR FOLATE-BINDING PROTEINS

The high affinity of folylpolyglutamate inhibitors for some of the enzymes of one-carbon metabolism (Section IV,A) has a number of regulatory implications. However, binding of folylpolyglutamates to cellular proteins would be expected to reduce the availability of some of these compounds and consequently modify their potential for the regulation of pathways (Zamierowsky and Wagner, 1977a).

Rat liver contains five major folate-binding proteins (Zamierowsky and Wagner, 1977a,b; Wagner, 1986). The two mitochondrial proteins, sarcosine and dimethylglycine dehydrogenases, contain primarily bound H_4PteGlu$_5$ (Wittwer and Wagner, 1981). Dimethylglycine dehydrogenase has a similar affinity for mono- and pentaglutamate folates (K_i 0.4 μM versus 0.2 μM), and its isolation with bound pentagluta-mate probably reflects the folylpolyglutamate distribution in rat liver mitochondria.

The major cytoplasmic folate-binding protein, glycine methyltrans-ferase, is present in high concentrations (approximately 40 μM mono-mers) and contains bound 5-methyl-H_4PteGlu$_5$, which is an inhibitor of the enzyme (Cook and Wagner, 1984; Wagner et al., 1985). The pentaglutamate is the most effective inhibitor (K_i 0.5 μM; Wagner and Cook, 1986).

Rat liver contains two additional cytoplasmic folate-binding proteins of M_r 210,000 and 25,000 (Wagner, 1986). The larger protein has been purified to homogeneity and contains bound H_4PteGlu$_5$ (Cook

and Wagner, 1982). This protein has recently been identified as formyltetrahydrofolate dehydrogenase–hydrolase (Min *et al.*, 1988), and
its ability to bind folates is consistent with the high affinity of
folylpolyglutamates for this protein. In folate deficiency, tight binding
of $H_4PteGlu_n$ to this protein (Zamierowsky and Wagner, 1977a) may
make $H_4PteGlu_n$ unavailable for other enzymes of one-carbon metabolism.

The isolation of proteins as major folate-binding proteins presumably reflects the abundance of some of these proteins and also the
affinities of folates for the proteins. Serine hydroxymethyltransferase
is also a high-abundance protein (approximately 20 μM monomers) but
has not been identified as a folate-binding protein. Many other proteins of one-carbon metabolism are present in the 1–5 μM range in
liver, while the proteins of the methionine cycle and folylpolyglutamate synthetase are minor proteins (approximately 50 nM). Based on
the affinities reported for folylpolyglutamates for these enzymes, it is
probable that a significant proportion, if not most, of the intracellular
folate is associated with proteins under physiological conditions, although the association may not survive tissue extraction and protein
purification procedures.

D. Folate Transport and Retention

Folate transport by mammalian tissues and cells has been recently
reviewed (Henderson, 1986) and is beyond the scope of this chapter.
Pteroylmonoglutamates are transported by a carrier-mediated,
energy-dependent process. In recent years, studies on a high-affinity
plasma, folate-binding protein and a membrane-associated, folate-
binding protein have demonstrated extensive homology between the
two proteins (McHugh and Cheng, 1979; Antony *et al.*, 1981, 1985;
Selhub and Franklin, 1984; Kane *et al.*, 1986b; Wagner, 1986; Price
and Freisheim, 1987), and they may differ only in extent of fatty acid
acylation (Luhrs *et al.*, 1987). The membrane-associated binding protein may be the folate transport carrier, although affinities of pteroylmonoglutamates for this protein suggest considerably tighter binding
than is suggested by the K_t for transport of these compounds by cells,
and the increased affinity of polyglutamates of methotrexate is inconsistent with the inability of these compounds to be transported by cells
(Elwood *et al.*, 1986). Folate and methotrexate binding by the membrane protein and cellular uptake is increased when cells are cultured
in folate-deficient medium (Kane *et al.*, 1986a) and, based on the time
dependence of internalization of bound folate, it has been suggested

that folates are transported by a receptor-mediated, endocytotic mechanism (Kamen and Capdevila, 1986), although this proposal remains to be verified. The level of the binding protein may also be regulated by cell differentiation (Sirotnak et al., 1986). Antisera to the binding protein inhibit folate uptake and reduce intracellular folate accumulation in erythroid progenitor cells (Antony et al., 1987), which is consistent with a role for the protein in folate transport. However, although the cells were megaloblastic, cell replication rates increased, which is a puzzling observation. The role of the soluble, extracellular folate-binding protein has not been established. Several distinct mechanisms have been identified for methotrexate efflux by mammalian cells (Henderson and Tsuji, 1987).

Pteroylmonoglutamates, primarily 5-methyl-H_4PteGlu, are the circulating forms of folate, and mammalian cells are not believed to transport polyglutamates of chain length three or above, although this has received little study. CHO mutants lacking folylpolyglutamate synthetase activity (AUX B1) transport folates normally, and low intracellular folate concentrations in this mutant are due to an inability to retain folates (McBurney and Whitmore, 1974a). AUX B3, a CHO mutant with a defective folylpolyglutamate synthetase, contains short-chain-length folates, presumed to be triglutamates, and is also defective in folate accumulation (McBurney and Whitmore, 1974a). However, it is not clear whether defective folate retention by this mutant is due to an inability to retain pteroyltriglutamates or to a slow rate of synthesis of pteroyltriglutamate. Folate retention by AUX B1 cells transfected with the *Escherichia coli* folylpolyglutamate synthetase gene (*folC*) has recently been investigated (C. Osborne and B. Shane, unpublished observations). AUX B1-*folC* transfectants contain pteroyltriglutamates, reflecting the substrate specificity of the *E. coli* folylpolyglutamate synthetase. Retention of triglutamates by these transfectants is similar to that of the longer-chain-length folates, primarily hexa- and heptaglutamates, in wild-type CHO cells. Labeled intracellular pteroyltri-, hexa-, and heptaglutamate are slowly released by cells chased with high levels of unlabeled folate and at similar rates, while mono- and diglutamates are rapidly released. These data suggest that metabolism of folate to the triglutamate is sufficient to allow normal retention of folates and that long-chain-length polyglutamates slowly cross the cell membrane. No detectable loss of labeled intracellular tri-, hexa-, or heptaglutamate is observed when cells are incubated in the absence of an unlabeled folate chase. Under these conditions, about half of the intracellular pteroylmonoglutamate in AUX B1 cells is rapidly released, but the remainder remains in the cell. These data suggest that under normal physiological conditions a slow release of folylpolyglutamates is prevented by intracellular binding of these derivatives, and, in the absence of polyglutamates, binding of some pteroylmonoglutamate to proteins can prevent its efflux.

Similarly, the half-life of labeled folates, primarily folylpolyglutamates, in cultured cells is similar to the generation time of the cells when cells accumulate levels of folate that support normal rates of growth, while the half-life is reduced, indicative of folate efflux, when cells contain high levels of folate (Steinberg et al., 1983). Studies on the retention of antifolates by a variety of cell lines also indicate a rapid efflux of mono- and diglutamate forms of aminopterin and methotrexate and a greatly reduced or negligible efflux of longer-chain derivatives (Jolivet et al., 1982; Fabre et al., 1984; McGuire et al., 1985; Samuels et al., 1985). Folylpolyglutamates do turn over in liver under physiological conditions (Thenen et al., 1973), although it is not known whether this involves release of intact folylpolyglutamates or their hydrolysis to pteroylmonoglutamates prior to release (Section VI,D).

E. ASSESSMENT OF *in Vivo* EFFECTS

As described earlier, CHO AUX B1 cells, which lack folylpolyglutamates, are auxotrophic for glycine, thymidine, and purines, although the thymidine requirement can be partially overcome by high levels of medium folate (McBurney and Whitmore, 1974a; Sussman et al., 1986a). Wild-type CHO cells will grow, albeit at a reduced rate, in the absence of methionine, provided the medium is supplemented with homocysteine, vitamin B_{12}, and very high levels of folate. Under identical conditions, AUX B1 cells will not grow (Taylor and Hanna, 1975).

Recently, a number of *in vivo* systems have been developed to explore whether specific folylpolyglutamate chain lengths are favored for different cycles of one-carbon metabolism under physiological conditions. As pointed out above, *in vitro* studies with purified enzymes cannot be used to ascertain any specific effects of folylpolyglutamates that influence the functioning of potential multiprotein complexes in tissues, distinct from their roles as substrates or inhibitors of the individual enzymes. In addition, *in vitro* studies may suffer from artifacts introduced by the assay conditions employed, for example, the choice of buffer.

1. *Thymidylate Cycle*

The functioning of the thymidylate cycle has been studied in murine L1210 cells permeabilized with dextran sulfate (Kalman, 1986), a procedure that allows folylpolyglutamates to enter the cell while macromolecules are retained in the cell. In this novel approach, the permeable cells were incubated with PteGlu$_n$, serine, NADPH, and 5-[^{3}H]dUMP, and the activity of the thymidylate cycle was monitored by the release of the tritium label that occurs when dUMP is metabolized to dTMP. The activity obtained reflects the functioning of serine hydroxymethyltransferase, thymidylate synthase, and dihydrofolate reductase. The apparent K_m for PteGlu$_6$ was less than 1 μM, and maximal activity was obtained at the physiologically relevant concentration of about 5 μM. The apparent K_m for the monoglutamate substrate was above 10 μM, and the maximal activity, observed with about 50 μM substrate, was about 6-fold lower than with the hexaglutamate substrate. V_{max}/K_m(app) of PteGlu$_n$, compared to monoglutamate (equals 1), increased significantly with the di- (14-fold) and triglutamate (40-fold), less steeply with the tetraglutamate (62-fold), and little effect of further chain elongation was noted (penta-, hexa-, and heptaglutamate 56-, 56-, and 51-fold, respectively). Replacement of serine with formaldehyde, which excludes serine hydroxymethyltransferase from the cycle, did not affect the qualitative differences observed with polyglutamate chain length, but quantitative differences were less pronounced. These data suggest that pteroyltetraglutamates and longer-chain derivatives are the optimal substrates for the hydroxymethyltransferase and for thymidylate synthase *in vivo* and that the major increases in substrate efficacy are due to extension of the chain from the mono- to the triglutamate. In general, these conclusions agree fairly well with data obtained in *in vitro* studies with the isolated enzymes (Section IV,A,2), although the pig liver thymidylate synthase does not show a pronounced preference for polyglutamate substrates.

Inhibition of the thymidylate cycle in L1210 cells by methotrexate polyglutamates also shows an effect of polyglutamate chain length (Kalman, 1986). The IC$_{50}$ is reduced from 60 μM with the monoglutamate to 1 μM with the tetraglutamate, and most of this change occurs between the mono- and triglutamates.

Permeabilized cells appear to be very useful for studying the effects of folate substrates and inhibitors under physiological conditions, and it is possible to modify experimental conditions to make different enzymes in metabolic cycles rate limiting. A potential confounding parameter in this type of study is the use of a buffer to mimic the intracellular milieu.

Mammalian cell mutants have also been used to study the effect of changes in folylpolyglutamate distributions on one-carbon metabolism. CHO AUX B3 mutants, which appear to contain pteroyltriglutamates, will grow in the absence of thymidine and purines but require higher levels of medium folate to achieve the same growth rates as wild-type cells, and will also grow, although poorly, in the absence of glycine, provided very high levels of folate are provided (McBurney and Whitmore, 1974a). It is not possible to assess whether the phenotype of AUX B3 cells is due to a reduced capacity of pteroyltriglutamates, compared to hexa- and heptaglutamates, as substrates of the enzymes of one-carbon metabolism and/or results from the decreased accumulation of folate by these cells.

This question has recently been addressed by measuring intracellular folate levels that support half-maximal doubling times of AUX B1 transfectants cultured in medium lacking thymidine. The transfectants used were AUX B1-*folC*, which express *E. coli* folylpolyglutamate synthetase and contain primarily pteroyltriglutamates (C. Osborne and B. Shane, unpublished observations), and AUX B1-human, which express various levels of human folylpolyglutamate synthetase, and contain folate distributions ranging from primarily pentaglutamate to longer distributions than are found in wild-type CHO cells (Sussman *et al.*, 1986b). In the absence of thymidine, a similar intracellular folate concentration supports similar growth rates of AUX B1-*folC* and wild-type cells, although the maximal growth rate is slightly depressed in the transfectant, while intracellular pteroylmonoglutamate over 100-fold higher support a depressed rate of thymidine synthesis in AUX B1 cells. In CHO cells, pteroyltriglutamates function approximately as well as longer-chain-length derivatives in the thymidylate cycle, and the increased folate requirement of AUX B3 cells in medium lacking thymidine probably reflects a decreased ability to accumulate folate.

2. *Purine Cycle*

Similar intracellular folate concentrations also support purine biosynthesis in AUX B1-*folC,* AUX B1-human, and wild-type CHO cells, while greatly elevated intracellular pteroylmonoglutamate concentrations do not support growth of AUX B1 cells in the absence of hypoxanthine (C. Osborne, K. Lowe, and B. Shane, unpublished observations). It appears that pteroyltriglutamates are sufficient for whichever enzyme(s) is rate limiting for *de novo* purine biosynthesis *in vivo*. The folate-dependent enzymes involved in this cycle are serine hydroxymethyltransferase, methylenetetrahydrofolate dehydrogenase, cyclohydrolase, GAR and AICAR transformylases, and also dihydrofolate reductase, as oxidized folate was supplied in the medium. *In vitro* substrate specificity studies suggest limited or no folylpolyglutamate preference for the dehydrogenase and reductase and a triglutamate or longer preference for the hydroxymethyltransferase. The transformylases show a strong preference for polyglutamate substrates, but differences between individual chain lengths have not been assessed. The data obtained *in vivo* are consistent with *in vitro* derived data.

3. *Glycine Synthesis*

Preliminary studies suggest that the glycine requirement of CHO AUX B1-human transfectants, which contain modified folylpolyglutamate distributions ranging from the pentaglutamate to the hexaglutamate, is met by similar intracellular folate concentrations to wild-type CHO cells (K. Lowe and B. Shane, unpublished observations), while AUX B1 cells do not grow in the absence of glycine, even when they contain greatly elevated pteroylmonoglutamate concentrations. AUX B1-*folC* transfectants grow very poorly in medium lacking glycine and require over 100-fold higher levels of intracellular folate to achieve growth rates similar to those in wild-type cells. The inability of pteroyltriglutamates to support glycine synthesis for growth in CHO cells is surprising in light of the apparently normal functioning of triglutamates in the thymidylate and purine cycles, both of which involve serine hydroxymethyltransferase. As discussed previously (Section II,B,3), mammalian cells require mitochondrial glycine synthesis to provide glycine for protein synthesis. The glycine requiring CHO mutants *glyB* and *glyC* (AUX B2) are defective in mitochondrial glycine synthesis, although both have normal mitochondrial serine hydroxymethyltransferase activities (Taylor and Hanna, 1982). Mitochondrial folylpolyglutamates are greatly reduced in *glyB* mutants but appear to be normal in *glyC* mutants. The actual defects in these cells have not been elucidated but appear to involve defects in mitochondrial folate transport or recycling (Taylor and Hannah, 1982). The inability of pteroyltriglutamates to support glycine synthesis in AUX B1-*folC* transfectants is probably due to a lack of folylpolyglutamates in the mitochondria. Conclusive evidence for this proposal must await identification of subcellular folates in this transfectant. Mitochondria appear to contain folylpolyglutamate synthetase activity (Section V,A), and it is likely that folylpolyglutamates do not cross the mitochondrial membrane. If this is the case, mammalian cells transfected with the *E. coli folC* gene would not be expected to contain pteroyltriglutamates, as the *E. coli* protein would lack the leader sequence required for mitochondrial protein import. A mutation in the leader sequence of the *glyB* folylpolyglutamate synthetase could also explain the phenotype of this mutant.

4. *Other Metabolic Pathways*

Although mammalian tissues contain primarily pteroylpenta-, hexa-, or longer-glutamate chain-length folates, pteroyltriglutamates, or possibly tetraglutamates, appear to possess sufficiently long polyglutamate chains to allow normal thymidylate and purine biosyntheses, and possibly glycine biosynthesis, *in vivo* and also to allow normal retention of folates by cells. Do the longer-chain-length derivatives confer any additional advantages to the cell? *In vitro* studies with folylpolyglutamate inhibitors (Section IV,A) suggest some regulatory effects of polyglutamates, but most of the advantages of long-chain derivatives are achieved by extension of the chain to the triglutamate derivative.

Channeling of folates through the bifunctional formiminotransferase–cyclodeaminase from pig liver requires at least the tetraglutamate and is optimal with the pentaglutamate (Paquin *et al.*, 1985). Although channeling is incomplete with the tetraglutamate, it is also incomplete with the hexaglutamate, the major polyglutamate species in pig liver, and there does not seem to be any specific advantage of the hexaglutamate over the tetraglutamate.

The only metabolic cycle with enzymes that show a clear-cut preference for long-chain-length folates *in vitro* is the methionine cycle. The committed enzyme, methylenetetrahydrofolate reductase, from pig liver shows a marked preference for the hexaglutamate substrate and for long-glutamate chain-length inhibitors (Matthews and Baugh, 1980). The effects of modified folylpolyglutamate distributions on the methionine cycle *in vivo* remain to be investigated. However, the accumulation of the long-glutamate chain-length folates typically found in mammalian tissues may reflect a requirement for methionine synthesis.

Different endogenous folate one-carbon distributions for different polyglutamate chain lengths, with the $H_4PteGlu_n$ distribution favoring slightly longer chain lengths than the 5-methyl-$H_4PteGlu_n$ distribution, have been reported for rat liver and brain (Brody *et al.*, 1976, 1982). In another study, differences in one-carbon distributions in rat liver were also observed, but the 10-formyl-$H_4PteGlu_n$ distribution was longer than the other one-carbon forms (Eto and Krumdieck, 1982a). These observations are suggestive of differences in one-carbon metabolism with different-chain-length polyglutamates. However, no changes in one-carbon distribution with chain length were noted in human fibroblast folate pools (Foo *et al.*, 1982). Methionine administration to nitrous oxide-treated rats significantly diminishes 5-methyl-$H_4PteGlu_{5-7}$, indicating that penta-, hexa-, and heptaglutamates are metabolically active (Brody *et al.*, 1982). Labeled histidine also labels the 5-methyl-$H_4PteGlu_{5,6}$ pools in rat liver, indicating that the metabolic pathways linking formiminoglutamate with 5-methyl-$H_4PteGlu_n$ function with both penta- and hexaglutamates (T. Brody and E. L. R. Stokstad, personal communication).

V. FOLYLPOLYGLUTAMATE SYNTHESIS AND DEGRADATION

The synthesis of folylpolyglutamates, and factors that regulate this synthesis, would be expected to play a major role in the regulation of folate homeostasis and one-carbon metabolism. Mammalian cells possess two types of enzyme activities that can potentially directly regulate this process: folylpolyglutamate synthetase, which catalyzes the synthesis of folylpolyglutamates, and γ-glutamylhydrolase, a peptidase that can hydrolyze the folate polypeptide chain. The general properties of both of these activities have been the subject of a recent review (McGuire and Coward, 1984).

A. FOLYLPOLYGLUTAMATE SYNTHETASE

1. *Distribution and General Properties*

Folylpolyglutamate synthetase catalyzes the general reaction:

$$MgATP + folate(glu_n) + glutamate \rightarrow MgADP + folate(glu_{n+1}) + phosphate$$

Because of the marked lability and low abundance of the protein, the mammalian enzyme has only received detailed study in the last few years. After preliminary characterization of crude enzyme preparations from sheep liver (Gawthorne and Smith, 1973) and partially purified enzyme from CHO cells (Taylor and Hanna, 1977), McGuire *et al.* (1980) extensively characterized a 70-fold purified preparation from rat liver. Following this, the enzymes from mouse (Moran and Colman, 1984a), beef (Pristupa *et al.*, 1984), and pig liver (Cichowicz *et al.*, 1981; Bognar *et al.*, 1983) were partially purified and characterized. The human liver enzyme, which has been purified about 100-fold, has low activity in crude extracts and is very unstable (C. Cody, G. Milman, and B. Shane, unpublished observations). Some properties of 6-fold purified human liver enzyme have been recently reported (Clarke and Waxman, 1987). The pig liver enzyme has recently been purified to homogeneity (Cichowicz and Shane, 1987a). Although pig liver is a richer source of the enzyme than other mammalian tissues, purification required about a 50,000-fold enrichment, and the synthetase is present at a concentration of about 50 nM in pig liver. In most respects the properties of the pig liver enzyme are similar to those reported for partially purified enzymes from other mammalian sources. Bacterial folylpolyglutamate synthetases have been purified to homogeneity from *Corynebacterium* (Shane, 1980a), *L. casei* (Bognar and Shane, 1983), and *E. coli* (Bognar *et al.*, 1985), and the *E. coli* gene has been cloned and sequenced (Bognar *et al.*, 1985, 1987). The bacterial enzymes differ markedly from the mammalian enzymes in their substrate specificities, and the *Corynebacterium* and *E. coli* proteins also possess dihydrofolate synthetase activity, an activity not associated with the mammalian enzyme. Consequently, the bacterial enzyme is a poor model for assessing regulatory factors that may play a role in the regulation of mammalian folate metabolism.

The turnover number of the pig liver enzyme with H_4PteGlu as the substrate (2.5 per second) is slightly higher than that found with the preferred substrates of the bacterial enzymes (Shane, 1980b; Bognar and Shane, 1983; Bognar *et al.*, 1985). The low levels of folylpolyglutamate synthetase activity commonly found in mammalian tissues, especially when compared to most bacterial sources, are due to the low concentration of this protein in mammalian sources rather than to a decreased catalytic rate for the mammalian protein.

Synthetase activity is highest in liver, and appreciable levels are found in most mammalian tissues, although it appears to be absent or present in only negligible amounts in muscle tissue (McGuire *et al.*, 1979; Moran and Colman, 1984b). Most synthetase activity is present in the cytoplasm of cells, although some activity is found in the mitochondrial fraction (Gawthorne and Smith, 1973; McGuire *et al.*, 1979). It is not known whether a separate mitochondrial enzyme exists or whether the mitochondrial activity differs in its specificity from the cytoplasmic enzyme. The reversion frequency of the CHO folylpolyglutamate synthetase mutant AUX B1 is consistent with a single genetic lesion, and AUX B1 cells lack both cytoplasmic and mitochondrial folylpolyglutamates (McBurney and Whitmore, 1974a; Taylor and Hannah, 1982). AUX B1 extracts cannot use H_4PteGlu$_{2,3}$ as a substrate, and the degree of activity restored in revertants is similar with mono- and diglutamate substrates, suggesting that a single enzyme is responsible for the conversion of folates to polyglutamate forms and that the mutant phenotype is due to a mutation in the folylpolyglutamate synthetase structural gene (Taylor and Hannah, 1977, 1979). Similarly, AUX B1 transfectants expressing the *E. coli* folylpolyglutamate synthetase gene contain triglutamate derivatives, characteristic of *E. coli,* and lack a separate activity for the further extension of the glutamaté chain (unpublished observations). The pig liver enzyme metabolizes $H_4PteGlu$ *in vitro* to similar folate derivatives to those found *in vivo* with the hexaglutamate predominating, indicating that a single enzyme can account for the folylpolyglutamate distribution in pig liver (Cichowicz and Shane, 1987a; Cook *et al.,* 1987). *Escherichia coli* contains a separate activity that can add additional glutamate moieties in α-peptide bond linkage to pteroyltriglutamates (Ferone *et al.,* 1986a,b). The accumulation of pteroyltriglutamates in AUX B1-*folC* transfectants suggests that mammalian cells lack this activity.

The human gene for folylpolyglutamate synthetase has been assigned to chromosome 9 (Jones *et al.,* 1980) and the mouse gene to chromosome 2 (Fournier and Moran, 1983) by examining chromosomes retained in AUX B1-human and AUX B1-mouse cell and microcell hybrids grown in selective media. The chromosomal assignment of the CHO gene is unknown, although it has been reported to be tightly linked to the CHO dihydrofolate reductase gene (Spandidos and Siminovitch, 1977). This would position the CHO synthetase gene on chromosome 2 (Urlaub *et al.,* 1983). However, the human dihydrofolate reductase gene is located on a different chromosome to the synthetase gene (Maurer *et al.,* 1984).

General characteristics of folylpolyglutamate synthetases from pig, mouse, rat, and beef liver have been described (McGuire *et al.,* 1980; Moran and Colman, 1984a; Pristupa *et al.,* 1984; Cichowicz and Shane, 1987a). All have native molecular weights of 60,000–70,000. The pig enzyme and all purified bacterial synthetases (Shane, 1980a; Bognar and Shane, 1983; Bognar *et al.,* 1985) are monomeric proteins. The pig liver enzyme was purified as two species, both of $M_r^.$ 62,000, with indistinguishable catalytic properties (Cichowicz and Shane, 1987a). It is not clear whether the two species exist in tissues or whether they arose during purification. Mammalian folylpolyglutamate synthetases are very susceptible to proteolytic modification and inactivation. The possibility that the two species represent separate isozymes seems unlikely in light of the genetic evidence for a single locus.

There is an absolute requirement for a monovalent cation which is met most effectively by K^+ (K_d 2–3 mM). NH_4^+ and Rb^+ will also activate the enzyme but to a lesser extent. The enzyme appears to contain a separate inhibitory binding site for monovalent ions in general. High levels of monovalent ions inhibit enzyme activity and the extent of inhibition is proportional to ionic radius. An enzymatic requirement for the divalent cation Mg^{2+} is for generation of the nucleotide substrate $MgATP^{2-}$. Free ATP is a potent inhibitor of the reaction.

Mammalian folylpolyglutamate synthetases have an absolute requirement for a reducing agent which is distinct from the reducing agent required for protection of the reduced folate substrate. Mercaptoethanol (K_d 3–5 mM) or dithiothreitol (K_d 1 mM) activates the pig (Cichowicz and Shane, 1987a) and beef liver (Pristupa *et al.*, 1984) enzymes, while the K_d for the rat liver enzyme is higher (McGuire *et al.*, 1980), with maximal activation at 10 mM and 100 mM, respectively. High concentrations of these agents inhibit most of the synthetases.

The pH optimum for all folylpolyglutamate synthetases is high, ranging from pH 8.4 to 9.5. The lower values in this range probably reflect time-dependent inactivation at the higher pH, as enzyme activity for most of the synthetases is higher at pH 9 than at pH 8.5 when assays are carried out for a short time period. The K_m for L-glutamate decreases with increasing pH, and a very sharp alkaline pH optimum is observed, with little activity at physiological pH at low glutamate concentrations. At high glutamate concentrations (k_{cat} conditions), enzyme activity at physiological pH is only slightly decreased from that observed at high pH (Cichowicz and Shane, 1987a). This pH effect, and the ability of high glutamate concentrations to overcome it at physiological pH, suggest that the free amine of glutamate is the form of the substrate that binds to the enzyme. Plots of $k_{cat}/K_{m(glutamate)}$ against pH indicate a p$K_{glutamate}$ of about 8.5, which is lower than the pK of the amino group of glutamate (Cichowicz and Shane, 1987a). It is possible that this pK reflects titration of a functional group on the enzyme that aids in the binding or deprotonation of glutamate, although the ability of high levels of glutamate to overcome the poor activity at lower pH values suggests that this is unlikely.

Pteroic acid (Pte), which is not a substrate, has been reported to stimulate beef liver folylpolyglutamate synthetase activity in the physiological pH range (Vickers *et al.*, 1985). The physiological significance of this observation is not clear, as Pte is not known to occur in mammalian tissues.

2. *Kinetic Properties and Catalytic Mechanism*

Kinetic studies on folylpolyglutamate synthetase are complicated by the ability of folate products to act as substrates for further glutamate chain elongation. The kinetic mechanism of the hog liver enzyme was investigated using aminopterin as the folate substrate, as the diglutamate of aminopterin is a very poor substrate (Cichowicz and Shane,

1987b). The data were consistent with the following ordered Ter Ter mechanism:

MgATP	aminopterin	glutamate	MgADP	aminopterin(glu-2)	phosphate
↓	↓	↓	↑	↑	↑

This type of mechanism would preclude the sequential addition of glutamate to enzyme-bound folate and is consistent with the observed metabolism of labeled folate doses in mammalian tissues described above and with *in vitro* metabolism studies using mammalian enzymes. As would be predicted for a reaction in which products can compete with the initial substrate of the enzyme for the substrate-binding site, the CHO (Taylor and Hannah, 1977), rat (McGuire *et al.*, 1980), mouse (Moran and Colman, 1984a), beef (Pristupa *et al.*, 1984), and pig (Cichowicz and Shane, 1987a,b) liver enzymes metabolize high concentrations of $H_4PteGlu$ primarily to the diglutamate *in vitro*, while multiple glutamate moieties are added when low substrate concentrations are used.

Although it is possible that the kinetic mechanism might be different with folylpolyglutamate substrates, an identical mechanism was observed with bacterial folylpolyglutamate synthetases when H_4Pte-Glu and 5,10-methylene-$H_4PteGlu_2$ were used as substrates (Shane, 1980b; Bognar and Shane, 1983). The folylpolyglutamate synthetase reaction resembles the glutamine synthetase reaction (Meister, 1978), with folate replacing the glutamate substrate and glutamate replacing ammonia. By analogy, it has been suggested that the folylpolyglutamate synthetase reaction proceeds via phosphorylation of the γ-carboxyl of folate, followed by nucleophilic attack by the free amine of glutamate on the acyl-phosphate intermediate (Shane, 1980b; Tang and Coward, 1983), as shown in Fig. 4. Recent studies demonstrating transfer of ^{18}O from [α,γ-^{18}O]methotrexate or [α,γ-^{18}O]folate to phosphate provide more direct evidence for an acyl-phosphate intermediate (Banerjee *et al.*, 1986).

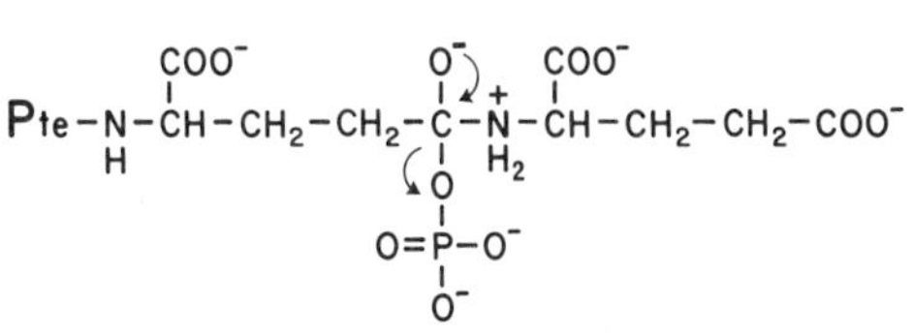

FIG. 4. Proposed reaction intermediate for the folylpolyglutamate synthetase reaction.

3. Substrate Specificity

a. Pteroylmonoglutamates. Kinetic constants for pteroylmonoglutamate substrates of the pig and mouse liver enzymes are shown in
Table III (Moran and Colman, 1984a; Cichowicz and Shane, 1987b).
For an ordered Ter Ter mechanism, K_m values are a function of k_{cat}
and the "on" rate of the folate substrate, and do not necessarily reflect
affinity for the enzyme. k_{cat}/K_m, the pseudo-first-order rate constant,
can be used as a comparison of substrate effectiveness under physiological conditions, as pteroylmonoglutamate concentrations in tissues
are considerably below the K_m values shown in Table III. For an ordered Ter Ter mechanism, k_{cat}/K_m is also the on rate for the folate
substrate (Fromm, 1975).

The most effective substrates for the pig liver enzyme are $H_4PteGlu$,
$H_2PteGlu_n$, and 10-formyl-$H_4PteGlu$, while 5,10-methylene-H_4Pte-
Glu, 5-methyl-$H_4PteGlu$, and PteGlu are very poor substrates
(Cichowicz and Shane, 1987b). The mouse liver enzyme shows a similar specificity, except that 5,10-methylene-$H_4PteGlu$ is a good substrate (Moran and Colman, 1984a).

The specificities for pteroylmonoglutamate derivatives shown in
Table III are generally similar to those reported for partially purified
enzyme preparations from rat (McGuire *et al.*, 1980) and beef liver
(Pristupa *et al.*, 1984) in studies in which substrates were compared at
one or two fixed concentrations. 5,10-Methylene-$H_4PteGlu$ is also a
good substrate for the rat liver enzyme. 5-Formyl-$H_4PteGlu$ is an ef-

TABLE III

KINETIC CONSTANTS OF PTEROYLMONOGLUTAMATES
FOR FOLYLPOLYGLUTAMATE SYNTHETASE[a]

Substrate	Pig liver			Mouse liver		
	K_m (μM)	k_{cat}	k_{cat}/K_m	K_m (μM)	k_{cat}	k_{cat}/K_m
$H_4PteGlu$	7.7	100	100	7.0	100	100
$H_2PteGlu$	5.0	101	156	8.6	120	93
PteGlu	115	95	6.4	137	76	3.3
10-Formyl-$H_4PteGlu$	2.2	27	95	(3.9)	95	147
5,10-Methylene-$H_4PteGlu$	57	39	5.2	4.8	89	87
5-Methyl-$H_4PteGlu$	54	39	5.6	(87)	99	6.7
5-Formyl-$H_4PteGlu$	—	—	—	(8.1)	74	53

[a] Values in parentheses are for mixed isomers. k_{cat} and k_{cat}/K_m are relative to
$H_4PteGlu$. [Data are from Cichowicz and Shane (1987b) and Moran and Colman
(1984a).]

fective substrate for the enzymes from mouse and beef liver but is a poor substrate for the pig and rat liver enzymes.

With the pig enzyme, the on rates for H_4PteGlu, H_4PteGlu, and 10-formyl-H_4PteGlu are identical, while H_2PteGlu binds about 50% faster, so these compounds represent the optimal configurations for binding. The on rates for 5-methyl-H_4PteGlu, 5,10-methyl-H_4PteGlu, and PteGlu are about 20-fold lower than that for H_4PteGlu. k_{cat} values are highest with PteGlu, H_2PteGlu, and H_4PteGlu, which implies that these compounds represent the optimal configurations for catalysis and that the 5- and 10-substitutions of naturally occurring folates hinder catalysis.

b. Pteroylpolyglutamates. Kinetic constants for pteroylpolygluta-mate substrates of the pig liver enzyme are shown in Table IV (Cicho-wicz and Shane, 1987b). k_{cat} values for H_4PteGlu$_n$, H_2PteGlu$_n$, and PteGlu$_n$ decrease with increasing glutamate chain length. k_{cat} values for H_2PteGlu$_n$ are almost identical to the H_4PteGlu$_n$ series for the mono- and diglutamates but fall off faster with longer glutamate de-rivatives, such that the pentaglutamate is essentially inactive as a substrate (Cook *et al.*, 1987). The PteGlu$_n$ series also shows a drop in k_{cat} with extension of the polyglutamate chain. However, although the k_{cat} for PteGlu is identical to that of H_4PteGlu, the value for PteGlu$_2$ is slightly higher than that for H_4PteGlu$_2$, and the value for PteGlu$_3$ is 4-fold higher than that for H_4PteGlu$_3$. k_{cat} values for H_2PteGlu$_3$ and PteGlu$_3$ are also decreased compared to their monoglutamate forms with the mouse liver enzyme (Moran and Colman, 1984a).

Addition of glutamate moieties to H_4PteGlu does not affect the on

TABLE IV

KINETIC CONSTANTS OF PTEROYLPOLYGLUTAMATES SUBSTRATES FOR PIG LIVER FOLYLPOLYGLUTAMATE SYNTHETASE[a]

	H_4PteGlu			H_2PteGlu			PteGlu		
glu$_n$	K_m (μM)	k_{cat}	k_{cat}/K_m	K_m (μM)	k_{cat}	k_{cat}/K_m	K_m (μM)	k_{cat}	k_{cat}/K_m
1	7.7	100	100	5.0	101	156	115	95	6.4
2	3.4	45	102	2.6	51	152	62	60	7.4
3	1.1	8.8	62				119	33	2.2
4	2.0	4.5	17						
5	2.7	1.6	4.6						

[a] k_{cat} and k_{cat}/K_m are relative to H_4PteGlu. [Data are from Cichowicz and Shane (1987b).]

rate for the diglutamate, but the on rate decreases with further extension of the glutamate chain. $H_2PteGlu_2$ and $PteGlu_2$ also have on rates identical to those of their monoglutamates, while the rate decreases for $PteGlu_3$. These data demonstrate little discrimination in initial binding between these pteroylmono- and diglutamates and moderate decreases in initial binding with longer-chain-length derivatives. The fastest on rate for any folate substrate, $4.3 \times 10^5/M/sec$, is observed with $H_2PteGlu_{1,2}$. This slow rate is several orders of magnitude lower than the diffusion-controlled limit and may reflect a conformational change in the protein on substrate binding (Cichowicz and Shane, 1987b).

The conformation of the folate molecule and substitutions of the pterin moiety optimal for catalysis can be quite different from that required for binding to the protein. Increasing the glutamate chain length of the folate molecule causes a decrease in catalytic rate, presumably reflecting an increased difficulty in positioning the γ-carboxyl of the terminal glutamate residue at the active site. In addition, the substrate specificity of the enzyme for pteroylmonoglutamate derivatives is not a good indicator of which compounds are the most effective substrates *in vivo*. An effective *in vivo* substrate would have to be converted to long-chain polyglutamate derivatives. For the hog liver enzyme, little or no substrate activity is detected with $H_4PteGlu_6$, $H_2PteGlu_5$, and 10-formyl-$H_4PteGlu_3$, although their monoglutamate derivatives are all excellent substrates (Cook *et al.*, 1987). 5-Methyl-$H_4PteGlu$ is a relatively poor substrate and its diglutamate derivative is essentially inactive. The accumulation of hexaglutamate derivatives *in vivo* in hog liver is due primarily to the very low k_{cat} values with hexaglutamate substrates and appears to reflect the substrate effectiveness of $H_4PteGlu_n$ rather than other one-carbon forms of folate. Similarly, the accumulation of pentaglutamates in rat liver can be explained by the extremely poor substrate activity of $H_4PteGlu_5$ for the rat liver synthetase, although this compound still retains fairly good affinity for the enzyme (McGuire *et al.*, 1980).

   c. Folate Analogs. 4-Aminofolates (e.g., aminopterin, methotrexate) are much more effective substrates of folylpolyglutamate synthetase than their parent 4-oxo-pteroylmonoglutamate derivatives (McGuire *et al.*, 1980; Moran *et al.*, 1984; Schoo *et al.*, 1985; George *et al.*, 1987) due to increases in their on rates. However, the 4-amino substitution significantly impairs catalysis with polyglutamate derivatives. The diglutamate of methotrexate is a fairly good substrate for the mouse liver enzyme (Moran *et al.*, 1984) but is a poor substrate for the beef (Schoo *et al.*, 1985) and pig (George *et al.*, 1987; Cook *et al.*,

1987) liver enzymes. The triglutamate is essentially inactive as a substrate for the rat (McGuire et al., 1983a) and beef liver enzymes. However, long-glutamate chain-length methotrexate derivatives retain apparent affinity for the beef liver enzyme (Schoo et al., 1985). Some 5,8-dideazafolate derivatives are also very good substrates for the enzyme, with similar activities to (6S)-H_4PteGlu (McGuire et al., 1983b, 1987; Hynes et al., 1986), indicating that a pyrazine ring is not required for substrate binding or catalysis.

A large number of pteroylmonoglutamate analogs with modified glutamate residues have been tested as substrates or inhibitors of the enzyme. Nearly all modifications lead to loss of substrate activity and also apparent affinity for the enzyme (McGuire et al., 1983b; Bognar et al., 1983; Moran et al., 1985; George et al., 1987), suggesting tight specificity for the L-glutamate moiety. The only modification that retains reasonable activity is the 4-fluoroglutamate derivative (Galivan et al., 1985a). Replacement of glutamate with homocysteate, cysteate, or glutamine or replacement of the γ-carboxyl of glutamate with a phosphonate (Rosowsky et al., 1984a,b, 1986a; Cichowicz et al., 1985; George et al., 1987) eliminates substrate activity but not affinity for the enzyme, suggesting a less stringent specificity around the δ carbon of the glutamate moiety. Some interaction around the δ carbon is still evident, as the affinity of Pte-2-aminobutyrate is reduced and Pte-2-aminovalerate lacks measurable affinity (George et al., 1987).

Pte-ornithine analogs have greatly enhanced affinity for all folylpolyglutamate synthetases and are the only potent inhibitors of the synthetase thus far developed (Cichowicz et al., 1985; McGuire et al., 1986; Rosowsky et al., 1986b; George et al., 1987; Clarke et al., 1987). Although the reason for the high affinity of the ornithine analogs is not understood, the potent inhibition observed with enzymes from different sources suggests that the ω-amino group is interacting with a conserved functional group of the enzyme that is presumably essential for substrate binding or catalysis and that the compounds may act as analogs of reaction intermediates. Nucleophilic attack by the free amine of glutamate on a folyl acylphosphate intermediate would be expected to result in protonation of the entering amino nitrogen (Fig. 4). Catalysis would require removal of a proton from the amine and donation of a proton to the phosphate-leaving group. The protonated ω-amino group of Pte-ornithine may be interacting with a base on the enzyme that stabilizes the transition state and/or abstracts the proton.

Limited studies with pteroyldiglutamate analogs modified in the terminal glutamate residue suggest a similar specificity to that found with pteroylmonoglutamate analogs (Bognar et al., 1983; Moran et al.,

1984; George *et al.,* 1987). The binding specificity for the internal glutamate of pteroyldiglutamates is qualitatively similar, if not identical, to the terminal residue, although modified internal glutamate analogs still retain substrate activity (Bognar *et al.,* 1983; Moran *et al.,* 1984; George *et al.,* 1987). Modifications of internal glutamate moieties cause large decreases in on rates but relatively minor changes in k_{cat} (George *et al.,* 1987).

    d. Mechanism of Binding. Pterins have low, but detectable, affinity for the enzyme, while *p*-aminobenzoylmonoglutamate is a substrate for some folylpolyglutamate synthetases with a greatly decreased on rate but an apparently normal k_{cat} (George *et al.,* 1987). This suggests that binding of folates to the enzyme reflects a cooperative effect resulting from two low-affinity events, the initial binding of the pterin or pteroate moiety followed by the binding of a glutamate residue. High-affinity binding would then result from a conformational change in the protein, suggested by the low on rates for folate substrates (Cichowicz and Shane, 1987b). It was initially proposed that folate binding involved the pterin and terminal glutamate moieties (Cichowicz *et al.,* 1981) and that internal glutamate residues loop out of the active site (Moran *et al.,* 1984). The similar binding specificities for the internal and terminal glutamate residues of pteroyldiglutamate, however, suggest that initial binding involves the pterin moiety and the internal glutamate residue of pteroyldiglutamates, as shown in Fig. 5 (George *et al.,* 1987). Movement of glutamate residues through this single, low-affinity glutamate-binding site would occur until the terminal glutamate residue is bound. The conformational change required for tight binding would not occur when an internal glutamate residue is bound, due to interference by the nonbound carboxyterminal residues. This mechanism is consistent with the retention of affinity by PteGluNH$_2$, which can be considered an analog of pteroate with an internal glutamate residue and an unsubstituted carboxy terminus. Decreased on rates with longer-chain-length derivatives might result from random movement of the polyglutamate chain and the consequent decreased likelihood of the terminal residue being positioned in the site, or by the increased difficulty in moving the internal residues out of the site, due to steric effects. This mechanism would also presumably position the terminal glutamate residue in the appropriate position for catalysis.

    If the pterin moiety remains bound throughout catalysis, steric constraints on the ability to loop out internal glutamate residues would explain the large differences in catalytic effectiveness between pteroylpolyglutamates differing in their pterin moieties, despite relatively

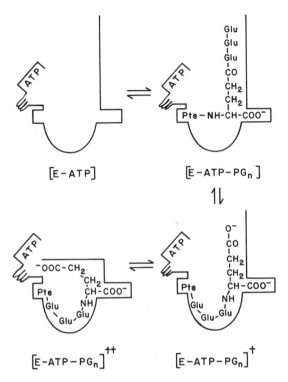

FIG. 5. Proposed mechanism for binding of folylpolyglutamates to folylpolyglutamate synthetase.

minor differences in k_{cat} between the equivalent pteroylmonogluta-mates.

e. Nucleotides. MgATP is the most effective nucleotide substrate for mammalian folylpolyglutamate synthetases (Taylor and Hanna, 1977; McGuire *et al.*, 1980; Cichowicz and Shane, 1987b) with K_m values in the range of 10–70 µM. MgdATP is also a fairly effective substrate and some activity is observed with inosine triphosphate. Uridine triphosphate and 5-amino-4-imidazolecarboximide riboside 5'-triphosphate also function as substrates for the pig liver enzyme. The relatively slow on rates with MgATP ($1.3 \times 10^5/M$/sec for the pig liver enzyme) may be due to a conformational change on nucleotide binding. A conformational change would explain why MgATP protects the *Corynebacterium* enzyme from proteolytic inactivation (Shane, 1983).

A variety of nucleotide derivatives are potent inhibitors of the reaction with affinities similar to that of MgATP (K_i 3 µM). These include

β,γ-methylene-ATP, β,γ-imido-ATP, ATP-γ-S, Ap$_5$A, and Ap$_6$A (Cichowicz and Shane, 1987b).

f. Glutamate. With H$_4$PteGlu as the folate substrate and at optimal assay pH, K_m values for L-glutamate range from about 0.3 to 1 mM, depending on the source of the mammalian enzyme (McGuire *et al.*, 1980; Pristupa *et al.*, 1984; Cichowicz and Shane, 1987b). The K_m is considerably higher at physiological pH and also varies depending on the particular folate used as the substrate (Cichowicz and Shane, 1987b; Schoo *et al.*, 1985).

Almost all modifications of the L-glutamate molecule lead to loss of affinity for the mammalian enzyme. The only exceptions are compounds that are alternate substrates, such as homocysteate and 4-fluoroglutamate. These compounds are less effective substrates than glutamate (McGuire and Coward, 1985; Cichowicz and Shane, 1987b; Cook *et al.*, 1987). Ornithine and glutamine are not enzyme inhibitors.

B. γ-GLUTAMYLHYDROLASES

Mammalian tissues contain γ-glutamylhydrolases that can hydrolyze the polyglutamate chain of folates. The properties of these enzymes have been extensively documented in a recent review (McGuire and Coward, 1984). The hydrolases lack specificity for the pterin moiety and will hydrolyze pABAglu$_n$ with equal efficacy and probably also poly(γ-glutamate). Longer-chain folylpolyglutamates are usually much better substrates than the shorter-glutamate chain-length derivatives. Glutamylhydrolase in most mammalian tissue is located in the lysosome and has an acid pH optimum. The bovine liver enzyme is an endopeptidase which cleaves folylpolyglutamates randomly at internal peptide bonds (Silink *et al.*, 1975). A second distinct lysosomal hydrolase has been isolated from beef liver which also appears to be an endopeptidase (Vickers *et al.*, 1986). This enzyme appears to be identical in properties to a previously described rat liver folylpolyglutamate–amino acid transpeptidase that catalyzes transfer of a variety of amino acids to PteGlu$_n$ (n = 2–7), with formation of PteGlu-amino acid and a polyglutamate peptide (Brody and Stokstad, 1982). The transpeptidase activity may reflect the ability of isolated peptidases to catalyze nonphysiological, synthetic reactions and the enzyme appears to be an endopeptidase that attacks the first γ-peptide bond and hydrolases folates directly to the monoglutamate derivative. An interesting feature of the transpeptidase activity is its physiological pH optimum (Brody and Stokstad, 1982). If this activity functions *in vivo*, the PteGlu-amino acid product would not be a substrate for folylpolyglutamate synthetase and would not be retained by tissues. The pteroyldipeptide analog would, however, be hydrolyzed to pteroylmonoglutamate by plasma glutamylhydrolase.

The glutamylhydrolases from mouse liver (Priest *et al.*, 1982b) and rat intestinal mucosal cells (Elsenhans *et al.*, 1984) are lysosomal endopeptidases that specifically cleave folates to the monoglutamate derivative, while the human jejunal enzyme appears to be a random endopeptidase (Wang *et al.*, 1986). Human intestinal brush border membranes also contain a membrane-bound glutamylhydrolase with exopeptidase activity (Chandler *et al.*, 1986). This enzyme, and other hydrolases found in the gut, are the only hydrolases that function well at neutral pH, and this appears to be related to their specialized role in the hydrolysis of dietary folates prior to folate absorption by the intestinal mucosa.

The role of lysosomal glutamylhydrolases in folate homeostasis has not been established and will be discussed further in Section VI,D. Folate is excreted primarily as cleavage products, and it has been suggested that nonenzymatic cleavage of labile tissue folylpolyglutamates to pABAglu$_n$ represents the first step in folate catabolism, and the lysosomal hydrolase may play a role in the hydrolysis of these cleavage products (Murphy *et al.*, 1976). There is no compelling evidence for the existence of cytoplasmic hydrolases that function at physiological pH, although this cannot be excluded, as the possibility has not been rigorously addressed.

VI. Factors That Affect Folylpolyglutamate Distributions and Folate Levels

A. Substrate Specificity of Folylpolyglutamate Synthetase

The retention and concentration of folates by mammalian tissues require their conversion to polyglutamate derivatives. The pig liver folylpolyglutamate synthetase has been used as a model *in vitro* system for studying factors that may regulate folate retention and distributions in tissues (Cook *et al.*, 1987). When H$_4$PteGlu and other substrates, at concentrations that approximate those expected in mammalian tissues, are incubated with purified enzyme, at about 10% of the *in vivo* concentration, the hexaglutamate and smaller amounts of the heptaglutamate accumulate, which resembles the folate distribution found *in vivo*. Under similar conditions, shorter derivatives are formed with H$_2$PteGlu and 10-formyl-H$_4$PteGlu as the substrates and

5-methyl-H_4PteGlu and aminopterin are converted primarily to the diglutamate derivatives (Cook *et al.*, 1987). Products that accumulated in these studies are very poor substrates for the enzyme, and the distributions obtained in metabolism studies can be modeled using kinetic constants obtained with individual folate substrates of folylpolyglutamate synthetase (Cichowicz and Shane, 1987b; Cook *et al.*, 1987; Table V). The accumulation of hexaglutamate derivatives *in vivo* and *in vitro* is due to the very slow catalytic turnover of the enzyme with pteroylhexaglutamate substrates. The absence of very long-chain-length derivatives such as octa- and nonaglutamates in *in vitro* studies, although small amounts of these compounds are found *in vivo*, is due to the lengthy times required for their synthesis. The formation of these derivatives *in vivo* would be expected to be a very slow process (Table V). The primary factor in determining the predominant folyl-polyglutamate in pig liver is the substrate specificity of its folylpolyglutamate synthetase. Similarly, CHO cell transfectants expressing the human (Sussman *et al.*, 1986b) or *E. coli* (C. Osborne and B. Shane, unpublished observations) folylpolyglutamate synthetase

TABLE V

TURNOVER TIMES FOR FOLYLPOLYGLUTAMATE
SYNTHETASE SUBSTRATES[a]

Substrate	Enzyme turnover[b] (per hr)	Substrate turnover[c] (hr)
H_4PteGlu	98	0.04
H_4PteGlu$_2$	99	0.04
H_4PteGlu$_3$	57	0.07
H_4PteGlu$_4$	16	0.25
H_4PteGlu$_5$	4.4	0.9
H_4PteGlu$_6$	0.4	11
H_4PteGlu$_7$	0.1	30
5-Methyl-H_4PteGlu	5.5	0.72
PteGlu	6.3	0.63
PteGlu$_5$	0.005	>800
Methotrexate	3.4	1.2

[a] Data are from Cook *et al.* (1987).

[b] Enzyme turnover is catalytic turnovers per hour at optimal assay conditions, with 100 nM folate as substrate.

[c] Substrate turnover is the time taken for complete conversion of 100 nM folate(glu) to folate(glu + 1), assuming initial rate conditions, under expected physiological conditions (50 nM enzyme, half-saturating glutamate).

gene contain folylpolyglutamate distributions characteristic of human cells or *E. coli,* respectively, provided the enzyme activity expressed is similar to the normal level in CHO cells. Pentaglutamates are the major folates in rat liver, and this tissue also contains smaller amounts of hexaglutamate and trace amounts of heptaglutamate. After administration of a pulse dose of labeled folate to the rat, pentaglutamates accumulate as the major labeled hepatic folates after about 6 hours, significant proportions of labeled hexaglutamate are formed by 2–3 days, and significant labeling of the heptaglutamate fraction occurs after about 4 weeks (Leslie and Baugh, 1974; Shane, 1982; Eto and Krumdieck, 1982a).

B. FOLYLPOLYGLUTAMATE SYNTHETASE ACTIVITY

The effect of folylpolyglutamate synthetase activity on folate accumulation and retention has been investigated using CHO transfectants (AUX B1-human) which express the human folylpolyglutamate synthetase gene at various levels (Sussman *et al.,* 1986b). Large decreases in enzyme activity (14- and 50-fold) result in only relatively minor decreases in folate accumulation (2- and 4-fold) and only minor shifts in the major folate derivatives, although the proportion of very long-chain-length derivatives is greatly diminished. Similarly, AUX B1 revertants with very low enzyme activities accumulate folates almost as well as wild-type cells and have only slightly reduced growth rates in media lacking glycine, thymidine, and purines (Taylor *et al.,* 1985). *In vitro* studies with the purified pig synthetase have also shown that with substrates that turn over at a rapid rate, such as $H_4PteGlu$, relatively large reductions in enzyme concentration cause relatively minor changes in the predominant folate that accumulates, i.e., hexaglutamate, although the appearance of longer-chain derivatives, which are formed at a very slow rate, is greatly suppressed (Cook *et al.,* 1987).

These observations suggest that folate accumulation by tissues may not be very responsive to differences in enzyme levels, as normal levels of enzyme activity are sufficient to allow rapid metabolism of folate to polyglutamates that are of considerably longer chain length than that required for folate retention. This excess enzyme capacity, in terms of folate accumulation, and the normal metabolism of folates to chain lengths longer than that required for retention, may represent a safety margin to ensure that folate is well retained. However, although only low levels of enzyme are required to metabolize folates to derivatives that are retained by mammalian cells, the higher levels are needed to generate the long-chain-length derivatives that are normally observed in these cells.

The greatly decreased formation of very long-chain-length derivatives, with decreases in enzyme activity, reflects that formation of these derivatives occurs at a slow rate and can be considered rate limiting in folylpolyglutamate synthesis. In addition, as multiple glutamate residues are added to pteroylmonoglutamates to generate folylpolyglutamates, a reduction in folylpolyglutamate synthetase activity would be expected to have a larger effect on the formation of long-chain-length than on short-chain-length derivatives.

Maximal retention of 4-aminofolates by mammalian cells requires their conversion to tri- or tetraglutamates, depending on the particular cell type (Samuels *et al.*, 1985; Section IV,D). Although 4-aminofolates are fairly good substrates of folylpolyglutamate synthetase, their di- and/or triglutamate derivatives are extremely poor substrates (McGuire *et al.*, 1983a; Moran *et al.*, 1984; Schoo *et al.*, 1985; George *et al.*, 1987; Cook *et al.*, 1987). The metabolism of 4-aminofolates to potentially retainable polyglutamate derivatives would be a relatively slow process in mammalian cells compared to reduced folates. Consequently, differences in folylpolyglutamate synthetase levels would be expected to have a large effect on the retention of antifolates. As the metabolism of pteroyldiglutamates to triglutamates is a relatively slow process in CHO AUX B1-*folC* transfectants, these cells can be considered a model for the expected effects of changes in synthetase levels on antifolate accumulation by mammalian cells. Folate accumulation by these transfectants is directly proportional to synthetase levels (C. Osborne and B. Shane, unpublished observations), which differs markedly from the limited effects of changes in enzyme levels noted with transfectants expressing the human enzyme.

The diglutamate of methotrexate is the major metabolite detected in *in vitro* metabolism studies with the rat (McGuire *et al.*, 1983a), beef (Schoo *et al.*, 1985), and hog liver enzymes (Cook *et al.*, 1987). The diglutamate is also the major product of methotrexate metabolism in primary rat hepatocyte cultures (Rhee and Galivan, 1986) and of aminopterin metabolism in a human leukemia cell line (Samuels *et al.*, 1985), but 4-aminofolates that accumulate in cultured mammalian cells are usually of longer glutamate chain length, ranging from tri- to pentaglutamates (Jolivet *et al.*, 1982; Fabre *et al.*, 1984; McGuire *et al.*, 1985; Samuels *et al.*, 1985). These longer derivatives, which are still of shorter glutamate chain length than are folates in these cells, are more prevalent after prolonged exposure to the drug or after further incubation of cultured cells in drug-free medium. The different *in vivo* and *in vitro* distributions can be explained by the slow metabolism of antifolates to retainable forms (Cook *et al.*, 1987). If the drug is metabolized to a retainable form, with prolonged exposure further chain extension of the drug would be expected, even if the rate of metabolism is very slow. With increased culture time, the longer-chain-length derivatives formed would become more prominent as the levels of shorter-chain-length derivatives would be expected to reach a steady state based on their rates of synthesis and efflux.

Similarly, the longer polyglutamate distributions found after further incubation in drug-free medium (McGuire *et al.*, 1985) would be predicted, as shorter derivatives would be lost from the cell and only chain extension of retainable forms would occur. This implies that antifolate retention by tissues, and consequently cytotoxicity, would be very sensitive to relatively minor differences in folylpolyglutamate synthetase levels, in efflux rates for di- and triglutamate derivatives, and in differences in substrate specificity of synthetases from different sources, especially with di- and/or triglutamate derivatives (Cook *et al.*, 1987). A methotrexate-resistant human breast cancer cell line has been described in which the major cause of resistance appears to be an almost total inability to synthesize, or retain, methotrexate polyglutamates, although synthetase activity appears normal, with monoglutamate substrates at least (Cowan and Jolivet, 1984). Labeled folate accumulation is also impaired in these cells, but not nearly to the same extent, and folylpolyglutamates distributions are slightly longer than those in the parent cell line.

C. SUBSTRATE COMPETITION AND FOLATE-BINDING PROTEINS

Long-chain folylpolyglutamates retain affinity for folylpolyglutamate synthetase, which has led to the suggestion that competition between substrates may regulate folylpolyglutamate synthesis (McGuire *et al.*, 1980; Foo and Shane, 1982). The long-chain derivatives would act as pseudocompetitive inhibitors because of their extremely low k_{cat} values (Cichowicz and Shane, 1987b). However, under physiological conditions the maximum rate reduction would be about 2-fold, and probably considerably less, as most of the intracellular folate would be bound to folate-dependent enzymes (Cook *et al.*, 1987). This would have the same effect as reducing folylpolyglutamate synthetase levels by a factor of 2 which, as discussed above, would not significantly affect folate accumulation but could have an effect on antifolate accumulation.

Folate and methotrexate accumulation by cultured cells is approx-

imately proportional to the medium folate or methotrexate content
(Hilton et al., 1979; Foo and Shane, 1982; Foo et al., 1982; Watkins and
Cooper, 1983; Steinberg et al., 1983; McGuire et al., 1985; Cook et al.,
1987). Mammalian cells can transport high levels of folate because the
K_t for PteGlu transport is very high (Sirotnak, 1985; Henderson, 1986;
Henderson et al., 1986). The K_t for reduced folates is considerably
lower, and the levels of reduced folate in the medium required to
support growth and similar intracellular folate concentrations are
much lower than with PteGlu (McBurney and Whitmore, 1974a; Taylor and Hanna, 1975; Foo and Shane, 1982; Foo et al., 1982; Watkins
and Cooper, 1983). The capacity to accumulate high levels of folate
demonstrates that the conversion of high levels of folate to retainable
polyglutamate derivatives is not limited under these conditions. Polyglutamate distributions are slightly shortened in mammalian cells
cultured in the presence of high folate, and short-chain derivatives do
not accumulate. However, there is an almost complete loss of very
long-chain-length derivatives (Cook et al., 1987).

This effect of high folate concentrations is also seen in in vitro
metabolism studies and can be explained by the slower metabolic fractional turnover of folates when folate levels are high (Table V), which
becomes significant with derivatives that turn over at a slow rate. Any
reduction in turnover rate would have a greater effect on the formation of long-chain derivatives, as more catalytic turnovers are required
for their synthesis. Competition with medium-chain-length derivatives may also play a role in the loss of long-chain derivatives under
these conditions but, as discussed above, this would only be expected at
very high folate levels and is unlikely to have any physiological
relevance.

Endogenous folate levels are reduced in folate-depleted hepatoma
cells (Priest et al., 1983) and in the livers of folate-depleted animals
(Cassady et al., 1980), but the chain lengths of endogenous folylpolyglutamates are increased. This could suggest an increased rate of polyglutamate synthesis under these conditions. However, as the predominant folates in cells are synthesized at a relatively rapid rate, while
long-chain-length derivatives are formed only slowly, a reduction or a
removal of entering pteroylmonoglutamate would be expected to gradually change the distribution of any retained intracellular folylpolyglutamates to longer-chain-length derivatives.

Folate and methotrexate accumulation by mammalian cells is increased by prior folate depletion (Foo and Shane, 1982; Nimec and
Galivan, 1983; Galivan et al., 1983), and polyglutamate formation is
more rapid in dividing cultures (Nimec and Galivan, 1983). Increased

net accumulation of a labeled folate dose occurs in the regenerating rat liver (Marchetti *et al.*, 1980), while endogenous folate levels drop slightly and slightly longer endogenous polyglutamates are found (Eto and Krumdieck, 1982b). A reduction in competing folate may explain increased methotrexate polyglutamate formation under these conditions. However, reduction of competition by intracellular folate is unlikely to be responsible for the increased folate accumulation. These data may reflect the increased capacity of mammalian cells cultured in the presence of limited folate to transport folate (Kane *et al.*, 1986a; Kamen and Capdevila, 1986; Section IV,D).

D. FOLYLPOLYGLUTAMATE TURNOVER

Folylpolyglutamates turn over in mammalian cells and tissues, albeit at a slow rate (Thenen *et al.*, 1973; Steinberg *et al.*, 1983; Section IV,D), but the mechanism of turnover has not been established. When a pulse dose of labeled folate is given to the rat, the small amount of labeled folate retained in liver 4 weeks after the dose is primarily hexa- and heptaglutamates (Leslie and Baugh, 1974; Section VI,A). This overshoot of the endogenous polyglutamate distribution after a lengthy time interval represents the same phenomenon as the appearance of longer polyglutamate distributions in folate-depleted cells and tissues and is consistent with the very poor substrate activity of longer-chain-length folylpolyglutamates for folylpolyglutamate synthetase. This overshoot, and the ability to mimic *in vivo* folate metabolism using *in vitro* conditions, suggest that extension of the polyglutamate chain is a one-way process in cells and implies that folate turnover in tissues does not involve hydrolysis of the polyglutamate chain or, alternately, that any hydrolyzed folate is released and does not equilibrate with the folylpolyglutamate pool. A slow efflux of folylpolyglutamates without hydrolysis, turnover by direct cleavage to nonfolate derivatives (Murphy *et al.*, 1976), or direct hydrolysis to short-chain-length folates and their consequent release from the cell would be consistent with the data. Mammalian γ-glutamylhydrolases and transpeptidases that can hydrolyze folylpolyglutamates directly to the mono- or diglutamate derivatives, which would not be retained by tissues, have been discussed previously (Section V,B).

E. ONE-CARBON DISTRIBUTIONS

The distribution of folylpolyglutamates in hog liver reflects the substrate effectiveness of $H_4PteGlu_n$ for folylpolyglutamate synthetase rather than other one-carbon forms of folate (Cook *et al.*, 1987). The lack of substrate activity of relatively short-polyglutamate chain-length derivatives of some folate one-carbon forms does not preclude further chain elongation, but these compounds have to be converted to $H_4PteGlu_n$ before chain extension occurs. Folate retention and distributions would be expected to be regulated by physiological and nutritional factors which affect the proportion of folate present as the $H_4PteGlu_n$ form.

If the interconversion of different folate one-carbon forms via the metabolic pathways of one-carbon metabolism occurs at a faster rate than the addition of glutamate moieties to folate, a decrease in the proportion of cellular folate derivatives that are effective substrates for the enzyme would have the same effect on the rate of polyglutamate synthesis as an equivalent decrease in enzyme level. As discussed above, this would not be expected to significantly affect folate accumulation. However, metabolic interconversion of different pteroylmonoglutamates may be quite slow, as many of the enzymes of one-carbon metabolism would preferentially bind polyglutamate substrates (Section IV,A). Although $H_2PteGlu$ and 10-formyl-$H_4PteGlu$ are metabolized to shorter-chain-length products than $H_4PteGlu$, their initial metabolism *in vivo* to retainable polyglutamates would be quite rapid, and an increase in the proportion of these forms of the vitamin is unlikely to have a significant effect on the accumulation of cellular folate. However, metabolism of 5-methyl-$H_4PteGlu$ to the diglutamate is fairly slow (Table V), conversion of the latter compound to the triglutamate is extremely slow (Cichowicz and Shane, 1987b; Cook *et al.*, 1987), and an inability to convert this compound via methionine synthase to $H_4PteGlu$ would result in its loss from the cell and consequently a decrease in cellular folate levels.

In humans and experimental animals, methionine synthase activity is reduced in vitamin B_{12} deficiency, and a functional folate deficiency results due to accumulation of 5-methyl-$H_4PteGlu_n$, a substrate for methionine synthase, at the expense of other folate one-carbon forms, including $H_4PteGlu_n$ (Matthews, 1984; Shane and Stokstad, 1985; Wilson and Horne, 1986). In addition, tissue levels of folate are reduced up to 60%, due to an impaired ability to retain folate rather than impaired tissue uptake of the vitamin (Shane and Stokstad, 1985; Shane *et al.*, 1977). The impaired retention of folate can be explained by the decreased level of $H_4PteGlu_n$ under these conditions, the poor substrate activity of 5-methyl-$H_4PteGlu$ for folylpolyglutamate synthetase, and the almost complete lack of substrate activity with polyglutamate forms of this compound.

F. Other Regulatory Factors

The high K_m for the glutamate substrate of folylpolyglutamate synthetase at physiological pH, which is similar to the concentration of glutamate in hepatic tissue and higher than that in peripheral tissues, suggests that folylpolyglutamate synthesis *in vivo* may be regulated in part by intracellular glutamate levels. Methotrexate polyglutamate accumulation by Ehrlich ascites tumor cells is dependent on the glutamate or glutamine concentration in the culture medium (Fry *et al.*, 1983).

Insulin and dexamethasone stimulate methotrexate polyglutamate formation by cultured mammalian cells, while cyclic adenosine monophosphate has the opposite effect (Kennedy *et al.*, 1983; Galivan, 1984; Galivan *et al.*, 1986). The mechanism by which these changes occur has not been established but does not appear to involve modifications of folylpolyglutamate synthetase, adenosine triphosphate, or glutamate levels (Galivan *et al.*, 1985b).

Variations in the methionine concentration in the media of tissue culture cells cause changes in the polyglutamate chain-length distribution of intracellular folates. High levels of methionine significantly decrease folate accumulation, and shorter polyglutamates are found in CHO cells (Foo and Shane, 1982) and in primary human fibroblasts (Foo *et al.*, 1982), suggesting a greatly decreased rate of folylpolyglutamate synthesis. Intracellular methionine regulates the proportion of 5-methyl-H_4PteGlu$_n$ and H_4PteGlu$_n$, and longer-polyglutamate chain derivatives are found under conditions in which the proportion of H_4PteGlu$_n$ would be expected to be increased. Although variations in 5-methyl-H_4PteGlu$_n$ could explain the data, this particular mechanism was not explicitly studied.

Folylpolyglutamate synthetase levels in CHO cells are unaffected by modulation of medium vitamin B_{12}, methionine, glycine, purines, thymidine, folate concentration or type, or cell density (Taylor and Hanna, 1977). In rat hepatoma cells, however, methionine restriction decreases enzyme levels (T. Johnson and J. Galivan, personal communication), which may explain the stimulation by methionine of methotrexate polyglutamate formation in this cell line (Nimec and Galivan, 1983). This effect may be cell type specific, as omission of methionine from the medium of primary hepatocyte cultures increases methotrexate polyglutamylation (Galivan *et al.*, 1986).

Folylpolyglutamates distributions in CHO cells are not affected by growth under folate-dependent and -independent conditions, i.e., in medium containing or lacking thymidine, purines, and glycine (Foo and

Shane, 1982). This differs from bacteria in which addition of purines to culture media causes a decrease in the polyglutamate chain-length distribution of intracellular folates, which results from a purine-induced rearrangement of folate one-carbon forms favoring 10-formyl-$H_4PteGlu_n$, an ineffective substrate for bacterial folylpolyglutamate synthetases (Shane et al., 1983).

VII. Changes in Folylpolyglutamate Distributions as a Regulatory Mechanism

It has been proposed that one-carbon metabolism may be regulated under different physiological and nutritional conditions by changing the glutamate chain length of folates in the cell, thus affecting the flux of one-carbon units through the different metabolic reactions of one-carbon metabolism (Krumdieck et al., 1977). As discussed above, modulations of the glutamate chain length of folates have been observed in mammalian cells and tissues in response to folate, methionine, and vitamin B_{12} status and to changes in growth rates, although distributions in mouse hepatoma cells are unchanged throughout the cell cycle (Priest et al., 1982a).

Direct modulation of folylpolyglutamate distributions would require regulation of folylpolyglutamate synthetase and/or glutamylhydrolase activities. Decreases in rat liver folylpolyglutamate activity have been reported under conditions of nitrous oxide-induced B_{12} deficiency (Perry et al., 1985) and folate depletion (Tolomelli et al., 1987b), while activity increases in regenerating liver (Tolomelli et al., 1987a). As discussed above, modulation of synthetase levels would not be expected to significantly affect folate accumulation but would affect the proportion of very long-chain-length folates. Changes in glutamylhydrolase levels occur in the rat uterus at different stages of the reproductive cycle (Krumdieck et al., 1976), and levels also vary in response to the phase of tumor cell growth (Samuels et al., 1986) and to changes in growth rates (Sur et al., 1985). As mentioned previously, glutamylhydrolase is one of a large number of folate-dependent enzymes that increase in response to increased replication rates (Rowe et al., 1979), and modest changes observed in endogenous folate distributions with changes in growth rate do not correlate with changes in glutamylhydrolase activity (Sur et al., 1985). A recent study showing that 2-mercaptomethylglutaric acid, a glutamylhydrolase inhibitor, causes an increased accumulation of longer-chain-length methotrexate polyglutamates in human lymphocytes and fibroblasts (Whitehead *et al.*, 1987) is the only direct evidence that glutamylhydrolase may play a role in this process.

Most of the observed changes in folylpolyglutamate distributions *in vivo* can be explained by the substrate specificity and affinities of folates for folylpolyglutamate synthetase, and can be mimicked *in vitro* using purified enzyme. Thus, most changes in polyglutamate distribution probably reflect a secondary effect, due to variations in the folate one-carbon distribution and/or the folate level in the cell. These changes would occur at a slow rate, and such a regulatory mechanism would be incapable of responding immediately to changing needs for specific products of one-carbon metabolism.

It is possible that the changes observed may reflect a long-term mechanism for the regulation of one-carbon metabolism. For example, folate depletion or hepatectomy causes an increase in the proportion of folylpolyglutamates of chain lengths longer than those for the major species in the tissue. The studies described in Section IV suggest that these very long-chain-length derivatives would not be any more effective than the predominant folate species as substrates for folate-dependent enzymes. However, the possibility remains that partitioning of the one-carbon flux through the different cycles of one-carbon metabolism may be changed with these longer derivatives (Section IV,E,3).

VIII. Summary

The physiological importance of folylpolyglutamates is now well established. These derivatives are the intracellular substrates and regulators of one-carbon metabolism, and their synthesis is required for normal folate retention by tissues. Over the last few years, a considerable amount of information has been obtained on the mechanism by which these compounds are synthesized, on how this synthesis is regulated, and on the effects of the polyglutamate chain on the interaction of folate substrates and inhibitors with folate-dependent enzymes. Many regulatory implications have been suggested by these studies, but the physiological relevance of some of these observations remains to be explored.

Folates in mammalian tissues are metabolized to polyglutamates of chain lengths considerably longer than that required for folate retention, but the metabolic advantages of this are not entirely clear. Several *in vivo* model systems have been developed to explore the functioning of specific folylpolyglutamate chain lengths in metabolic cycles of one-carbon metabolism, and these are likely to shed further light on this point.

The role of folate-binding proteins in folate transport, the metabolic role of glutamylhydrolases, and the role of folylpolyglutamates in putative multifunctional protein complexes are also areas that are being actively pursued at present and are likely to produce new insights in the future.

Recent studies on the retention of antifolates by cells and on their substrate efficacy for folylpolyglutamate synthetases have also suggested mechanisms for the differential cytotoxicity of these agents for different tissues.

ACKNOWLEDGMENTS

Some of the described studies were supported in part by National Cancer Institute Grant CA41991, Department of Health and Human Services. I would like to thank John McGuire (Roswell Park Memorial Institute), Jim Coward and Rowena Matthews (University of Michigan), Richard Moran (University of Southern California), Andy Bognar (University of Toronto), Bob Stokstad (University of California–Berkeley), and John Galivan (New York State Department of Health–Albany) for helpful discussions and for making available prepublication information.

REFERENCES

Allegra, C. J., Chabner, B. A., Drake, J. C., Lutz, R., Rodbard, D., and Jolivet, J. (1985a). Enhanced inhibition of thymidylate synthase by methotrexate polyglutamates. *J. Biol. Chem.* **260,** 9720–9726.

Allegra, C. J., Drake, J. C., Jolivet, J., and Chabner, B. A. (1985b). Inhibition of phosphoribosylaminoimidazolecarboxamide transformylase by methotrexate and dihydrofolic acid polyglutamates. *Proc. Natl. Acad. Sci. U.S.A.* **82,** 4881–4885.

Allegra, C. J., Drake, J. C., Jolivet, J., and Chabner, B. A. (1985c). Inhibition of folate-dependent enzymes by methotrexate polyglutamates. *In* "Proceedings of the Second Workshop on Folyl and Antifolyl Polyglutamates" (I. D. Goldman, ed.), pp. 348–359. Praeger, New York.

Allegra, C. J., Hoang, K., Yeh, G. C., Drake, J. C., and Baram, J. (1987). Evidence for direct inhibition of *de novo* purine synthesis in human MCF-7 breast cells as a principal mode of metabolic inhibition by methotrexate. *J. Biol. Chem.* **262,** 13520–13526.

Allen, J. R., Lasser, G. W., Goldman, D. A., Booth, J. W., and Mathews, C. K. (1983). T4 phage deoxyribonucleotide-synthesizing enzyme complex. *J. Biol. Chem.* **258,** 5746–5753.

Antony, A. C., Utley, C., Van Horne, K. C., and Kolhouse, J. F. (1981). Isolation and characterization of a folate receptor from human placenta. *J. Biol. Chem.* **256,** 9684–9692.

Antony, A. S., Kane, M. A., Portillo, R. M., Elwood, P. C., and Kolhouse, J. F. (1985). Studies of the role of a particulate folate-binding protein in the uptake of 5-methyltetrahydrofolate by cultured human KB cells. *J. Biol. Chem.* **260,** 14911–14917.

Antony, A. C., Bruno, E., Briddell, R. A., Brandt, J. E., Verma, R. S., and Hoffman, R. (1987). Effect of perturbation of specific folate receptors during in vitro erythropoiesis. *J. Clin. Invest.* **80**, 1618–1623.

Ayusawa, D., Shimizu, K., Koyama, H., Takeishi, K., and Seno, T. (1983). Unusual aspects of human thymidylate synthase in mouse cells introduced by DNA-mediated gene transfer. *J. Biol. Chem.* **258**, 48–53.

Baggot, J. E., and Krumdieck, C. L. (1979). Folylpoly-γ-glutamates as cosubstrates of 10-formyltetrahydrofolate : 5′-phosphoribosyl-5-amino-4-imidazolecarboxamide formyltransferase. *Biochemistry* **18**, 1036–1041.

Baggot, J. E., Vaughn, W. H., and Hudson, B. B. (1986). Inhibition of 5-aminoimidazole-4-carboxamide ribotide transformylase, adenosine deaminase and 5′-adenylate deaminase by polyglutamates of methotrexate and oxidized folates and by 5-aminoimidazole-4-carboxamide riboside and ribotide. *Biochem. J.* **236**, 193–200.

Banerjee, R., McGuire, J. J., Shane, B., and Coward, J. K. (1986). Folylpolyglutamate synthetase: Direct evidence for an acyl phosphate intermediate in the enzyme-catalyzed reaction. *Fed. Proc., Fed. Am. Soc. Exp. Biol.* **45**, 1609.

Benkovic, S. J. (1984). Transformylase enzymes in *de novo* biosynthesis. *Trends Biochem. Sci.* **9**, 320–322.

Bognar, A. L., and Shane, B. (1983). Purification and properties of *Lactobacillus casei* folylpoly-γ-glutamate synthetase. *J. Biol. Chem.* **258**, 12574–12581.

Bognar, A. L., Cichowicz, D. J., and Shane, B. (1983). Purification and characterization of folylpolyglutamate synthetase from *Lactobacillus casei* and hog liver. In "Chemistry and Biology of Pteridines" (J. A. Blair, ed.), pp. 627–632. de Gruyter, Berlin.

Bognar, A. L., Osborne, C., Shane, B., Singer, S. C., and Ferone, R. (1985). Folylpoly-γ-glutamate synthetase–dihydrofolate synthetase. Cloning and high expression of the *Escherichia coli folC* gene and purification and properties of the gene product. *J. Biol. Chem.* **260**, 5625–5630.

Bognar, A. L., Osborne, C., and Shane, B. (1987). Primary structure of the *Escherichia coli folC* gene and its folylpolyglutamate synthetase–dihydrofolate synthetase produce and regulation of expression by an upstream gene. *J. Biol. Chem.* **262**, 12337–12343.

Brody, T., and Stokstad, E. L. R. (1982). Folate oligoglutamate: Amino acid transpeptidase. *J. Biol. Chem.* **257**, 14271–14279.

Brody, T., Shane, B., and Stokstad, E. L. R. (1975). Identification and subcellular distribution of folates in rat brain. *Fed. Proc., Fed. Am. Soc. Exp. Biol.* **34**, 905.

Brody, T., Shin, Y. S., and Stokstad, E. L. R. (1976). Rat brain folate identification. *J. Neurochem.* **47**, 409–413.

Brody, T., Shane, B., and Stokstad, E. L. R. (1979). Separation and identification of pteroylpolyglutamates by polyacrylamide gel chromatography. *Anal. Biochem.* **92**, 501–509.

Brody, T., Watson, J. E., and Stokstad, E. L. R. (1982). Folate pentaglutamate and folate hexaglutamate mediated one-carbon metabolism. *Biochemistry* **21**, 276–282.

Caperelli, C. A. (1985). Mammalian glycinamide ribonucleotide transformylase: Purification and some properties. *Biochemistry* **24**, 1316–1320.

Caperelli, C. A., Benkovic, P. A., Chettur, G., and Benkovic, S. J. (1980). Purification of a complex catalyzing folate cofactor synthesis and transformylation in *de novo* purine biosynthesis. *J. Biol. Chem.* **255**, 1885–1890.

Case, G. L., and Steele, R. D. (1987). Resolution of rat liver 10-formyl-tetrahydrofolate dehydrogenase/hydrolase activities. *Fed. Proc., Fed. Am. Soc. Exp. Biol.* **46**, 1003.

Cassady, I. A., Budge, M. M., Healy, M. J., and Nixon, P. F. (1980). An inverse relationship of rat liver folate polyglutamate chain length to nutritional folate sufficiency. *Biochim. Biophy. Acta* **633**, 258–268.

Chabner, B. A., Allegra, C. J., Curt, G. A., Clendeninn, N. J., Baram, J., Koizumi, S., Drake, J. C., and Jolivet, J. (1985). Polyglutamation of methotrexate. Is methotrexate a prodrug? *J. Clin. Invest.* **76**, 907–912.

Chan, V. T., and Baggott, J. E. (1982). Polyglutamyl folate coenzymes and inhibitors of chicken liver glycinamide ribotide transformylase. *Biochim. Biophys. Acta* **702**, 99–104.

Chandler, C. J., Wang, T. T. Y., and Halsted, C. H. (1986). Pteroylpolyglutamate hydrolase from human jejunal brush borders. Purification and characterization. *J. Biol. Chem.* **261**, 928–933.

Chasin, L. A., Feldman, A., Konstam, M., and Urlaub, G. (1974). Reversion of a Chinese hamster cell auxotrophic mutant. *Proc. Natl. Acad. Sci. U.S.A.* **71**, 718–722.

Cheng, F. W., Shane, B., and Stokstad, E. L. R. (1975). Pentaglutamate derivatives of folate as substrates for rat liver tetrahydropteroylglutamate methyltransferase and 5,10-methylenetetrahydrofolate reductase. *Can. J. Biochem.* **53**, 1020–1027.

Chiu, C.-S., Cook, K. S., and Greenberg, G. R. (1982). Characteristics of a bacteriophage T4-induced complex synthesizing deoxyribonucleotides. *J. Biol. Chem.* **257**, 15087–15097.

Cichowicz, D. J., and Shane, B. (1987a). Mammalian folylpoly-γ-glutamate synthetase. 1. Purification and general properties of the hog liver enzyme. *Biochemistry* **26**, 504–512.

Cichowicz, D. J., and Shane, B. (1987b). Mammalian folylpoly-γ-glutamate synthetase. 2. Substrate specificity and kinetic properties. *Biochemistry* **26**, 513–521.

Cichowicz, D. J., Foo, S. K., and Shane, B. (1981). Folylpoly-γ-glutamate synthesis by bacteria and mammalian cells. *Mol. Cell. Biochem.* **39**, 209–228.

Cichowicz, D. J., Cook, J., George, S., and Shane, B. (1985). Hog liver folylpolyglutamate synthetase: substrate specificity and regulation. *In* "Proceedings of the Second Workshop on Folyl and Antifolylpolyglutamates" (I. D. Goldman, ed.), pp. 7–13. Praeger, New York.

Clarke, L., and Waxman, D. J. (1987). Human liver folylpolyglutamate synthetase: Biochemical characterization and interactions with folates and folate antagonists. *Arch. Biochem. Biophys.* **256**, 585–596.

Clarke, L., Rosowsky, A., and Waxman, D. J. (1987). Inhibition of human liver folylpolyglutamate synthetase by non-γ-glutamylatable antifolate analogs. *Mol. Pharmacol.* **31**, 122–127.

Cohen, L., and MacKenzie, R. E. (1978). Methylenetetrahydrofolate dehydrogenase–methenyltetrahydrofolate cyclohydrolase–formyltetrahydrofolate synthetase from porcine liver. Interaction between the dehydrogenase and cyclohydrolase activities of the multifunctional enzyme. *Biochim. Biophys. Acta* **522**, 311–317.

Cook, J. D., Cichowicz, D. J., George, S., Lawler, A., and Shane, B. (1987). Mammalian folylpoly-γ-glutamate synthetase. 4. In vitro and in vivo metabolism of folates and analogues and regulation of folate homeostasis. *Biochemistry* **26**, 530–539.

Cook, R. J., and Wagner, C. (1982). Purification and partial characterization of rat liver folate binding protein: Cytosol. I. *Biochemistry* **21**, 4427–4434.

Cook, R. J., and Wagner, C. (1984). Glycine-*N*-methyltransferase is a folate binding protein of rat liver cytosol. *Proc. Natl. Acad. Sci. U.S.A.* **81**, 3631–3634.

Cossins, E. A. (1984). Folates in biological materials. *In* "Folates and Pterins" (R. L. Blakley and S. J. Benkovic, eds.), Vol. 1, pp. 1–59. New York.

Cowan, K. H., and Jolivet, J. (1984). A methotrexate-resistant human breast cancer cell line with multiple defects, including diminished formation of methotrexate polyglutamates. *J. Biol. Chem.* **259**, 10793–10800.

Coward, J. K., Parameswaran, K. N., Cashmore, A. R., and Bertino, J. R. (1974). 7,8-Dihydropteroyl oligo-γ-L-glutamates: Synthesis and kinetic studies with purified dihydrofolate reductase from mammalian sources. *Biochemistry* **13**, 3899–3903.

Coward, J. K., Chello, P. L., Cashmore, A. R., Parameswaran, K. N., DeAngelis, L. M., and Bertino, J. R. (1975). 5-Methyl-5,6,7,8-tetrahydropteroyl oligo-γ-L-glutamates: Synthesis and kinetic studies with methionine synthetase from bovine brain. *Biochemistry* **14**, 1548–1552.

Cybulski, R. L., and Fisher, R. R. (1976). Intramitochondrial localization and proposed metabolic significance of serine transhydroxymethylase. *Biochemistry* **15**, 3183–3186.

Cybulski, R. L., and Fisher, R. R. (1981). Uptake of oxidized folates by rat liver mitochondria. *Biochim. Biophys. Acta* **646**, 329–333.

Daubner, S. C., and Benkovic, S. J. (1985). Characterization of mammalian phosphoribosylglycineamide formyltransferase from transformed cells. *Cancer Res.* **45**, 4990–4997.

Daubner, S. C., and Matthews, R. G. (1982). Purification and properties of methylenetetrahydrofolate reductase from pig liver. *J. Biol. Chem.* **257**, 140–145.

Daubner, S. C., Schrimsher, J. L., Schendel, F. J., Young, M., Henikoff, S., Patterson, D., Stubbe, J., and Benkovic, S. J. (1985). A multifunctional protein possessing glycinamide ribonucleotide synthetase, glycinamide ribonucleotide transformylase, and aminoimidazole ribonucleotide synthetase activities in de novo purine biosynthesis. *Biochemistry* **24**, 7059–7062.

Dolnick, B. J., and Cheng, Y.-C. (1978). Human thymidylate synthetase. II. Derivatives of pteroylmono- and -polyglutamates as substrates and inhibitors. *J. Biol. Chem.* **253**, 3563–3567.

Drury, E. J., Bazar, L. S., and MacKenzie, R. E. (1975). Formiminotransferase–cyclodeaminase from porcine liver. Purification and physical properties of the enzyme complex. *Arch. Biochem. Biophys.* **169**, 662–668.

Eichler, H.-G., Hubbard, R., and Snell, K. (1981). The role of serine hydroxymethyltransferase in cell proliferation: DNA synthesis from serine following mitogenic stimulation of lymphocytes. *Biosci. Rep.* **1**, 101–106.

Elsenhans, B., Ahmad, O., and Rosenberg, I. H. (1984). Isolation and characterization of pteroylpolyglutamate hydrolase from rat intestinal mucosa. *J. Biol. Chem.* **259**, 6364–6368.

Elwood, P. C., Kane, M. A., Portillo, R. M., and Kolhouse, J. F. (1986). The isolation, characterization, and comparison of the membrane-associated and soluble folate-binding proteins from human KB cells. *J. Biol. Chem.* **261**, 15416–15423.

Eto, I., and Krumdieck, C. L. (1982a). Determination of three different pools of reduced one-carbon-substituted folates. III. Reversed-phase high-performance liquid chromatography of the azo dye derivatives of *p*-aminobenzoylpoly-γ-glutamates and its application to the study of unlabeled endogenous pteroylpolyglutamates of rat liver. *Anal. Biochem.* **120**, 323–329.

Eto, I., and Krumdieck, C. L. (1982b). Changes in the chain length of folylpolyglutamates during liver regeneration. *Life Sci.* **30**, 183–189.

Fabre, G., Fabre, I., Matherly, L. H., Cano, J.-P., and Goldman, I. D. (1984). Synthesis and properties of 7-hydroxymethotrexate polyglutamyl derivatives in Ehrlich ascites tumor cells *in vitro*. *J. Biol. Chem.* **259**, 5066–5072.

Farnham, P. J., and Schimke, R. T. (1985). Transcriptional regulation of mouse dihydrofolate reductase in the cell cycle. *J. Biol. Chem.* **260**, 7675–7680.

Ferone, R., Hanlon, M. H., Singer, S. C., and Hunt, D. F. (1986a). α-Carboxyl-linked glutamates in the folylpolyglutamates of *Escherichia coli. J. Biol. Chem.* **261**, 16356–16362.

Ferone, R., Singer, S. C., and Hunt, D. F. (1986b). *In vitro* synthesis of α-carboxyl-linked folylpolyglutamates by an enzyme preparation from *Escherichia coli. J. Biol. Chem.* **261**, 16363–16371.

Foo, S. K., and Shane, B. (1982). Regulation of folylpoly-γ-glutamate synthesis in mammalian cells. *In vivo* and *in vitro* synthesis of pteroylpoly-γ-glutamates by Chinese hamster ovary cells. *J. Biol. Chem.* **257**, 13587–13592.

Foo, S. K., McSloy, R. M., Rousseau, C., and Shane, B. (1982). Folate derivatives in human cells: Studies on normal and 5,10-methylenetetrahydrofolate reductase-deficient fibroblasts. *J. Nutr.* **112**, 1600–1608.

Fournier, R. E. K., and Moran, R. G. (1983). Complementation mapping in microcell hybrids: Localization of *Fpgs* and *Ak-1* on *Mus musculus* chromosome 2. *Somatic Cell Genet.* **9**, 69–84.

Frasca, V., Riazzi, B. S., and Matthews, R. G. (1986). *In vitro* inactivation of methionine synthase by nitrous oxide. *J. Biol. Chem.* **261**, 15823–15826.

Fromm, H. J. (1975). Initial rate enzyme kinetics. *Mol. Biol. Biochem. Biophys.* **22**, 41–60.

Fry, D. W., Gewirtz, D. A., Yalowich, J. C., and Goldman, I. D. (1983). Characteristics of the accumulation of methotrexate polyglutamate derivatives in Ehrlich tumor cells and isolated rat hepatocytes. *Adv. Exp. Med. Biol.* **163**, 215–234.

Fujiwara, K., Okamura-Ikeda, K., and Motokawa, Y. (1984). Mechanism of the glycine cleavage reaction. Further characterization of the intermediate attached to H-protein and of the reaction catalyzed by T-protein. *J. Biol. Chem.* **259**, 10664–10668.

Galivan, J. (1984). Hormonal alteration of methotrexate and folate polyglutamate formation in cultured hepatoma cells. *Arch. Biochem. Biophys.* **230**, 355–362.

Galivan, J., Nimec, Z., and Balinska, M. (1983). Regulation of methotrexate polyglutamate accumulation *in vitro:* Effects of cellular folate content. *Biochem. Pharmacol.* **32**, 3244–3247.

Galivan, J., Inglese, J., McGuire, J. J., Nimec, Z., and Coward, J. K. (1985a). γ-Fluoromethotrexate: Synthesis and biological activity of a potent inhibitor of dihydrofolate reductase with greatly diminished ability to form poly-γ-glutamates. *Proc. Natl. Acad. Sci. U.S.A.* **82**, 2598–2602.

Galivan, J., Nimec, Z., Coward, J. K., and McGuire, J. J. (1985b). Glutamylation of methotrexate in hepatoma cells *in vitro:* Regulation and the development of specific inhibitors. *Adv. Enzyme Regul.* **23**, 13–23.

Galivan, J., Pupons, A., and Rhee, M. S. (1986). Hepatic parenchymal cell glutamylation of methotrexate studied in monolayer culture. *Cancer Res.* **46**, 670–675.

Gawthorne, J. M., and Smith, R. M. (1973). The synthesis of pteroylpolyglutamates by sheep liver enzymes *in vitro. Biochem. J.* **136** 295–301.

George, S., Cichowicz, D. J., and Shane, B. (1987). Mammalian folylpoly-γ-glutamate synthetase. 3. Specificity for folate analogues. *Biochemistry* **26**, 522–529.

Green, J. M., Ballou, D. P., and Matthews, R. G. (1988). Methylenetetrahydrofolate reductase does not play a role in the incorporation of methyltetrahydrofolate into cellular metabolism. *FASEB J.* **2**, 42–47.

Henderson, G. B. (1986). Transport of folate compounds into cells. *In* "Folates and

Pterins" (R. L. Blakley and V. M. Whitehead, eds.), Vol. 3, pp. 207–250. Wiley, New York.

Henderson, G. B., and Tsuji, J. M. (1987). Methotrexate efflux in L1210 cells. Kinetic and specificity properties of the efflux system sensitive to bromosulfophthalein and its possible identity with a system which mediates the efflux of 3′,5′-cyclic AMP. *J. Biol. Chem.* **262**, 13571–13578.

Henderson, G. B., Suresh, M. R., Vitols, K. S., and Huennekens, F. M. (1986). Transport of folate compounds in L1210 cells: Kinetic evidence that folate influx proceeds via the high-affinity transport system for 5-methyltetrahydrofolate and methotrexate. *Cancer Res.* **46**, 1639–1643.

Henikoff, S., Keene, M. A., Sloane, J. S., Bleskan, J., Hards, R., and Patterson, D. (1986). Multiple purine pathway enzyme activities are encoded at a single genetic locus in *Drosophila. Proc. Natl. Acad. Sci. U.S.A.* **83**, 720–724.

Hilton, J. G., Cooper, B. A., and Rosenblatt, D. S. (1979). Folate polyglutamate synthesis and turnover in cultured human fibroblasts. *J. Biol. Chem.* **254**, 8398–8403.

Hopkins, S., and Schirch, V. (1984). 5,10-Methenyltetrahydrofolate synthetase. Purification and properties of the enzyme from rabbit liver. *J. Biol. Chem.* **259**, 5618–5622.

Hynes, J. B., Cichowicz, D. J., and Shane, B. (1986). 5,8-Dideazafolates as substrates for folylpoly-γ-glutamate synthetase from pig liver. *In* "Chemistry and Biology of Pteridines 1986" (B. A. Cooper and V. M. Whitehead, eds.), pp. 997–1000. de Gruyter, Berlin.

Jencks, D. A., and Matthews, R. G. (1987). Allosteric inhibition of methylenetetrahydrofolate reductase by adenosylmethionine. Effects of adenosylmethionine and NADPH on the equilibrium between active and inactive forms of the enzyme and on the kinetics of approach to equilibrium. *J. Biol. Chem.* **262**, 2485–2493.

Jolivet, J., Schilsky, R. L., Bailey, B. D., Drake, J. C., and Chabner, B. A. (1982). Synthesis, retention, and biological activity of methotrexate polyglutamates in cultured human breast cancer cells. *J. Clin. Invest.* **70**, 351–360.

Jones, C., Kao, F.-T., and Taylor, R. T. (1980). Chromosomal assignment of the gene for folylpolyglutamate synthetase to human chromosome 9. *Cytogenet. Cell Genet.* **28**, 181–194.

Kalman, T. I. (1986). Effects of polyglutamylation on folate cofactor and antifolate activity in the thymidylate synthase cycle of permeabilized murine leukemia L1210 cells. *In* "Chemistry and Biology of Pteridines 1986" (B. A. Cooper and V. M. Whitehead, eds.), pp. 763–766. de Gruyter, Berlin.

Kamen, B. A., and Capdevila, A. (1986). Receptor-mediated folate accumulation is regulated by the cellular folate content. *Proc. Natl. Acad. Sci. U.S.A.* **83**, 5983–5987.

Kane, M. A., Portillo, R. M., Elwood, P. C., Antony, A. C., and Kolhouse, J. F. (1986a). The influence of extracellular folate concentration on methotrexate uptake by human KB cells. Partial purification of a membrane-associated methotrexate binding protein. *J. Biol. Chem.* **261**, 44–49.

Kane, M. A., Elwood, P. C., Portillo, R. M., Antony, A. C., and Kolhouse, J. F. (1986b). The interrelationship of the soluble and membrane-associated folate-binding proteins in human KB cells. *J. Biol. Chem.* **261**, 15625–15631.

Kennedy, D. G., Clarke, R., van den Berg, H. W., and Murphy, R. F. (1983). The kinetics of methotrexate polyglutamate formation and efflux in a human breast cancer cell line (MDA.MB.436): The effect of insulin. *Biochem. Pharmacol.* **32**, 41–46.

Kikuchi, G. (1973). The glycine cleavage system: Composition, reaction mechanism, and physiological significance. *Mol. Cell. Biochem.* **1**, 169–187.

Kisliuk, R. L. (1981). Pteroylpolyglutamates. *Mol. Cell. Biochem.* **39**, 331–345.

Kisliuk, R. L., Gaumont, Y., and Baugh, C. M. (1974). Polyglutamyl derivatives of folate as substrates and inhibitors of thymidylate synthetase. *J. Biol. Chem.* **249**, 4100–4103.

Kisliuk, R. L., Gaumont, Y., Lafer, E., Baugh, C. M., and Montgomery, J. A. (1981). Polyglutamyl derivatives of tetrahydrofolate as substrates for *Lactobacillus casei* thymidylate synthase. *Biochemistry* **20**, 929–934.

Krebs, H. A., Hems, R., and Tyler, B. (1976). The regulation of folate and methionine metabolism. *Biochem. J.* **158**, 341–353.

Krumdieck, C. L., Boots, L. R., Cornwell, P. E., and Butterworth, C. E., Jr. (1976). Cyclic variations in folate composition and pteroylpolyglutamyl hydrolase (conjugase) activity of the rat uterus. *Am. J. Clin. Nutr.* **29**, 288–294.

Krumdieck, C. L., Cornwell, P. E., Thompson, R. W., and White, W. E., Jr. (1977). Studies on the biological role of folic acid polyglutamates. *In* "Folic Acid" (Food and Nutrition Board, ed.), pp. 25–42. Nat. Acad. Press, Washington, D.C.

Krumdieck, C. L., Tamura, T., and Eto, I. (1983). Synthesis and analysis of the pteroylpolyglutamates. *Vitam. Horm. (N.Y.)* **40**, 45–104.

Kutzbach, C., and Stokstad, E. L. R. (1968). Partial purification of a 10-formyltetrahydrofolate: NADP oxidoreductase from mammalian liver. *Biochem. Biophys. Res. Commun.* **30**, 111–117.

Kutzbach, C., and Stokstad, E. L. R. (1971). Mammalian methylenetetrahydrofolate reductase. Partial purification, properties, and inhibition by S-adenosylmethionine. *Biochim. Biophys. Acta* **250**, 459–477.

Leslie, G. I., and Baugh, C. M. (1974). The uptake of pteroyl[^{14}C]-glutamic acid into rat liver and its incorporation into the natural pteroyl poly-γ-glutamates of that organ. *Biochemistry* **13**, 3957–4961.

London, R. E., Gabel, S. A., and Funk, A. (1987). Metabolism of excess methionine in the liver of intact rat: An in vivo ^{2}H NMR study. *Biochemistry* **26**, 7166–7172.

Lu, Y.-Z., Aiello, P. D., and Matthews, R. G. (1984). Studies on the polyglutamate specificity of thymidylate synthase from fetal pig liver. *Biochemistry* **23**, 6870–6876.

Luhrs, C. A., Pitiranggon, P., Da Costa, M., Rothenberg, S. P., Slomiany, B. L., Brink, L., Tous, G. I., and Stein, S. (1987). Purified membrane and soluble folate binding proteins from cultured KB cells have similar amino acid compositions and molecular weights but differ in fatty acid acylation. *Proc. Natl. Acad. Sci. U.S.A.* **84**, 6546–6549.

MacKenzie, R. E. (1984). Biogenesis and interconversion of substituted tetrahydrofolates. *In* "Folates and Pterins" (R. L. Blakley, and S. J. Benkovic, eds.), Vol. 1, pp. 255–306. Wiley, New York.

MacKenzie, R. E., and Baugh, C. M. (1980). Tetrahydropteroylpolyglutamate derivatives as substrates of two multifunctional proteins with folate-dependent enzyme activities. *Biochim. Biophys. Acta* **611**, 187–195.

MacKenzie, R. E., Aldridge, M., and Paquin, J. (1980). The bifunctional enzyme formiminotransferase–cyclodeaminase is a tetramer of dimers. *J. Biol. Chem.* **255**, 9474–9478.

Marchetti, M., Tolomelli, B., Formiggini, G., Bovina, C., and Barbiroli, B. (1980). Distribution of pteroylpolyglutamates in rat liver after partial hepatectomy. *Biochem. J.* **188**, 553–556.

Matthews, R. G. (1984). Methionine biosynthesis. *In* "Folates and Pterins" (R. L. Blakley, and S. J. Benkovic, eds.), Vol. 1, pp. 497–554. Wiley, New York.

Matthews, R. G., and Baugh, C. M. (1980). Interactions of pig liver methylenetetrahydrofolate reductase with methylenetetrahydropteroylpolyglutamate substrates and with dihydropteroylpolyglutamate inhibitors. *Biochemistry* **19**, 2040–2045.

Matthews, R. G., and Haywood, B. J. (1979). Inhibition of pig liver methylenetetrahydrofolate reductase by dihydrofolate: Some mechanistic and regulatory implications. *Biochemistry* **18**, 4845–4851.

Matthews, R. G., Ross, J., Baugh, C. M., Cook, J. D., and Davis, L. (1982). Interactions of pig liver serine hydroxymethyltransferase with methyltetrahydropteroylpolyglutamate inhibitors and with tetrahydropteroylpolyglutamate substrates. *Biochemistry* **21**, 1230–1238.

Matthews, R. G., Ghose, C., Green, J. M., Matthews, K. D., and Dunlap, R. B. (1987). Folylpolyglutamates as substrates and inhibitors of folate-dependent enzymes. *Adv. Enzyme Regul.* **26**, 157–171.

Maurer, B. J., Barker, P. E., Masters, J. N., Ruddle, F. H., and Attardi, G. (1984). Human dihydrofolate reductase gene is located in chromosome 5 and is unlinked to the related pseudogenes. *Proc. Natl. Acad. Sci. U.S.A.* **81**, 1484–1488.

McBurney, M. W., and Whitmore, G. F. (1974a). Isolation and biochemical characterization of folate deficient mutants of Chinese hamster cells. *Cell (Cambridge, Mass.)* **2**, 173–182.

McBurney, M. W., and Whitmore, G. F. (1974b). Characterization of a Chinese hamster cell with a temperature-sensitive mutation in folate metabolism. *Cell (Cambridge, Mass.)* **2**, 183–188.

McClain, L. D., Carl, G. F., and Bridgers, W. F. (1975). Distribution of folic acid coenzymes and folate dependent enzymes in mouse brain. *J. Neurochem.* **24**, 719–722.

McGuire, J. J., and Bertino, J. R. (1981). Enzymatic synthesis and function of folylpolyglutamates. *Mol. Cell. Biochem.* **38**, 19–48.

McGuire, J. J., and Coward, J. K. (1984). Pteroylpolyglutamates: Biosynthesis, degradation, and function. *In* "Folates and Pterins" (R. L. Blakley and S. J. Benkovic, eds.), Vol. 1, pp. 135–190. Wiley, New York.

McGuire, J. J., and Coward, J. K. (1985). DL-*threo*-4-Fluoroglutamic acid. A chain-terminating inhibitor of folylpolyglutamate synthesis. *J. Biol. Chem.* **260**, 6747–6754.

McGuire, J. J., Kitamoto, Y., Hsieh, P., Coward, J. K., and Bertino, J. R. (1979). Characterization of mammalian folylpolyglutamate synthetases. *Dev. Biochem.* **4**, 471–476.

McGuire, J. J., Hsieh, P., Coward, J. K., and Bertino, J. R. (1980). Enzymatic synthesis of folylpolyglutamates. Characterization of the reaction and its products. *J. Biol. Chem.* **255**, 5776–5788.

McGuire, J. J., Hsieh, P., Coward, J. K., and Bertino, J. R. (1983a). In vitro methotrexate polyglutamate synthesis by rat liver folylpolyglutamate synthetase and inhibition by bromosulfophthalein. *Adv. Exp. Med. Biol.* **163**, 199–214.

McGuire, J. J., Mini, E., Hsieh, P., and Bertino, J. R. (1983b). Folylpolyglutamate synthetase: Relation to methotrexate action and as a target for new drug treatment. *Prog. Cancer Res. Ther.* **28**, 97–106.

McGuire, J. J., Mini, E., Hsieh, P., and Bertino, J. R. (1985). Role of methotrexate polyglutamates in methotrexate- and sequential methotrexate-5-fluorouracil-mediated cell kill. *Cancer Res.* **45**, 6395–6400.

McGuire, J. J., Hsieh, P., Franco, C. T., and Piper, J. R. (1986). Folylpolyglutamate synthetase inhibition and cytotoxic effects of methotrexate analogs containing 2,φ-diaminoalkanoic acids. *Biochem. Pharmacol.* **35**, 2607–2613.

McGuire, J. J., Sobrero, A. F., Hynes, J. B., and Bertino, J. R. (1987). Mechanism of action of 5,8-dideazaisofolic acid and other quinazoline antifols in human colon carcinoma cells. *Cancer Res.* **47,** 5975–5981.

McHugh, M., and Cheng, Y.-C. (1979). Demonstration of a high affinity folate binder in human cell membranes and its characterization in cultured human KB cells. *J. Biol. Chem.* **254,** 11312–11318.

Meister, A. (1978). Inhibition of glutamine synthetase and γ-glutamylcysteine synthetase by methionine sulfoximine and related compounds. *In* "Enzyme-Activated Irreversible Inhibitors" (N. Seiler, M. J. Jung, and J. Koch-Weser, eds.), pp. 187–210. Elsevier, Amsterdam.

Mejia, N. R., and MacKenzie, R. E. (1985). NAD-dependent methylenetetrahydrofolate dehydrogenase is expressed by immortal cells. *J. Biol. Chem.* **260,** 14616–14620.

Min, H., Shane, B., and Stokstad, E. L. R. (1988). Identification of 10-formyltetrahydrofolate dehydrogenase-hydrolase as a major folate binding protein in liver cytosol. *Biochim. Biophys. Acta* **967,** 348–353.

Moran, R. G., and Colman, P. D. (1984a). Mammalian folyl polyglutamate synthetase: Partial purification and properties of the mouse liver enzyme. *Biochemistry* **23,** 4580–4589.

Moran, R. G., and Colman, P. D. (1984b). Measurement of folylpolyglutamate synthetase in mammalian tissues. *Anal. Biochem.* **140,** 326–342.

Moran, R. G., Werkheiser, W. C., and Zakrzewski, S. F. (1976). Folate metabolism in mammalian cells in culture. I. Partial characterization of the folate derivatives present in L1210 mouse leukemia cells. *J. Biol. Chem.* **251,** 3569–3575.

Moran, R. G., Colman, P. D., Forsch, R. A., and Rosowsky, A. (1984). A mechanism for the addition of multiple moles of glutamate by folylpolyglutamate synthetase. *J. Med. Chem.* **27,** 1263–1267.

Moran, R. G., Colman, P. D., Rosowsky, A., Forsch, R. A., and Chan, K. K. (1985). Structural features of 4-amino antifolates required for substrate activity with mammalian folylpolyglutamate synthetase. *Mol. Pharmacol.* **27,** 156–166.

Mueller, W. T., and Benkovic, S. J. (1981). On the purification and mechanism of action of 5-aminoimidazole-4-carboxamide-ribonucleotide transformylase from chicken liver. *Biochemistry* **20,** 337–344.

Murphy, M., Keating, M., Boyle, P., Weir, D. G., and Scott, J. M. (1976). The elucidation of the mechanism of folate catabolism in the rat. *Biochem. Biophys. Res. Commun.* **71,** 1017–1024.

Navalgund, L. G., Rossana, C., Muench, A. J., and Johnson, L. F. (1980). Cell cycle regulation of thymidylate synthetase gene expression in cultured mouse fibroblasts. *J. Biol. Chem.* **255,** 7386–7390.

Nimec, Z., and Galivan, J. (1983). Regulatory aspects of the glutamylation of methotrexate in cultured hepatoma cells. *Arch. Biochem. Biophys.* **226,** 671–680.

Nixon, P. F., Slutsky, G., Nahas, A., and Bertino, J. R. (1973). The turnover of folate coenzymes in murine lymphoma cells. *J. Biol. Chem.* **248,** 5932–5936.

Ogawa, H., and Fujioka, M. (1982). Purification and properties of glycine *N*-methyltransferase from rat liver. *J. Biol. Chem.* **257,** 3447–3452.

Okamura-Ikeda, K., Fujiwara, K., and Motokawa, Y. (1982). Purification and characterization of chicken liver T-protein, a component of the glycine cleavage system. *J. Biol. Chem.* **257,** 135–139.

Okamura-Ikeda, K., Fujiwara, K., and Motokawa, Y. (1987). Mechanism of the glycine cleavage reaction. *J. Biol. Chem.* **262,** 6746–6749.

Palese, M., and Tephley, T. R. (1975). Metabolism of formate in the rat. *J. Toxicol. Environ. Health* **1,** 13–24.

Paquin, J., Baugh, C. M., and MacKenzie, R. E. (1985). Channeling between the active sites of formiminotransferase–cyclodeaminase. Binding and kinetic studies. *J. Biol. Chem.* **260**, 14925–14931.

Patey, C. A. H., and Shaw, G. (1973). Purification and properties of an enzyme duet, phosphoribosylaminoimidazole carboxylase and phosphoribosylaminoimidazolesuccinocarboxamide synthetase, involved in the biosynthesis of purine nucleotides *de novo. Biochem. J.* **135**, 543–545.

Paukert, J. L., Strauss, L. D., and Rabinowitz, J. C. (1976). Formyl-methenyl-methylenetetrahydrofolate synthetase-(combined). An ovine protein with multiple catalytic activities. *J. Biol. Chem.* **251**, 5104–5111.

Perry, J., Chanarin, I., Deacon, R., and Lumb, M. (1985). Folate polyglutamate synthetase activity in the cobalamin-inactivated rat. *Biochem. J.* **227**, 73–77.

Pfendner, W., and Pizer, L. I. (1980). The metabolism of serine and glycine in mutant lines of Chinese hamster ovary cells. *Arch. Biochem. Biophys.* **200**, 503–512.

Porter, D. H., Cook, R. J., and Wagner, C. (1985). Enzymatic properties of dimethylglycine dehydrogenase and sarcosine dehydrogenase from rat liver. *Arch. Biochem. Biophys.* **2**, 396–407.

Price, E. M., and Freisheim, J. H. (1987). Photoaffinity analogues of methotrexate as folate antagonist binding probes. 2. Transport studies, photoaffinity labeling, and identification of the membrane carrier protein for methotrexate from murine L1210 cells. *Biochemistry* **26**, 4757–4763.

Priest, D. G., Happel, K. K., Mangum, M., Bednarek, J. M., Doig, M. T., and Baugh, C. M. (1981). Tissue folylpolyglutamate chain-length characterization by electrophoresis as thymidylate synthetase–fluorodeoxyuridylate ternary complexes. *Anal. Biochem.* **115**, 163–169.

Priest, D. G., Doig, M. T., and Ledford, B. E. (1982a). Cell cycle patterns of thymidylate synthetase and 5,10-methylenetetrahydrofolate polyglutamates in cultured mouse hepatoma cells. *Experientia* **38**, 88–89.

Priest, D. G., Veronee, C. D., Mangum, M., Bednarek, J. M., and Doig, M. T. (1982b). Comparison of folylpolyglutamate hydrolases of mouse liver, kidney, muscle and brain. *Mol. Cell. Biochem.* **43**, 81–87.

Priest, D. G., Doig, M. T., and Magnum, M. (1983). Response of mouse hepatoma cell methylenetetrahydrofolate polyglutamates to folate deprivation. *Biochim. Biophys. Acta* **756**, 253–257.

Pristupa, Z. B., Vickers, P. J., Sephton, G. B., and Scrimgeour, K. G. (1984). Folylpolyglutamate synthetase from beef liver: Assay, stabilization, and characterization. *Can. J. Biochem. Cell Biol.* **62**, 495–506.

Reddy, G. P. V., and Pardee, A. B. (1980). Multienzyme complex for metabolic channeling in mammalian DNA replication. *Proc. Natl. Acad. Sci. U.S.A.* **77**, 3312–3316.

Reddy, G. P. V., and Pardee, A. B. (1982). Coupled ribonucleoside diphosphate reduction, channeling, and incorporation into DNA of mammalian cells. *J. Biol. Chem.* **257**, 12526–12531.

Rhee, M. S., and Galivan, J. (1986). Conversion of methotrexate to 7-hydroxymethotrexate and 7-hydroxymethotrexate polyglutamates in cultured rat hepatic cells. *Cancer Res.* **46**, 3793–3797.

Rios-Orlandi, E. M., Zarkadas, C. G., and MacKenzie, R. E. (1986). Formyltetrahydrofolate dehydrogenase–hydrolase from pig liver: Simultaneous assay of the activities. *Biochim. Biophys. Acta* **871**, 24–35.

Rosowsky, A., Forsch, R. A., Freisheim, J. H., Moran, R. G., and Wick, M. (1984a). Methotrexate analogues. 19. Replacement of the glutamate side chain in classical antifolates by L-homocysteic acid and L-cysteic acid: Effect on enzyme inhibition and antitumor activity. *J. Med. Chem.* **27,** 600–604.

Rosowsky, A., Moran, R. G., Forsch, R., Colman, P., Uren, J., and Wick, M. (1984b). Methotrexate analogues—XVII. Antitumor activity of 4-amino-4-deoxy-N^{10}-methylpteroyl-D,L-homocysteic acid and its dual inhibition of dihydrofolate reductase and folyl polyglutamate synthetase. *Biochem. Pharmacol.* **33,** 155–161.

Rosowsky, A., Moran, R. G., Forsch, R. A., Radike-Smith, M., Colman, P. D., Wick, M. M., and Freisheim, J. H. (1986a). Methotrexate analogues—27. Dual inhibition of dihydrofolate reductase and folylpolyglutamate synthetase by methotrexate and aminopterin analogues with a γ-phosphonate group in the side chain. *Biochem. Pharmacol.* **35,** 3327–3333.

Rosowsky, A., Freisheim, J. H., Moran, R. G., Solan, V. C., Bader, H., Wright, J. E., and Radike-Smith, M., (1986b). Methotrexate analogues. 26. Inhibition of dihydrofolate reductase and folylpolyglutamate synthetase activity and *in vitro* tumor cell growth by methotrexate and aminopterin analogues containing a basic amino acid side chain. *J. Med. Chem.* **29,** 655–660.

Ross, J., Green, J., Baugh, C. M., MacKenzie, R. E., and Matthews, R. G. (1984). Studies on the polyglutamate specificity of methylenetetrahydrofolate dehydrogenase from pig liver. *Biochemistry* **23,** 1790–1801.

Rowe, P. B., McCairns, E., Madsen, G., Sauer, D., and Elliott, H. (1978). *De novo* purine synthesis in avian liver. Co-purification of the enzymes and properties of the pathway. *J. Biol. Chem.* **21,** 7711–7721.

Rowe, P. B., Tripp, E., and Craig, G. C. (1979). Folate metabolism in lectin activated human peripheral blood lymphocytes. *Dev. Biochem.* **4,** 587–592.

Samuels, L. L., Moccio, D. M., and Sirotnak, F. M. (1985). Similar differential for total polyglutamylation and cytotoxicity among various folate analogues in human and murine tumor cells *in vitro. Cancer Res.* **45,** 1488–1495.

Samuels, L. L., Goutas, L. J., Priest, D. G., Piper, J. R., and Sirotnak, F. M. (1986). Hydrolytic cleavage of methotrexate γ-polyglutamates by folylpolyglutamyl hydrolase derived from various tumors and normal tissues of the mouse. *Cancer Res.* **46,** 2230–2235.

Schirch, L. (1984). Folates in serine and glycine metabolism. *In* "Folates and Pterins" (R. L. Blakley, and S. J. Benkovic, eds.), Vol. 1, pp. 399–432. Wiley, New York.

Schirch, L., and Peterson, D. (1980). Purification and properties of mitochondrial serine hydroxymethyltransferase. *J. Biol. Chem.* **16,** 7801–7806.

Schoo, M. M. J., Pristupa, Z. B., Vickers, P. J., and Scrimgeour, K. G. (1985). Folate analogues as substrates of mammalian folylpolyglutamate synthetase. *Cancer Res.* **45,** 3034–3041.

Scrutton, M. C., and Beis, I. (1979). Inhibitory effects of histidine and their reversal. *Biochem. J.* **177,** 833–846.

Selhub, J., and Franklin, W. A. (1984). The folate-binding protein of rat kidney. Purification, properties, and cellular distribution. *J. Biol. Chem.* **259,** 6601–6606.

Shane, B. (1980a). Pteroylpoly(γ-glutamate) synthesis by *Corynebacterium* species. Purification and properties of folylpoly(γ-glutamate) synthetase. *J. Biol. Chem.* **255,** 5655–5662.

Shane, B. (1980b). Pteroylpoly(γ-glutamate) synthesis by *Corynebacterium* species. Studies on the mechanism of folylpoly(γ-glutamate) synthetase. *J. Biol. Chem.* **255,** 5663–5667.

Shane, B. (1982). High performance liquid chromatography of folates: Identification of poly-γ-glutamate chain lengths of labeled and unlabeled folates. *Am. J. Clin. Nutr.* **35,** 599–608.

Shane, B. (1983). Properties of *Corynebacterium species* dihydrofolate synthetase–folylpolyglutamate synthetase. *In* "Chemistry and Biology of Pteridines" (J. A. Blair, ed.), pp. 621–626. de Gruyter, Berlin.

Shane, B., and Stokstad, E. L. R. (1984). Folates in the synthesis and catabolism of histidine. *In* "Folates and Pterins" (R. L. Blakley and S. J. Benkovic, eds.), Vol. 1, pp. 433–456. Wiley, New York.

Shane, B., and Stokstad, E. L. R. (1985). Vitamin B_{12}–folate interrelationships. *Annu. Rev. Nutr.* **5**, 115–141.

Shane, B., Watson, J. E., and Stokstad, E. L. R. (1977). Uptake and metabolism of [^{3}H]folate by normal and by vitamin B-12 and methionine-deficient rats. *Biochim. Biophys. Acta* **497**, 241–252.

Shane, B., Bognar, A. L., Goldfard, R. D., and LeBowitz, J. H. (1983). Regulation of folylpoly-γ-glutamate synthesis in bacteria: In vivo and in vitro synthesis of pteroylpoly-γ-glutamates by *Lactobacillus casei* and *Streptococcus faecalis. J. Bacteriol.* **153**, 316–325.

Shannon, K. W., and Rabinowitz, J. C. (1986). Purification and characterization of a mitochondrial isozyme of C_1-tetrahydrofolate synthase from *Saccharomyces cerevisiae. J. Biol. Chem.* **261**, 12266–12271.

Shin, Y. S., Chan, C., Vidal, A. J., Brody, T., and Stokstad, E. L. R. (1976). Subcellular localization of γ-glutamyl carboxypeptidase and of folates. *Biochim. Biophys. Acta* **444**, 794–801.

Silink, M., Reddel, R., Bethel, M., and Rowe, P. B. (1975). γ-Glutamyl hydrolase (conjugase). Purification and properties of the bovine hepatic enzyme. *J. Biol. Chem.* **250**, 5982–5994.

Sirotnak, F. M. (1985). Obligate genetic expression in tumor cells of a fetal membrane property mediating "folate" transport: Biological significance and implications for improved therapy of human cancer. *Cancer Res.* **45**, 3992–4000.

Sirotnak, F. M., Jacobsen, D. M., and Yang, C.-H. (1986). Alteration of folate analogue transport following induced maturation of HL-60 leukemia cells. Early decline in mediated influx, relationship to commitment, and functional dissociation of entry and exit routes. *J. Biol. Chem.* **261**, 11150–11155.

Skiba, W. E., Taylor, M. P., Wells, M. S., Mangum, J. H., and Awad, W. M., Jr. (1982). Human hepatic methionine biosynthesis. Purification and characterization of betaine : homocysteine S-methyltransferase. *J. Biol. Chem.* **257**, 14944–14948.

Smith, D. D. S., and MacKenzie, R. E. (1985). Methylenetetrahydrofolate dehydrogenase–methenyltetrahydrofolate–cyclohydrolase–formyltetrahydrofolate synthetase. Affinity labelling of the dehydrogenase-cyclohydrolase active site. *Biochem. Biophys. Res. Commun.* **128**, 148–154.

Smith, G. K., Mueller, W. T., Wasserman, G. F., Taylor, W. D., and Benkovic, S. J. (1980). Characterization of the enzyme complex involving the folate-requiring enzymes of de novo purine biosynthesis. *Biochemistry* **19**, 4313–4321.

Smith, G. K., Benkovic, P. A., and Benkovic, S. J. (1981). L(−)-10-formyltetrahydrofolate is the cofactor for glycinamide ribonucleotide transformylase from chicken liver. *Biochemistry* **20**, 4034–4036.

Spandidos, D. A., and Siminovitch, L. (1977). Linkage of markers controlling consecutive biochemical steps in CHO cells as demonstrated by chromosome transfer. *Cell (Cambridge, Mass.)* **12**, 235–242.

Steinberg, S. E., Fonda, S., Campbell, C. L., and Hillman, R. S. (1983). Folate utilization in Friend erythroleukemia cells. *J. Cell. Physiol.* **114**, 252–256.

Strong, W., Joshi, G., Lura, R., Muthukumaraswamy, N., and Schirch, V. (1987). 10-formyltetrahydrofolate synthetase. *J. Biol. Chem.* **262**, 12519–12525.

Sugiyama, K., Kushima, Y., and Muramatsu, K. (1987). Effect of dietary glycine on methionine metabolism in rats fed a high-methionine diet. *J. Nutr. Sci. Vitaminol.* **33**, 195–205.

Sur, P., Priest, D. G., and Doig, M. T. (1985). Effects of growth rate and methotrexate on folate polyglutamates and folylpolyglutamate hydrolase activity in Krebs ascites cells. *Biochem. Cell Biol.* **64**, 363–367.

Sussman, D. J., Milman, G., Osborne, C., and Shane, B. (1986a). *In situ* autoradiographic detection of folylpolyglutamate synthetase activity. *Anal. Biochem.* **158**, 371–376.

Sussman, D. J., Milman, G., and Shane, B. (1986b). Characterization of human folylpolyglutamate synthetase expressed in Chinese hamster ovary cells. *Somatic Cell Mol. Genet.* **12**, 531–540.

Tan, L. U. L., and MacKenzie, R. E. (1977). Methylenetetrahydrofolate dehydrogenase, methenyltetrahydrofolate cyclohydrolase and formyltetrahydrofolate synthetase from porcine liver. Isolation of a dehydrogenase–cyclohydrolase fragment from the multifunctional enzyme. *Biochim. Biophys. Acta* **485**, 52–59.

Tan, L. U. L., Drury, E. J., and MacKenzie, R. E. (1977). Methylenetetrahydrofolate dehydrogenase–methenyltetrahydrofolate cyclohydrolase–formyltetrahydrofolate synthetase. A multifunctional protein from porcine liver. *J. Biol. Chem.* **252**, 1117–1122.

Tang, D.-C., and Coward, J. K. (1983). Synthesis of acyl phosphonate analogues of biologically important acyl phosphates: *N*-(2-amino-10-methylpteroyl)-5-amino-2-oxopentanephosphonic acid. *J. Org. Chem.* **48**, 5001–5006.

Taylor, R. T., and Hanna, M. L. (1975). Folate-dependent enzymes in cultured Chinese hamster ovary cells: Induction of 5-methyltetrahydrofolate homocysteine cobalamin methyltransferase by folate and methionine. *Arch. Biochem. Biophys.* **171**, 507–520.

Taylor, R. T., and Hanna, M. L. (1977). Folate-dependent enzymes in cultured Chinese hamster ovary cells: Folylpolyglutamate synthetase and its absence in mutants auxotrophic for glycine + adenosine + thymidine. *Arch. Biochem. Biophys.* **181**, 331–344.

Taylor, R. T., and Hanna, M. L. (1979). Folate-dependent enzymes in cultured Chinese hamster ovary cells: Evidence for mutant forms of folylpolyglutamate synthetase. *Arch. Biochem. Biophys.* **197**, 36–43.

Taylor, R. T., and Hanna, M. L. (1982). Folate-dependent enzymes in cultured Chinese hamster ovary cells: Impaired mitochondrial serine hydroxymethyltransferase activity in two additional glycine–auxotroph complementation classes. *Arch. Biochem. Biophys.* **217**, 609–623.

Taylor, R. T., and Weissbach, H. (1973). N^5-Methyltetrahydrofolate–homocysteine methyltransferases. *In* "The Enzymes" (P. D. Boyer, ed.), 3rd ed., Vol. 9, pp. 121–165. Academic Press, New York.

Taylor, R. T., Wu, R., and Hanna, M. L. (1985). Induced reversion of a Chinese hamster ovary triple auxotroph. Validation of the system with several mutagens. *Mutat. Res.* **151**, 293–308.

Thenen, S. W., and Stokstad, E. L. R. (1973). Effect of methionine on specific folate coenzyme pools in vitamin B_{12} deficient and supplemented rats. *J. Nutr.* **103**, 363–370.

Thenen, S. W., Shin, Y. S., and Stokstad, E. L. R. (1973). The turnover of rat-liver folate pools. *Proc. Soc. Exp. Biol. Med.* **142**, 638–641.

Tolomelli, B., Marchi Marchetti, M., Laffi, R., and Marchetti, M. (1987a). Folylpolyglutamate synthetase activity in regenerating rat liver. *Int. J. Vitam. Nutr. Res.* **57**, 169–172.

Tolomelli, B., Marchi Marchetti, M., Laffi, R., and Marchetti, M. (1987b). Liver folylpolyglutamate synthetase activity in folic acid-deficient rats. *Int. J. Vitam. Nutr. Res.* **57,** 285–287.

Urlaub, G., Kas, E., Carothers, A. M., and Chasin, L. A. (1983). Deletion of the diploid dihydrofolate reductase locus from cultured mammalian cells. *Cell (Cambridge, Mass.)* **33,** 405–412.

Utley, C. S., Marcell, P. D., Allen, R. H., Antony, A. C., and Kolhouse, J. F. (1985). Isolation and characterization of methionine synthetase from human placenta. *J. Biol. Chem.* **260,** 13656–13665.

Vickers, P. J., Di Cecco, R., Pristupa, Z. B., and Scrimgeour, K. G. (1985). Activation of folylpolyglutamate synthetase by pteroic acid. *Can. J. Biochem. Cell Biol.* **63,** 777–779.

Vickers, P. J., Di Cecco, R., Pristupa, Z. B., and Scrimgeour, K. G. (1986). Folylpolygluta-mate hydrolase from beef liver. *In* "Chemistry and Biology of Pteridines 1986" (B. A. Cooper and V. M. Whitehead, eds.), pp. 933–936. de Gruyter, Berlin.

Villar, E., Schuster, B., Peterson, D., and Schirch, V. (1985). C_1-Tetrahydrofolate syn-thetase from rabbit liver. Structural and kinetic properties of the enzyme and its two domains. *J. Biol. Chem.* **260,** 2245–2252.

Wagner, C. (1986). Proteins binding pterins and folates. *In* "Folates and Pterins" (R. L. Blakley and V. M. Whitehead, eds.), Vol. 3, pp. 251–296. Wiley, New York.

Wagner, C., and Cook, R. J. (1986). Studies on glycine N-methyltransferase. *In* "Chemis-try and Biology of Pteridines 1986" (B. A. Cooper and V. M. Whitehead, eds.), pp. 593–596. de Gruyter, Berlin.

Wagner, C., Briggs, W. T., and Cook, R. J. (1984). Covalent binding of folic acid to dimethylglycine dehydrogenase. *Arch. Biochem. Biophys.* **233,** 457–461.

Wagner, C., Briggs, W. T., and Cook, R. J. (1985). Inhibition of glycine N-methyl-transferase activity by folate derivatives: Implications for regulation of methyl group metabolism. *Biochem. Biophys. Res. Commun.* **127,** 746–752.

Wang, T. T. Y., Chandler, C. J., and Halsted, C. H. (1986). Intracellular pteroylpolyglu-tamate hydrolase from human jejunal mucosa. Isolation and characterization. *J. Biol. Chem.* **261,** 13551–13555.

Wasserman, G. F., Benkovic, P. A., Young, M., and Benkovic, S. J. (1983). Kinetic relationships between the various activities of the formyl-methenyl-methylenete-trahydrofolate synthetase. *Biochemistry* **22,** 1005–1013.

Watkins, D., and Cooper, B. A. (1983). A critical intracellular concentration of fully reduced non-methylated folate polyglutamates prevents macrocytosis and dimin-ished growth rate of human cell line K562 in culture. *Biochem. J.* **214,** 465–470.

Whitehead, V. M., Kalman, T. I., and Vuchich, M.-J. (1987). Inhibition of gamma-glutamyl hydrolases in human cells by 2-mercaptomethylglutaric acid. *Biochem. Biophys. Res. Commun.* **144,** 292–297.

Wilson, S. D., and Horne, D. W. (1986). Effect of nitrous oxide inactivation of vita-min B_{12} on the levels of folate coenzymes in rat bone marrow, kidney, brain, and liver. *Arch. Biochem. Biophys.* **244,** 248–253.

Wittwer, A. J., and Wagner, C. (1981). Identification of the folate-binding proteins of rat liver mitochondria as dimethylglycine dehydrogenase and sarcosine dehydrogenase. Purification and folate-binding characteristics. *J. Biol. Chem.* **256,** 4102–4108.

Zamierowski, M. M., and Wagner, C. (1977a). Effect of folacin deficiency on folacin-binding proteins in the rat. *J. Nutr.* **107,** 1937–1945.

Zamierowski, M. M., and Wagner, C. (1977b). Identification of folate binding proteins in rat liver. *J. Biol. Chem.* **252,** 933–938.

Biotin

KRISHNAMURTI DAKSHINAMURTI AND JASBIR CHAUHAN

Department of Biochemistry and Molecular Biology
Faculty of Medicine
University of Manitoba
Winnipeg, Manitoba, Canada R3E 0W3

I. Introduction

It is 25 years since the biochemistry of biotin was reviewed in *Vitamins and Hormones* (Mistry and Dakshinamurti, 1964). The major interest at that time was in the identification of biotin containing enzymes and in understanding the molecular mechanism of the action of biotin in biotin enzymes. In the intervening years the enzymology

337

and regulatory features of biotin enzymes have been reviewed (Alberts and Vagelos, 1972; Brownsey and Denton, 1987; Lane et al., 1974; Moss and Lane, 1971; Utter et al., 1975; Wood and Barden, 1977). An international conference considered biochemical, nutritional, and clinical aspects of biotin in 1984, and the proceedings of this conference have been published (Dakshinamurti and Bhagavan, 1985). The recognition of the biotin-responsive multiple carboxylase deficiency syndrome has been a major development, which has been reviewed by Sweetman and Nyhan (1986). Other recent reviews have dealt with the regulation of biotin enzymes (Dakshinamurti and Chauhan, 1988), non-avidin biotin-binding proteins (Dakshinamurti and Chauhan, 1989) and the use of monoclonal antibodies to biotin (Dakshinamurti and Rector, 1989). Interesting data continue to be reported on the enzymology and structure of the biotin carboxylases. Recombinant cDNA clones for three biotin enzymes have been isolated from mammalian sources and have been very useful in elucidating the process of regulation of these genes and factors involved (Bai et al., 1986; Freytag and Collier, 1984; Lamhonwah et al., 1986). This review deals, among other things, with the hypothesis that biotin might be involved in the synthesis of growth factors, highlighting a nonprosthetic group function for this vitamin. The uptake and transport of biotin are also discussed.

II. Biotin Structure and Biosynthesis

The discovery of biotin and the eventual elucidation of its structure, as well as its role in metabolism, involved diverse investigations spanning many decades. Kogl and Tonnis (1936) isolated crystalline biotin in 1936. Du Vigneaud et al. (1942b) determined its chemical structure, and Harris et al. (1943) chemically synthesized biotin. Biotin was shown to be cis-hexahydro-2-oxo-1H-thieno[3,4]imidazole-4-valeric acid. Only the (+)-stereoisomer of biotin exhibits significant biological activity (Fig. 1a).

Various biotin derivatives, analogs, and antagonists are known. Dethiobiotin, a sulfur-free analog of biotin, is the direct precursor of biotin during its biosynthesis in microorganisms (Guillerm et al., 1977). Biocytin (biotinyl lysine) is released upon the enzymatic digestion of biotin-containing proteins (Lynen, 1967). It is cleaved by biotinidase (EC 3.5.1.12) into biotin and lysine (Fig. 1b).

Biotin is produced by many microorganisms (McElroy and Jukes, 1940; Wegner et al., 1940). The earlier studies on biotin biosynthesis

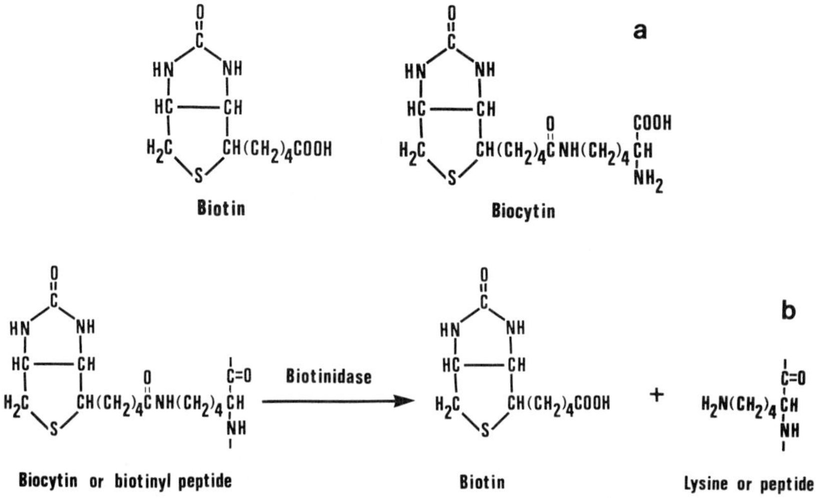

FIG. 1. (a) Structure of biotin and biocytin. (b) Hydrolysis of biocytin or biotinyl peptides by biotinidase.

involved the precursor–product relationship between pimelic acid and biotin and between dethiobiotin and biotin (Du Vigneaud *et al.*, 1942a; Eakin and Eakin, 1942; Tatum, 1945). The availability of biotin mutants of *Escherichia coli* K-12 helped Eisenberg and co-workers (Eisenberg, 1962, 1985; Rolfe and Eisenberg, 1968) to identify the intermediates in the biosynthetic pathway of biotin. The sequence of reactions in biosynthesis is shown in Fig. 2. Some of the enzymes involved in this pathway have been characterized (Eisenberg and Star, 1968; Izumi *et al.*, 1972a,b, 1973, 1975; Parry and Kunitani, 1976).

Biotin is degraded by microorganisms (Christner *et al.*, 1964) to yield urea, NH_4^+, HCO_3^-, and L-cysteine (Brady *et al.*, 1966). In animals biotin seems to be excreted in urine as such or in a form that can be used by *Lactobacillus arabinoseus*. Apart from biotin, biotin sulfone or sulfoxide derivatives have been reported to be excreted in urine. The carboxyl group of the biotin side chain is oxidized in animals (Mistry and Dakshinamurti, 1964; Baxter and Quastel, 1953).

III. BIOTIN-DEPENDENT ENZYMES

The best known and understood role of biotin is as the prosthetic group of several biotin-containing enzymes. The four major biotin-containing enzymes in higher organisms are propionyl-coenzyme A

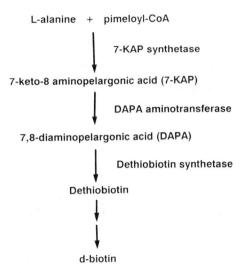

FIG. 2. Biosynthetic pathways for biotin in *E. coli*.

(CoA) carboxylase (PCC), pyruvate carboxylase (PC), β-methylcrotonyl-CoA carboxylase (MCC), and acetyl-CoA carboxylase (ACC). ACC is a cytosolic enzyme, whereas the other three are mitochondrial enzymes. Each of the biotin-dependent carboxylases catalyzes an adenosine triphosphate (ATP)-dependent CO_2 fixation reaction, and biotin functions as a CO_2 carrier on the surface of the enzyme. The role of biotin enzymes in intermediary metabolism is shown in Fig. 3.

ACC (EC 6.4.1.2) catalyzes the ATP-dependent carboxylation of acetyl-CoA, leading to the formation of malonyl-CoA, and is recognized to be the regulatory enzyme of lipogenesis. PC (EC 6.4.1.1) is a key regulatory enzyme of gluconeogenesis in the liver and the kidney, where it catalyzes the first step in the synthesis of glucose from pyruvate. It is also present in lipogenic tissues (i.e., liver, adipose, lactating mammary gland, and adrenal) and participates in fatty acid synthesis by transporting acetyl groups via citrate, and reducing groups via malate, from the mitochondria to cytosol (Ballard and Hanson, 1967). In all tissues it has an anapleurotic role in the formation of oxaloacetate. PCC (EC 6.4.1.3) is a key enzyme in the catabolic pathway of odd-chain fatty acids, isoleucine, threonine, methionine, and valine (Rosenberg, 1983). The enzyme catalyzes the conversion of propionyl-CoA to methylmalonyl-CoA, which in turn enters the tricarboxylic acid via succinyl-CoA. MCC (EC 6.4.1.4) catalyzes the conversion of β-meth-

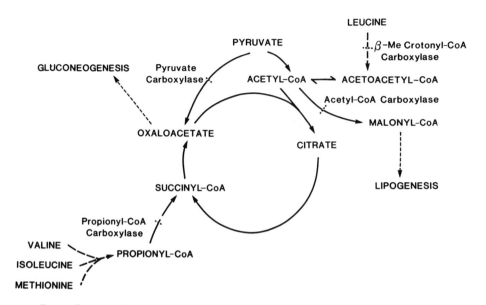

FIG. 3. Biotin carboxylase in cellular metabolism and accumulation on intermediary metabolites in individual carboxylase deficiencies.

ylcrotonyl-CoA to β-methylglutaconyl-CoA, a key reaction in the degradative pathway of leucine.

Biotin is covalently linked to the ε-amino group of lysine in all carboxylases. The amino acid sequences near the biotin of pyruvate carboxylase from sheep, chicken, and turkey livers (Rylatt et al., 1977), from transcarboxylase of *Propionibacterium shermanii* (Maloy et al., 1979), and ACC of *E. coli* (Sutton et al., 1977) show a great deal of homology in the sequences of this region. In all cases, an Ala-Met-Bct-Met (Bct for biocytin) sequence occurs, and in both PC and transcarboxylase the identity extends to Ala-Met-Bct-Met-Glu-Thr. It has been suggested that this conservation provides evidence that these biotin carboxylases and transcarboxylase may have evolved from a common ancestor (Wood and Barden, 1977). Furthermore, the sequence may be involved in activating biotin and/or orientating it so that it is an effective carboxyl carrier between the substrate sites. The sequence may also be important in designating the specific lysine of the protein that is to be biotinated posttranslationally by the apocarboxylase synthetase (Wood and Kumar, 1985).

Of the four mammalian biotin enzymes only two, ACC and PC, have regulatory features. Short- and long-term modulations of both enzyme activity and the amount of the enzyme protein by dietary factors and hormonal status are known to occur for these enzymes. The regulation of acetyl-CoA and PCCs is discussed in a recent review (Dakshinamurti and Chauhan, 1988).

Recombinant cDNA clones for three biotin enzymes have been isolated from mammalian sources and have been used in elucidating the regulation of these genes. Bai *et al.* (1986) recently isolated a 1.2-kb cDNA clone for ACC from rat mammary gland and demonstrated for the first time that the increased amount of ACC in rat liver occurring after eating a fat-free diet was mainly due to an increased amount of ACC mRNA. A cDNA clone for PC has been isolated and its gene was localized on the long arm of human chromosome 11 (Freytag and Collier, 1984). It was further demonstrated in 3T3-L1 cells that PC mRNA content increased 23-fold in 7 days after the onset of differentiation. Furthermore, cDNA clones coding for α and β polypeptides of human PCC have been isolated and assigned to independent chromosomes 13 and 3, respectively (Lamhonwah *et al.*, 1986).

IV. NONPROSTHETIC GROUP FUNCTIONS OF BIOTIN

A. PRESENCE OF BIOTIN IN CELL NUCLEI

Earlier work on the intracellular fractionation of biotin in various tissues of the rat and the chicken indicated that a significant amount of biotin was associated with the nuclear fraction (Dakshinamurti and Mistry, 1963a,b). The biotin content of biotin-deficient rat liver is about one tenth of that of normal rat liver, and a significant 20% of this was present in the nuclear fraction, suggesting that nuclear biotin was conserved in the deficient animal (Boeckx and Dakshinamurti, 1974, 1975). The presence of biotin in the nuclear fraction of rat and HeLa cells was further confirmed by Chalifour (1982), using a variety of subcellular fractionation procedures. Biotin-deficient rats were injected with [³H]biotin and were killed 24 hours later, and liver nuclei were prepared according to the method of Wray (1978), using a Percoll gradient. The nuclei, viewed under a phase contrast microscope, appeared intact and free of any contamination by membrane fragments and cellular organelles. Liver nuclei contained a significant amount of radioactivity. Nuclear biotin was noncovalently bound to protein. The biotin-binding protein has been isolated (Bhullar, 1985). Nuclei assayed negative for any of the biotin carboxylases, suggesting a function for nuclear biotin other than as a prosthetic group of the biotin-containing carboxylases.

B. Requirement for Biotin by Cells in Culture

A requirement for biotin by cells in culture would be expected in view of the obligatory involvement of biotin in the metabolism of carbohydrates and lipids and in the further utilization of deaminated residues of certain amino acids. However, various earlier reports have claimed that cells in culture do not require biotin (Eagle, 1955; Swim and Parke, 1958; Holmes, 1959; Dupree et al., 1962). Keranen (1972) reported that HeLA cells grown in a biotin-deficient medium contained more biotin than those grown in a biotin-supplemented medium, perhaps due to the ability of these transformed cells to synthesize biotin. Using biotin-depleted fetal bovine serum (Dakshinamurti and Chalifour, 1981) and Eagle's minimum essential medium, we demonstrated a requirement for biotin by HeLA cells, human fibroblasts, and Rous sarcoma virus-transformed baby hamster kidney cells based on the viability, biotin content, and activities of biotin-dependent and -independent enzymes (Chalifour and Dakshinamurti, 1982a,b). There was a drastic reduction in the viability of HeLa cells starting with the fourth passage, and following the sixth passage in this medium no further cell growth was observed (Fig. 4).

In a further study (Bhullar and Dakshinamurti, 1985) we have shown that there was a significant decrease in the incorporation of leucine into protein of the homogenate or cytosol of biotin-deficient HeLa cells as compared to cells grown in a biotin-supplemented medium. When biotin was added to the biotin-deficient medium there was a 2-fold increase in the incorporation of leucine into proteins. Based on experiments using puromycin and cordycepin, we concluded that the appearance of new RNA in the cytoplasm is an event brought about when biotin-deficient cells are supplemented with exogenous biotin.

Normal cells in G_1 arrest due to serine starvation start incorporating [^{3}H]thymidine into DNA as soon as serine is replaced in the medium. Biotin-deficient HeLa cells under similar conditions do not incorporate [^{3}H]thymidine into DNA even when serine is restored to the medium. However, within 4 hours of supplementation of biotin to the biotin-deficient medium, the incorporation of [^{3}H]thymidine into DNA reaches a maximum (Fig. 5). Cells cultured in a medium deficient in growth factor or nutrients do not multiply, owing to arrest of growth in the G_1 phase of the cell cycle (Allen and Moskowitz, 1973). Net synthesis of macromolecules during the G_1 phase is necessary for entry into the S phase. Progression through the cell cycle is dependent on the synthesis of specific proteins, and it is possible that the inhibition of the synthesis of such proteins would block the cell cycle. Significantly, the incorporation of thymidine into DNA reaches a maximum within

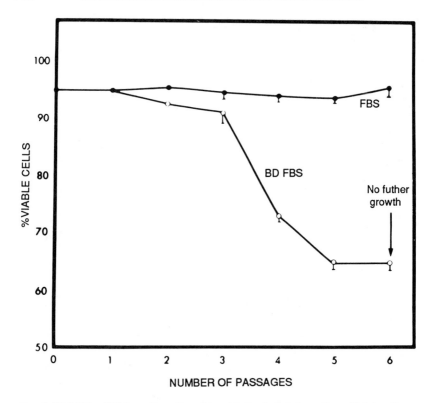

FIG. 4. Viability of HeLa cells cultured in a biotin-depleted medium. HeLA cells were subcultured in Eagle's minimum essential medium containing 5% fetal bovine serum (FBS) (●) or biotin-deficient FBS (○). The cells were carried through successive passages, and viability was determined using the trypan blue exclusion test. Results are the average of three experiments. Bars indicate 1 SD. (From Dakshinamurti and Chalifour, 1981. Used with permission of the publisher.)

4 hours of the addition of biotin to the deficient cells. By this time there is stimulation of protein synthesis. We speculate that these two phenomena are related and that the growth-promoting effect of biotin might be achieved through the stimulation of the synthesis of certain proteins.

Of the biotin-dependent carboxylases of significance in animals, ACC is required for lipogenesis and hence in membrane genesis. PC is essential for the generation of oxaloacetate, the maintenance of the tricarboxylic acid cycle (Nakano *et al.*, 1982), and gluconeogenesis. PCC and MCC are required for the further metabolism of certain amino acid residues. Thus, under culture conditions biotin should sub-

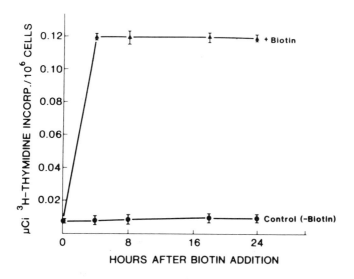

Fɪɢ. 5. Biotin-deficient cells were exposed to 2 ng/ml of biotin. The control deficient cells were left in the deficient medium. At various time intervals biotin-supplemented (●) and control biotin-deficient (▲) cells were removed, and the incorporation of [³H]thymidine into DNA was determined. (From Bhullar and Dakshinamurti, 1985. Used with permission of the publisher.)

serve the lipogenic and dicarboxylic acid needs of the cell. However, serum lipids are taken up by cells (Wisniesky *et al.,* 1973) and saturated fatty acids are without growth-promoting activity for cells such as simian virus-transformed 3T3 under conditions of biotin deficiency (Messmer and Young, 1977).

Cheng and Moscowitz (1982) have shown that G_1-arrested Rous sarcoma virus-transformed baby hamster kidney cells can be maintained in culture continuously in the basal medium supplemented with only biotin. Cells multiplied continuously in basal medium supplemented with delipidized serum and serum lipid extract but not in basal medium supplemented with serum lipid extract alone. Their results suggest that cell growth depended on some biotin-mediated activity whose level had decreased when cells were grown in a biotin-deficient medium. It has been claimed that RST cells growing in a biotin-containing medium produce a nondialyzable factor that stimulates cell multiplication (Moskowitz and Cheng, 1985). We have shown (Bhullar and Dakshinamurti, 1985) that the addition of biotin to the culture medium of HeLA cells results in enhanced protein synthesis, DNA synthesis, and cell growth. It is possible that the growth-promoting effect of biotin might be achieved through stimulation of the synthesis of certain proteins, highlighting the nonprosthetic group function of biotin.

A requirement for high-density lipoprotein (HDL) has been shown for the growth of Madin–Darby canine kidney cells exposed to Dulbecco's modified Eagle's medium (DMEM) supplemented with transferrin when cells were exposed to a mixture (1 : 1) of DMEM and F-12 medium (Cohen and Gospodarowicz, 1985; Gospodarowicz and Cohen, 1988). The components of the F-12 medium responsible for support of growth in the absence of HDL are biotin, which is absent in DMEM, and choline, which is present in insufficient concentration in DMEM. It is of particular significance in this context that the HDL fraction of plasma has a considerable amount of biotin associated with it (unpublished observations). This biotin is not dialyzable and is probably nonspecifically attached to the protein. Regardless of the nature of the association, this would then explain the HDL requirement, which can be replaced by biotin, as a specific requirement for biotin itself. Collins *et al.* (1987) reported that biotin is essential for the expression of the asialoglycoprotein receptor in HepG2 cells.

C. ROLE OF BIOTIN IN CELL DIFFERENTIATION

It is known that various transformed cell lines produce transforming growth factors that enable them to grow in a serum-free medium supplemented with transferrin and insulin (Kaplan *et al.*, 1982). The 3T3-L1 subline derived from 3T3 mouse fibroblast cell line has the capacity to differentiate in the resting state into a cell type having the characteristics of adipocytes (H. Green and Kehinde, 1974). When they reach confluence and start to differentiate, they greatly increase their rate of triglyceride synthesis and accumulate the product. The increase in lipogenic rate parallels a coordinate rise in the activities of the key enzymes of the fatty acid biosynthetic pathway (Mackall and Lane, 1977; Mackall *et al.*, 1976). The increases in many enzyme activities have been shown to result from specific translatable mRNA (Spiegelman and Farmer, 1982; Wise *et al.*, 1984). This increase correlated with a marked rise in nuclear run-off transcription rates for these mRNAs during differentiation (Bernlohr *et al.*, 1985). The process of differentiation can be accelerated in a number of ways, such as by increasing the amount of serum in the culture medium or by adding certain hormones, such as insulin, and other chemical agents, such as biotin, 1-methyl-3-isobutylxanthine, or dexamethasone (Rosen *et al.*, 1979). When the serum in the cultures was extensively dialyzed, the morphological and enzyme changes characteristic of adipocyte differentiation were induced without deposition of fat (Kuri-Harcuch et al., 1978). It was presumed that dialysis removed all biotin from the serum and the role of biotin was linked to the increase in ACC. However, it is not clear from their work why it would take 24–48 hours for the lipid-synthesizing enzymes to increase following the addition of biotin to the biotin-deficient cell culture medium. If this were only dependent on the synthesis of holoacetyl-CoA carboxylase from the apoenzyme, this would have been completed in 1 hour. The delay suggests that perhaps some factor required for the induction of the whole set of lipogenic enzymes (which, with the exception of ACC, are not biotin enzymes) might be formed under the influence of biotin. In addition, the 3T3-L1 subline had a greater capacity than did the very slowly differentiating M_2 subline to remove labeled palmitate from the culture medium and to incorporate it into triglyceride (Kasturi and Wakil, 1983). Esterification was the principal route of fatty acid utilization by both preadipose cells and cells committed to differentiation. The frequency of adipocyte conversion is a heritable condition. Genetic and epigenetic factors regulate the level of the lipogenic multienzyme system. To express differentiation, the attainment of confluency is accompanied by the presence of an adipogenic factor in the culture medium (Kuri-Harcuch and Green, 1978; Kuri-Harcuch and Marsch-Moreno, 1983). This is present in most animal sera but not in the domestic cat serum. It is significant that cat serum contains less than one tenth of the biotin content of bovine serum.

After interaction with the adipogenic factor, cells undergo DNA replication and cell division before they express the differentiated state. Cytosine arabinoside addition to the medium prevented cells from undergoing conversion. The molecular events initiated by the interaction of the cells with the adipogenic factor remain to be identified. The temporal relationship between DNA synthesis and differentiation after susceptible cells is stimulated with adipogenic serum, and the inhibition of differentiation by cytosine arabinoside supports the interpretation that DNA synthesis is required by 3T3-L1 cells for differentiation. As seen by us (Dakshinamurti and Chalifour, 1981) and by others (Baumgartner et al., 1985), biotin is not completely removed from fetal calf serum by extensive and repeated dialysis or by treatment with avidin–Sepharose. It is possible that at the low level present in extensively dialyzed serum, biotin is still available for the reactions that have to do with differentiation. Higher levels of biotin would, however, be required to biotinate acetyl-CoA apocarboxylase to form the holoenzyme. A monoclonal antibody to biotin (Dakshinamurti *et al.*, 1986) could be used to investigate whether the differentiation per se requires biotin.

D. ROLE OF BIOTIN IN THE INDUCTION OF GLUCOKINASE

The only protein which has been shown to be specifically induced by biotin is glucokinase. Biotin is not a part of this protein. Earlier work from this laboratory (Dakshinamurti and Cheah-Tan, 1968a,b) demonstrated that liver glucokinase activity was altered in response to the biotin status of rats. Biotin also plays a role in the precocious development of glucokinase in young rats (Dakshinamurti and Hong, 1969). In all of these experiments, an increase in enzyme activity was associated with protein synthesis. The synthesis of glucokinase is under developmental, nutritional, and hormonal control (Weinhowe, 1976; Meglasson and Matschnisky, 1984). Glucokinase activity in the liver decreases when rats are starved or fed a carbohydrate-free diet. Upon refeeding of a normal diet or glucose, there is a remarkable recovery, reaching essentially normal glucokinase levels within a few hours (Sharma *et al.*, 1963; Ureta *et al.*, 1970). Spence and Koudelka (1984), using primary cultures of rat hepatocytes, have shown that the addition of biotin to the culture medium at a concentration of 10^{-6} M resulted in a 4-fold increase in the glucokinase activity, which represented synthesis of the glucokinase protein. In our earlier work as well as in that of Spence *et al.* (1981), the effect on glucokinase synthesis was observed at pharmacological concentrations of biotin. We have shown that biotin enhances glucokinase activity in biotin-deficient rats. Spence *et al.* (1981) have indicated that biotin increased the amount of translatable mRNA coding for glucokinase.

E. BIOTIN AND TESTICULAR FUNCTION

In early work Shaw and Phillips (1942) reported that the testes of biotin-deficient rats were visually very small in relation to the size of the animal and that the seminiferous tubules were very small and showed signs of degeneration. Delost and Terroine (1956) performed a more systematic study and found that the testis size was smaller and weight was lower than those of normal animals. There was evidence of delayed spermatogenesis and a decreased number of spermatozoa. They reported that these disturbances in the testes were due to biotin deficiency alone, since animals on a restricted but normal diet did not show any of these abnormalities (Terroine, 1960). In a recent study (Paulose *et al.*, 1987) of testicular function in biotin-deficient male rats we found that serum and testis levels of testosterone were markedly decreased in these animals. The deficient testis was responsive to luteinizing hormone or biotin administration by increasing testosterone production. The morphological abnormalities of the biotin-deficient rat testes were reversed by biotin treatment alone, whereas continuous testosterone supply through implantation throughout the biotin-deficient period was without any effect. This paralleled the effects of biotin and testosterone on protein synthesis in the testes. The stimulation of testicular protein synthesis by testosterone required normal biotin status.

F. ROLE OF BIOTIN IN THE INDUCTION OF BIOTIN-BINDING PROTEINS OF EGG YOLK

It was demonstrated that biotin in egg yolk is bound to a nondialyzable, heat-denatured component (György and Rose, 1949). White and co-workers (Meslar et al., 1978) isolated heat-denaturable biotin-binding protein BBP1 and showed it to be distinct from avidin. In later work they demonstrated that the concentrations of BBP1 and a second biotin-binding protein (BBP2) in egg yolk were directly related to dietary biotin content (White and Whitehead, 1987). At low concentration of biotin BBP1 was the major transporter, while at higher concentration of biotin BBP2 predominated. It has been shown that avidin (Korpela, 1984) and BBP1 (Murty and Adiga, 1985) can be induced by various sex hormones. The induction of two egg yolk biotin-binding proteins by biotin (White and Whitehead, 1987) may suggest that biotin regulates biotin-binding proteins of egg yolk by transcriptional control that overrides hormonal control.

G. GUANYLATE CYCLASE AND RNA POLYMERASE II

Vesely and co-workers (Vesely, 1981, 1982; Vesely et al., 1984) reported that biotin and its analogs at micromolar concentration enhanced guanylate cyclase activity in various rat tissues and suggested a role for biotin in the activation of this enzyme. Spence and Koudelka (1984) studied the relationship between the biotin-mediated increase in glucokinase activity and the cellular level of cyclic guanosine monophosphate (cGMP) as well as the activity of guanylate cyclase. Increases in intracellular cGMP as well as in guanylate cyclase were reported. It should be noted that these effects were elicited at micromolar concentrations of biotin which are about two orders of magnitude higher than the normal cellular concentration of biotin.

The effects of biotin on cell growth are seen at physiological concentrations of this vitamin. We have examined the mechanism of action of biotin in cell growth (Singh and Dakshinamurti, 1988). The addition of physiological concentrations of biotin to the growth medium of biotin-deficient HeLa cells and fibroblasts resulted in increases in guanylate cyclase activity, as well as in the intracellular concentration of cGMP. The major role of cGMP in cells is connected with cell growth, DNA and RNA synthesis, and possibly malignant transformation of cells (Zeilberg and Goldberg, 1977). Using Novikoff hepatoma, Zeilberg and Goldberg (1977) showed that as the synchronized cells entered mitosis, cellular cGMP levels rose and cAMP levels decreased. Similar changes in cyclic nucleotide concentrations were observed after growth induction by fibroblast growth factor (Rudland et al., 1974). Agents that increase lymphocyte cGMP levels stimulate transformation of these cells (Goldberg et al., 1978). An increase in intracellular cGMP has been shown during rat liver regeneration, which is regulated by insulin and glucagon (Earp, 1980). In all of the above cases the growth factors produced an in vivo increase in the activity of guanylate cyclase. None of these factors stimulated the activity of guanylate cyclase in vitro. Their mode of action would seem to be distinct from the in vitro stimulatory effect of agents such as azide, nitroprusside, and nitrosamine (Braughler et al., 1979) as well as biotin and its analogs when used at pharmacological concentrations.

RNA polymerase II synthesizes mRNA precursors. The activity of this enzyme in nuclear lysate from biotin-deficient HeLa cells and fibroblasts was significantly lower than in similar preparations from biotin-supplemented cells. The addition of biotin to the culture medium at a concentration as low as 10^{-8} M resulted in a significant increase in enzyme activity, which reached a plateau by 4 hours following addition of biotin to the medium (Singh and Dakshinamurti, 1988).

Increased RNA polymerase II activity is found in rapidly growing mammalian cells. cGMP stimulation of nuclear DNA-dependent RNA polymerase has been shown in lymphocytes (Johnson and Haddon, 1975), rat mammary gland (Anderson et al., 1975), and fetal calf cells cultured in the presence of sheep erythropoietin (Canas and Congote, 1984; White and George, 1981). The addition of physiological concentrations of biotin to the growth medium of biotin-deficient cells results in the stimulation of guanylate cyclase activity and an increase in intracellular cGMP as well as RNA polymerase II activity. We contend that the stimulation of the synthesis of certain proteins (growth factors) by biotin might be mediated by its effect on cGMP.

V. Inherited Biotin Deficiencies—Single and Multiple Carboxylase Deficiencies

A. Single Carboxylase Deficiency

Biotin deficiency or dependency, an entity that was once virtually ignored in clinical medicine, is attracting much interest now because of the progress made in the study of inborn metabolic disorders (Tanaka, 1981). Since 1976 the incidence in infants of organic acidemia has been investigated with new analytical techniques. These conditions have been characterized as due to the lack of one or more of the biotin carboxylases (for a review, see Sweetman and Nyhan, 1986). Inherited disorders of individual biotin carboxylases have been reported and are distinct from the biotin-responsive multiple carboxylase deficiency, as these patients do not respond even to pharmacological doses of biotin. Figure 6 shows abnormal metabolites due to individual carboxylase deficiency. Of the four carboxylase deficiencies, only PCC deficiency has been studied in detail. The biochemical abnormalities include elevated concentrations of propionic and lactic acids in blood and elevated levels of secondary metabolites such as 3-hydroxypropionic acid, 2-methylcitrate, and propionylglycine in urine.

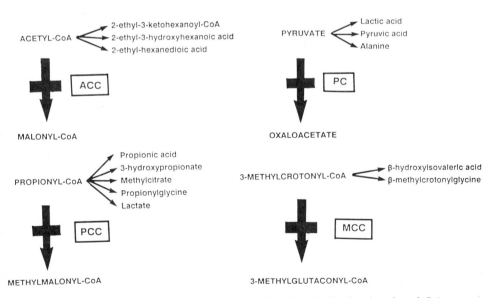

Fig. 6. Accumulation of intermediary metabolites in individual carboxylase deficiency. Acumulated metabolites are shown with multiple arrows.

Complementation studies between PCCs of deficient fibroblasts indicate that there is a considerable range of genetic heterogeneity (Gravel *et al.*, 1977; Wolf *et al.*, 1980). Two principal groups were identified by using complementation analysis and were designated *pccA* and *pccBC*, respectively. They represent defects in two different structural genes (Wolf, 1978; Wolf *et al.*, 1978). It was shown that mutants of the *pccA* group failed to complement each other but complemented mutants of all other groups. *pccBC* has been further divided into its subgroups *pccB* and *pccC*. These subgroups complemented each other in addition to *pccA* mutants, but they did not complement *pccBC* mutants (Gravel and Robinson, 1985; Wolf *et al.*, 1981). The occurrence of two complementation groups suggested involvement of two structural genes in the expression of α peptide by the *pccA* group and β peptide by the *pccBC* group. cDNA clones coding for α and β polypeptides of human PCC have been isolated (Kraus *et al.*, 1986a,b; Lamhonwah *et al.*, 1986). mRNA for PCC α and β chains, respectively, were 2.9 and 2.0 kb in length. PCC α- and β-chain genes have been assigned to independent chromosomes 13 and 3, respectively. This, together with the assignment of pyruvate carboxylase to chromosome 11, indicates the independent nature of the genes coding for the various biotin-dependent enzymes. It has been shown further that several *pccA* mutants were deficient in PCC α-chain mRNA but have normal β-chain mRNA (Lamhonwah *et al.*, 1986), strongly supporting the earlier observation that *pccA* mutants involve the defect at the *pcc* locus (Lamhonwah *et al.*, 1985).

B. Multiple Carboxylase Deficiency

Attention has recently been focused on the condition referred to as multiple carboxylase deficiency (MCD), in which deficiences of all three mitochondrial carboxylases are seen in the patient. Two distinct types of MCD have been recognized, based on the age of onset as well as the nature of clinical presentation (Sweetman, 1981; Wolf and Feldman, 1982; Wolf *et al.*, 1985; Sweetman *et al.*, 1985). There are differences in the serum–biotin concentrations of the patients with either type of MCD presentation. In addition, there are differences in the responses of the fibroblasts from patients of either group to varying levels of biotin in the medium. A deficiency of biotin holocarboxylase synthetase is generally regarded to be the prime biochemical lesion in the neonatal type of MCD (Burri *et al.*, 1981). The beneficial response of the affected infant to large doses of biotin administered prenatally suggests a defective holocarboxylase synthetase with a high K_m for biotin (Roth *et al.*, 1982). The late-onset (or juvenile) form of MCD is associated with low serum biotin values and is regarded to be associated with defective biotin absorption (Burri *et al.*, 1981). The characterization of the deficiency of biotinidase in the late-onset type of MCD (Sweetman, 1981; Wolf and Feldman, 1982; Wolf *et al.*, 1983a, 1985; Sweetman *et al.*, 1985; Burri *et al.*, 1981) has contributed much to an understanding of this disorder. Biotinidase specifically cleaves biocytin. It is possible that such a specific action of biotinidase in the gut is a prerequisite for the absorption of dietary protein-bound biotin in the gut. Biotinidase is also implicated in the renal resorption of biotin, as evidence has been presented for impaired absorption of biotin in both the gut and the kidney in the juvenile form of MCD. These patients have an increased renal clearance of biotin (Baumgartner *et al.*, 1985).

VI. BIOTIN-BINDING PROTEINS

Apart from the carboxylases in which biotin is attached covalently to the apocarboxylases, there is a group of proteins which bind to biotin noncovalently. Both avidin, the biotin-binding protein of raw egg white, and streptavidin, a bacterial protein, have exceedingly high affinities for biotin, with a K_d of 10^{-15} M. This is the strongest noncovalent binding between a protein and a small-molecular-weight ligand known. These proteins have been reviewed (Green, 1975). Apart from these there are other biotin-binding proteins, such as the egg yolk biotin-binding proteins, biotinidase, biotin-holocarboxylase synthetase, and nuclear biotin-binding protein with progressively lower affinities for biotin. Biotin-binding proteins vary considerably along the evolutionary scale. In *E. coli* biotin-holocarboxylase synthetase, a biotin-binding protein, has been shown to regulate the synthesis of the enzymes in the biotin biosynthesis pathway (Eisenberg, 1985).

A. AVIDIN–STREPTAVIDIN

Avidin, a biotin-binding protein from egg white, has served as a useful diagnostic tool in the identification and study of biotin-dependent enzymes. Avidin has been comprehensively reviewed (Green, 1975; Korpela, 1984). The interaction of avidin with biotin is the strongest noncovalent binding of biotin known, the dissociation constant of the binding sites being about 10^{-15} M (Green, 1963a). Avidin has been isolated from hen egg white (Eakin *et al.*, 1940; György *et al.*,

1941) and the oviduct of the avian species (Hertz and Sebrell, 1942). Avidin is a basic protein with an isoelectric point of 10 and M_r of 70,000 (s_{20} 4.7 S) (Woolley and Longsworth, 1942). It is a glycoprotein (Delange, 1970; Green and Toms, 1970) and has four identical subunits of M_r 17,000 (Green, 1963b, 1964b). The subunits of avidin have been sequenced; it is composed of 129 amino acid residues, four mannose residues, and three glucosamine residues, with alanine as the amino terminus. The exact physiological role of avidin in egg white is not known, but it is generally thought that avidin is a bacteriostat (Tranter and Board, 1982). Apart from this, avidin has been of considerable interest in immunological techniques as well as in labeling DNA and cell surface receptors. This aspect of avidin–biotin technology is covered in a *Methods in Enzymology* volume (Wilchek and Bayer, 1989).

In avidin–biotin interaction, importance has been attached to both tryptophanyl residues (four per subunit) (Green, 1962, 1964a,b; Green and Toms, 1970) and hydrogen bonding to the ureido ring in the binding process. This is supported both because binding of biotin causes a red shift in the absorption spectrum, which is characteristic of changes in the environment of tryptophan, and because each biotin bound protects four tryptophan residues from oxidation by N-bromosuccinimide (Green, 1962, 1964a). Destruction of two of the four tryptophans with N-bromosuccinimide essentially abolishes biotin-binding ability. Streptavidin is an acidic nonglycoprotein. cDNA representing streptavidin has recently been isolated and sequenced (Argarana *et al.*, 1986). The protein contains 159 amino acids, compared with 129 for avidin. Several regions of extensive homology were found between the two proteins. Of particular interest is the homology around the three tryptophan residues, suggesting that tryptophan residues are highly conserved in these two proteins.

B. Egg Yolk Biotin-Binding Proteins

In the egg-laying hen there are three biotin-binding proteins. In addition to avidin, present in albumen of the egg, there are two biotin-binding proteins in egg yolk. Other vitamins, such as riboflavin, have only one species of binding protein which is present in both egg albumen and yolk. The presence of distinct biotin-binding proteins for biotin suggests a specialized role for biotin in the regulation of the development of the embryo (White and Whitehead, 1987).

Of the two biotin-binding proteins in hen egg yolk, BBP1 and BBP2, the former has been well characterized (Mandella *et al.*, 1978; Meslar *et al.,* 1978). BBP1 constitutes about 0.03% of the total protein in egg yolk. It has a M_r of 74,300 and is a homotetramer. BBP1 is a glycoprotein with a pI of 4.6, and a high affinity for biotin with a K_d of 1×10^{-12} *M.* Differences in their isoelectric points, affinities for biotin, heat stability, amino-terminal amino acids, and immunological properties indicate that avidin and BBP1 are products of distinct genes rather than tissue-specific modifications of single-gene products (Mandella *et al.,* 1978). The identity of a plasma biotin-binding protein with BBP1 has been established on the basis of their degrees of saturation with biotin, denaturation temperatures, molecular weights, isoelectric points, and cross-reactivity with antibodies to the yolk BBP1 (White and Whitehead, 1987). The other egg yolk protein, BBP2, has not been purified.

The biotin content of eggs was shown to be directly related to the amount of biotin in the diet (Brewer and Edwards, 1972). After 2 weeks on a biotin-deficient diet, a hen lays eggs whose hatchability is reduced to zero and whose biotin content is 10% of that of a normal hen's egg (Couch *et al.,* 1949). Hen eggs contain about 10 μg of biotin. Of this, about 1 μg is in the albumen and bound to avidin, where it occupies 15% or less of the binding sites. The rest of the biotin is in egg yolk, bound to the two biotin-binding proteins, BBP1 and BBP2 (White and Whitehead, 1987). Both BBP1 and BBP2 are transported by the bloodstream to the ovary and are finally deposited in the developing oocyte. Since most of the biotin in egg yolk is bound to biotin-binding proteins, the physiological function of biotin-binding protein is undoubtedly to transport biotin to the egg for future use by the developing embryo.

C. BIOTINIDASE

Acid hydrolysis of biotin proteins releases free biotin, whereas proteolytic hydrolysis yields biotin peptides. The smallest among these is biocytin, ε-*N*-biotinyl-L-lysine. Thoma and Peterson (1954) described an enzyme from pig liver which liberated biotin from a peptic digest of liver. They proposed the name biotinidase (biotin-amide amidohydrolase, EC 3.5.1.12) for this enzyme, which also hydrolyzed the synthetic substrate *N*-(*d*-biotinyl)-*p*-aminobenzoic acid. At about the same time Wright *et al.* (1954) described an enzyme in blood plasma that hydrolyzed biocytin. After this initial description and partial purification from hog kidney (Knappe *et al.,* 1963), there had been very little interest in this enzyme until Wolf *et al.* (1983a, b) showed that biotinidase deficiency is the primary defect in patients with the late-onset variant of MCD. This enzyme has been partially purified from bacterial sources (Knappe *et al.*, 1963) as well as from hog liver (Pispa, 1965). More recently Craft *et al.* (1985) purified human plasma biotinidase to a specific activity of 361 U/mg of protein and we have purified human serum biotinidase to homogeneity (Chauhan and Dakshinamurti, 1986). The enzyme is a glycoprotein, a monomer with a M_r of 68,000. Sialic acid residues, however, are not required for enzyme activity. With biocytin, the natural substrate, the maximal activity of the enzyme was in the pH range 4.5–6.0, although with the most commonly used synthetic substrate, N-(d-biotinyl)-p-aminobenzoic acid, the optimum pH was in the range 6.0–7.5. Biotinidase is not a general proteolytic enzyme. It has specific structural requirements in the substrate for hydrolysis. Biotin inhibits biotinidase activity in the millimolar range (Chauhan and Dakshinamurti, 1986). The physiological significance of this inhibition is very little, as biotin is present in nanomolar concentration range in human plasma (Baker, 1985).

A biotinidase clone of 1.25 kb was isolated from a human liver λgt_{11} library (Chauhan and Dakshinamurti, 1988). The poly(A^+) RNA corresponding to the clone is 1.8 kb. This partial clone was further sequenced by the dideoxy-chain termination method. Although the predicted amino acid sequence from the biotinidase clone does not share extensive homology with avidin and streptavidin, there is conservation of sequence around tryptophan residues which have been shown to be critical for these biotin-binding proteins.

1. *Role of Biotinase as a Carrier Protein*

Based on investigations with HeLa cells and human fibroblasts, we suggested that biotin transport in mammalian cells may involve pinocytosis through the functioning of specific circulating proteins (Dakshinamurti and Chalifour, 1981; Chalifour and Dakshinamurti, 1983). Although earlier studies have indicated that human albumin and α and β globulin can bind biotin (Frank *et al.*, 1970), we found this binding to be nonspecific. It was reported that a glycoprotein in human serum can bind biotin (Vallotton *et al.*, 1965; Gehrig and Leuthardt, 1976). We have isolated this protein, using an agarose–biotin column, but it does not bind biotin specifically.

Human serum was fractionated on a Sephadex G-150 column and analyzed for biotinidase and biotin-binding activity (Chauhan and Dakshinamurti, 1988). Both activities coincided (Fig. 7), suggesting that biotinidase is the only protein that binds biotin in human serum. These findings were corroborated by binding studies on fractions of human serum analyzed on diethylaminoethyl (DEAE)–Sephacel,

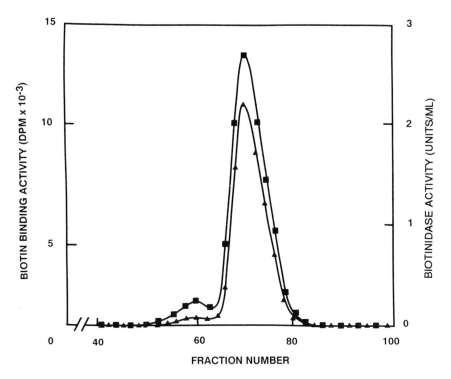

FIG. 7. Human serum (15 ml) was applied onto a Sephadex G-150 column (2.5 × 100 cm) and equilibrated with 0.05 M phosphate buffer, pH 6.0, containing 1 mM β-mercaptoethanol, 1 mM EDTA, 0.15 M NaCl, and 0.02% sodium azide. The same buffer was used for elution at the 20 ml/hr flow rate and 3-ml fractions were collected. Biotin-binding activity (■) and biotinidase activity (▲) were determined. (From Chauhan and Dakshinamurti, 1988. Used with permission of the publisher.)

hydroxylapatite, and octyl–Sepharose columns. On all column separations biotin-binding activity coincided with biotinidase activity. Biotin-binding studies with human serum support the notion that biotinidase might be a biotin-carrier protein in human serum.

We determined the binding of biotin to pure human serum biotinidase. Figure 8a shows concentration-dependent binding of [³H]d-biotin to biotinidase and the Scatchard transformation of the data (Scatchard, 1949). The Scatchard plot indicates two classes of biotin-binding sites, one of high and one of low affinity (0.5 nM and 50 nM, respectively). Biotin binding was also analyzed, using competitive inhibition; as shown in Fig. 8b, this also shows both low- and high-affinity binding sites. The high-capacity, low-affinity binding corresponds to that of other vitamin-binding proteins. For example,

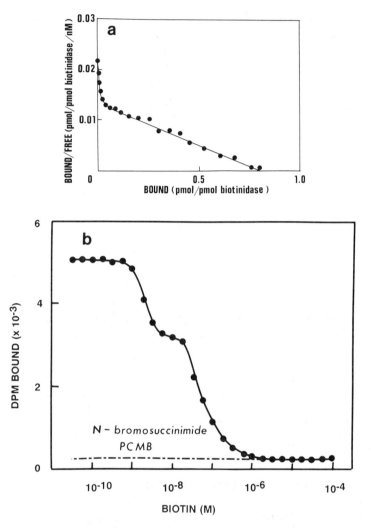

FIG. 8. Concentration-dependent binding of [³H]-d-biotin to purified human serum biotinidase. (a) Samples of purified biotinidase were incubated with increasing concentrations of [³H]d-biotin (0.1 nM–10 μM). A parallel set contained the amount of [³H]d-biotin plus a 1000-fold excess of cold d-biotin for the determination of nonspecific binding. Each point is the mean of duplicate determination. Linear regression of the points gave K_d of 0.5 and 50 nM. (b) Competitive inhibition of biotin binding to human serum biotinidase. Binding to human serum biotinidase with (●) 10^{-5} M N-bromosuccinimide or p-chloromercuribenzoate (PCMB; ———·———--). (From Chauhan and Dakshinamurti, 1988. Used with permission of the publisher.)

thiamine-binding protein binds thiamine with a K_d for thiamine of 5.5 × 10^{-7} M (Nishimura *et al.*, 1984). The biotin-binding activity of biotinidase can be completely inhibited by N-bromosuccinimide and p-chloromercuribenzoate (Fig. 8b), suggesting that tryptophan and cysteine residues are required for biotin binding. It is likely that the cysteine residues in biotinidase are required for the formation of enzyme–acyl complex for high-affinity, low-capacity binding. The formation of an enzyme–acyl complex was shown for biotinidase (Pispa, 1965).

Baumgartner *et al.* (1985) suggested that the decreased level of plasma biotin in biotinidase-deficient patients may be due to decreased levels of biotinidase or a specific biotin-binding protein in plasma. Other indirect evidence for the existence of a biotin-binding protein comes from the study of epileptic patients on long-term therapy with anticonvulsants (Krause *et al.*, 1985). Significantly low levels of biotin were observed in these patients, suggesting that these anticonvulsants probably compete with biotin for the biotin-binding protein in circulation. The anticonvulsants used in their study share with biotin the common structural feature of a cyclic carbamide group. It is this group of biotin that is involved in protein binding (Green, 1975). We have shown that all of these anticonvulsants competed with biotin for the biotin-binding activity of biotinidase (Chauhan and Dakshinamurti, 1988). Our results indicate that biotin in human serum is essentially noncovalently bound to protein(s) and that biotinidase is the only protein which exchanges with [^{3}H]d-biotin.

2. Role of Biotinidase in Intestinal Absorption of Biotin/Biocytin

There are conflicting reports on the intestinal absorption of biotin, with suggestions that the mode of uptake of biotin differs among the species. Earlier investigations using the everted sac technique (Turner and Hughes, 1962; Spencer and Brody, 1964) reported that biotin in the rat was absorbed through passive diffusion. Spencer and Brody (1964) observed that the hamster intestine transported biotin against a concentration gradient. In later work Berger *et al.* (1972) presented evidence for a sodium-dependent saturable process for the uptake of biotin by the proximal part of the hamster intestine. The K_m given for biotin transport (1.0 mM), however, was in the nonphysiological range.

The uptake of biotin by human cell lines was reported by us (Dakshinamurti and Chalifour, 1981; Chalifour and Dakshinamurti, 1982b, 1983) to be saturable. Based on the binding of avidin and avidin–biotin complex to rat liver plasma membrane (Chalifour and Dakshinamurti, 1983), we suggested that avidin in these systems was mimicking a natural biotin-binding carrier involved in biotin transport (Dakshinamurti *et al.*, 1985). This was corroborated by Cohen and Thomas (1982) in their study, using fully differentiated 3T3-L1 cells. Bowers-Komro and McCormick (1985) have indicated that biotin was transported in hepatocytes by a sodium-dependent process but was not associated with a definitive saturable process. Gore *et al.* (1986), who have used isolated rat mucosal cells in their study, concluded that at physiological concentrations the uptake of biotin by these cells was a passive phenomenon. However, both Bowman *et al.* (1986) and Said and Redha (1987) have concluded that at concentrations lower than 5 μM absorption of biotin by rat jejunal segments proceeded largely by a saturable process. Although a carrier has been proposed for biotin uptake, no attempt has been made to identify this carrier.

There are conflicting reports as to the source of biotin for intestinal absorption. It has been assumed that biotin synthesized by the colonic microflora makes a contribution to the host nutrition. Diverse studies (Bowman *et al.*, 1986; Said and Redha, 1987) show, however, that the transport of biotin was higher in the jejunum than in the ileum and was minimal in the colon. Along with the earlier observation (Sorrell *et al.*, 1971) that biotin was better absorbed when given orally than when instilled into the colon, this would suggest that, although biotin is synthesized by colonic microflora, such may not be a significant source of biotin nutrition for the host. Most of the biotin in foods such as meat and cereals is protein bound (György, 1939; Thomson *et al.*, 1941; Scheiner and DeRitter, 1975). The enzymatic hydrolysis in the gastrointestinal tract would release biocytin (or biotinyl peptides) rather than free biotin.

The uptake of biotin and biocytin in rat jejunal segments is shown in Fig. 9. The biphasic transport of biotin and biocytin in the rat small intestine observed in this study suggests that as the biotin concentration in the gut falls below 50 nM, the saturable uptake mechanism would operate to make enough biotin available to the animal (Dakshinamurti *et al.*, 1987). If such a system indeed operated in other mammals including humans, it would have tremendous advantage in the context of fluctuating amounts of biotin ingested in the diet. This is borne out by the rarity of primary biotin deficiency in humans. The late-onset type of MCD was shown to be due to the deficiency of biotinidase (Wolf *et al.*, 1983a). It has been suggested that in certain cases of late-onset MCD these patients lack the system for absorbing biotin in the nanomolar range (Thoene *et al.*, 1983). Furthermore, it has been shown these patients respond only to pharmacological doses of biotin (Roth, 1985), indicating that only the saturable portion of biotin transport system is defective in these patients.

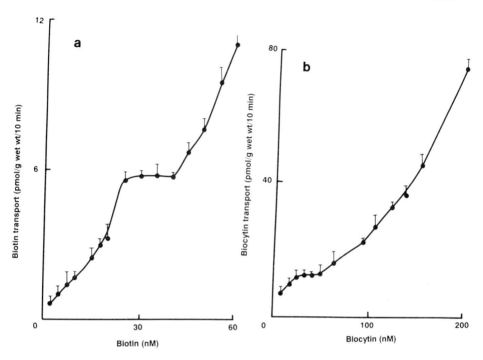

Fig. 9. Uptake of (a) biotin and (b) biocytin in jejunal segments. The uptake of biotin and biocytin in 2.0-cm jejunal segments was determined as a funtion of the concentration of biotin. The data shown are the means ± SE of three experiments. (From Dakshinamurti *et al.*, 1987. Used with permission of the publisher.)

In order to identify the nature of the biotin-binding carrier protein in the rat intestine, we fractionated solubilized brush border membrane and cytosol by sucrose density gradient centrifugation. Figure 10 shows the biotinidase activity and biotin-binding profiles of the separated proteins from the two preparations. In both fractions biotinidase activity migrated slightly ahead of albumin (68K). The biotin-binding activity in cytosol and brush border preparations migrated to a position identical to the biotinidase peak, and there was good correlation at each point between two activities. Furthermore, when we used N-bromosuccinimide and *p*-chloromercuribenzoate (inhibitors of biotinidase activity) (Chauhan and Dakshinamurti, 1986; Dakshinamurti and Chauhan, 1986; Craft *et al.*, 1985), both biotinidase and biotin-binding activities were inhibited, suggesting that tryptophan and cysteine residues were involved in biotin-binding activity. These results suggested that biotinidase is the only protein in brush border membrane that binds biotin. Based on this *in vitro* study, it is suggested that biotinidase *in vivo* may function in the transport of biotin.

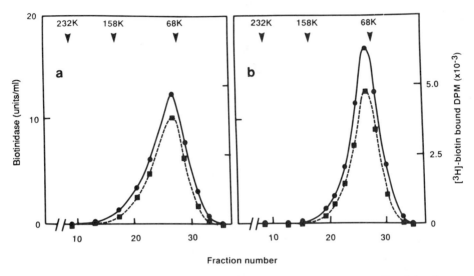

FIG. 10. (a) Cytosol and (b) the detergent-treated, dialyzed preparation of brush border proteins were separated by sucrose density gradient centrifugation. Cytosol and solubilized brush border proteins (0.3 ml) were layered in separate tubes on top of a 5–20% gradient of sucrose (12.5 ml) containing 0.1 M potassium phosphate buffer, pH 6.0, 1 mM 2-mercaptoethanol, and 1 mM EDTA. Centrifugation was at 3°C for 22 hours at 35,000 rpm in the Beckman SW-40 Ti rotor. At the end of the run, fractions were collected from the bottom of the gradient and analyzed for biotinidase (●) and biotin-binding activity (■). (From Dakshinamurti et al., 1987. Used with permission of the publisher.)

D. HOLOCARBOXYLASE SYNTHETASE

Biotin carboxylases are synthesized in the form of the apoproteins that undergo posttranslational covalent modification by the addition of biotin, the prosthetic group, to the ε-amino group of lysine of the apoproteins. This covalent attachment of biotin to a specific lysine in the apoenzyme is catalyzed by biotin-holocarboxylase synthetase in a two-step reaction [Eqs. (1) and (2)].

$$\text{ATP} + \text{biotin} \rightarrow 5'\text{-adenylate-biotin} \tag{1}$$

$$5'\text{-adenylate-biotin} + \text{apoenzyme} \rightarrow \text{holoenzyme} + \text{AMP} \tag{2}$$

Eisenberg et al. (1982) have purified this enzyme to homogeneity from E. coli and have shown that, apart from biotinating the apocarboxylases, this enzyme regulates the gene(s) for biotin biosynthesis. The reaction sequence for the biosynthesis of biotin by E. coli and genes involved has been reported by Eisenberg (1973, 1985). They have pointed out the similarities between the reactions involved in aminoacyl tRNA synthesis and biotin holoenzyme synthesis, in light of the regulatory role proposed for aminoacyl-tRNA. It was suggested that the holoenzyme synthetase with the bound biotinyl–5′-AMP functions as the corepressor for the biotin operon (Eisenberg et al., 1982). In the trp operon, the most extensively studied system (Yanofsky, 1981). trp-tRNA acts as a negative modulator at the attenuator site, terminating transcription of the trp operon under conditions of tryptophan excess or as a substrate for protein synthesis when the levels are low. In the biotin operon, the biotinyl–5′-AMP complex either inhibits initiation of transcription by binding to the operator site or utilizes the active form of biotin complex common to both reactions. The biotin operon in E. coli has been extensively studied and sequenced (Howard et al., 1985). Eisenberg et al. (1982) have shown that E. coli holocarboxylase synthetase is a single polypeptide of M_r 34,000. Biotin holocarboxylase synthetase can bind biotin with a K_d value of 1.3×10^{-7} M, and this value was decreased to 1.1×10^{-9} M with biotinyl-5′-adenylate, suggesting that the activated form of biotin binds much more tightly. Purification, assays, and properties of the bacterial biotin holocarboxylase synthetase are described in detail by Goss and Wood (1984).

The synthetase which biotinates the transcarboxylase (biotin--[methylmalonyl-CoA-carboxyltransferase] synthetase, EC 6.3.4.9) has been purified from P. shermanii by Wood and Harmon (1980). This reaction is fairly general in that the synthetase from one organism catalyzes biotination of apocarboxylases from heterologous sources. The synthetase from P. shermanii biotinates apopropionyl-CoA carboxylase from rat liver (Kosow et al., 1962). McAllister and Coon (1966) partially purified the holocarboxylase synthetase from rabbit liver and showed that it can biotinate apopropionyl-CoA carboxylase of rat liver and bacterial apo-β-methylcrotonyl-CoA carboxylase. No animal synthetases have yet been isolated and characterized.

E. NUCLEAR BIOTIN-BINDING PROTEIN

A biotin-binding protein has been isolated from pure preparations of rat liver nuclei (Bhullar, 1985). Polyacrylamide gel electrophoresis in sodium dodecyl sulfate provided an apparent subunit M_r of 60,000. The protein binds biotin in vitro in a reversible manner, with a maximum binding of 3.54 pmol of biotin per microgram of protein, and has a dissociation constant for biotin of 2.2×10^{-7} M. It is not known whether this protein functions in the transfer of biotin to the nuclei or whether it is important in expressing effects of biotin in the cell nucleus.

Such a function would be analagous to the effects of some hormones in enhancing expression of cellular protein synthesis. The mechanisms of action of steroid and thyroid hormones receptors have been extensively studied. In recent years similar action has been shown for certain classes of vitamins. Chambon and co-workers (Petkovich et al., 1987) have isolated cDNA coding for vitamin A receptor and have shown that the molecular mechanisms of the effect of retinoids on embryonic development, differentiation, and tumor cell growth are similar to those described for other members of nuclear receptor family. Similarly, O'Malley and co-workers (McDonnell et al., 1987) isolated cDNA coding for vitamin D_3 receptor and showed that vitamin D_3 upregulates its receptor via a direct increase in mRNA in 3T3 cells. In E. coli the biotin operon has been extensively studied and shown to be controlled by the biotin holocarboxylase synthetase (Eisenberg et al., 1982). However, such regulation and identification of biotin receptor in mammals are still to be identified.

VII. BIOTIN DEFICIENCY SYMPTOMS OF YET UNDETERMINED ETIOLOGY

A. SKIN LESIONS

The visible pathological changes in biotin-deficient animals and humans are scaly, seborrheic dermatoses, often accompanied by alopecia. The initial symptom of the deficiency in the rat is dermatitis in the groin, genitals, and neck and around the snout. In later stages of deficiency brown adherent scales, together with alopecia, are seen in and around the areas of inflammation. In mild cases the skin lesions may be limited to alopecia around the eye (spectacled eye). In the severe condition the dermatitis may involve the skin of the whole body (György and Langer, 1968). Seborrheic dermatitis in spontaneous cases of biotin deficiency has been described in very young infants and ascribed to the low content of biotin in human milk or possibly defective digestion or persistent diarrhea (Nisenson, 1969; Gauthier et al., 1957). Sweetman et al. (1979) have reported the case of an 11-year-old boy with hyperuricemia and mental retardation who developed alopecia totalis and a generalized erythematous scaly dermatitis. Since recognition of the MCD syndrome, characteristic dermatological features have been described in some afflicted children. Williams et al. (1983) have described three siblings with infantile-onset, biotin-responsive MCD. The characteristic dermatological manifestations included alopecia and peroral dermatitis. The dermatitis resolved completely within a few days in one of the infants treated orally with biotin. Munnich et al. (1980) described a 1-year-old child with features of MCD, including total alopecia and erythematous skin eruptions. In addition to a deficiency of mitochondrial carboxylases, there was also a deficiency of ACC. Interestingly, the concentration of linoleic acid in serum was also decreased in this child. There are also references to biotin deficiency as a complication of total parental nutrition. Deficiency symptoms such as skin lesions and alopecia have been reported in young as well as older patients on long-term total parenteral nutrition. These lesions responded to physiological doses of biotin (Mock et al., 1981; Innis and Sllardya, 1983).

Alopecia, dermatitis, and depigmentation, the signs of biotin deficiency in animals and humans, are also common to a deficiency of the essential fatty acids. The underlying cause of these dermal symptoms in biochemical terms is as yet unknown (Hansen et al., 1963). Kramer et al. (1984) have investigated the effect of biotin deficiency on polyunsaturated fatty acid metabolism in rats. To obviate the effects of generalized malnutrition, the profile of normalcy ratios of various fatty acids for biotin-deficient rats versus rats pair-fed a biotin-supplemented diet were calculated. The high ratios of odd-chain fatty acid (15 : 0 and 17 : 0) observed in liver phospholipids of deficient rats are explained on the basis of the accumulation of propionyl-CoA in deficiency and its utilization as the primer for odd-chain fatty acid synthesis. Similar increases of 15 : 0 and 17 : 0 saturated fatty acids in the plasma of a child with neonatal propionic acidemia have been reported (Hommes et al., 1968). In general, there was a decrease in the ω6 fatty acid series, specifically in 20 : 3 ω6 and 20 : 4 ω6 fatty acids. Mock et al. (1981) have reported decreased linoleic acid (9c.12c, 18 : 2) in the plasma of a biotin-deficient child with short gut syndrome. Munnich et al. (1980) also referred to a decrease in the concentration of linoleic acid in a 1-year-old child with MCD syndrome. Kramer et al. (1984) reported a very significant increase in the concentrations of ω3 fatty acids (9c.12c.15c, 18 : 3; 4c.7c.10c.13c.16c.19c.22c, 22 : 6) in liver phospholipids of biotin-deficient rats. These observations, particularly those of Kramer et al. (1984) on experimental biotin deficiency in the rat, pose the question about the difference in distribution between the ω6 and ω3 fatty acids. Inasmuch as the original source of the polyunsaturated fatty acids of both ω6 and ω3 series in rats is dietary safflower oil, why is there this profound difference in their tissue distribution? There is no information on whether both series of polyunsaturated fatty acids are absorbed in the intestinal tract to similar extents by the biotin-deficient rat. This area needs to be investigated further.

There have been other reports concerning the marked increase in the palmitoleate (9c, 16 : 1) to stearate (18 : 0) ratio in biotin deficiency (Balnave, 1971). This could be explained on the basis of the reported elevation in the desaturase activity in biotin-deficient rat tissues. However, the consequences of the elevation in tissue palmitoleic acid are not known.

The observations of decreased concentrations of linoleic acid in tissue of the biotin-deficient animal are significant, although the reason for this is not known. Watkins (1988) has reported that the conversion of linoleic acid to dihomo-т-linolenic acid (eicosatrienoic acid) is decreased in the biotin-deficient chick. Two linoleic acid derivatives (eicosatrienoic and eicosatetraenoic acids) are the precursors of prostaglandins of the 1 and 2 series, respectively.

The role of biotin deficiency in causing the observed skin lesions is only speculative at this time. The skin of all vertebrates produces a complex mixture of lipids found within the skin and on the skin surface. The surface lipids of mammals, in large part, are the products of the sebaceous glands. Quantitatively, the epidermal lipids contribute much less to total skin lipids, but physiologically they are very significant. The bulk of the sebaceous lipids is synthesized *de novo* by the cell. However, sebum seems not to be required for the health of the skin as human children and juvenile animals produce no sebum until the approach of sexual maturity, yet their skin and hair have excellent physical and cosmetic properties (Dowling *et al.*, 1983). The primary function of the epidermis is to generate a protective sheath, the stratum corneum, that protects the organism from both dessication and external assault (Elias, 1981). The stratum corneum is composed of anucleate corneocytes (bricks), consisting of a fibrous protein network and the intercellular matrix (mortar), composed mainly of neutral lipids. The composition of the stratum corneum lipids is markedly different from that of the lower cell layers of the viable epidermis. Phospholipids, a major component of the membrane lipids of the lower layers, is a minor component of the stratum corneum. Sterols, triglyceride, fatty acids, and hydrocarbons constitute 60–65% of the lipids of the stratum corneum. The predominance of neutral lipid-bearing long-chain saturated fatty acids is well suited for the provision of a hydrophobic barrier to water loss in the stratum corneum. In the essential fatty acid-deficient as well as the biotin-deficient rodent, the pelt is wet and matted due to a marked increase in transepidermal water loss, indicating a disturbance of epidermal barrier function (Menton, 1970). Linoleic acid itself constitutes as much as 5–10% of the fatty acids in the stratum corneum lipids. The molecular basis of the linoleic acid deficiency-induced lesions is not known. Whether it is the direct consequence of linoleate deficiency or the result of secondary epidermal hyperproliferation, due to diminished levels of prostanoids, is an area of current investigation. Evidence in favor of a direct role for linoleic acid in barrier function has been provided (Elias, 1981). Although topical prostaglandins correct the scaling of the skin of essential fatty acid-deficient animals, they do not reverse the defect in barrier function as effectively as topically applied linoleic acid. Moreover, the defect in barrier function can be corrected over cyclooxygenase and lipooxygenase blockades (Williams and Elias, 1987). Thus, the combined defects, such as the decreases in the synthesis of long-chain fatty acids, in tissue linoleic acid, and in the conversion of linoleic acid to eicosatrienoic and eicosatetraenoic acids in the biotin-deficient animal, could all contribute to a defective composition of the stratum corneum lipids, resulting in impaired barrier function. This could explain the similarity of the skin lesions in both biotin deficiency and essential fatty acid deficiency. Further work designed to verify this hypothesis is warranted.

B. IMMUNE DYSFUNCTION

The early work of Axelrod and co-workers (Prazansky and Axelrod, 1955; Axelrod, 1978; Kumar and Axelrod, 1978) led to the recognition that the immune system is impaired in the biotin-deficient animal. They found that lack of biotin prevented normal primary humoral immune response. Generalized forms of severe malnutrition, such as kwashiorkor and marasmus, are known to affect immunocompetence. These forms of generalized malnutrition are also accompanied by specific micronutrient deficiencies as well. Beisel (1982) has suggested a reevaluation of this area in its broader perspective. The mechanism of action for most of the vitamins on the host's immune response is not known.

Kung et al. (1979) studied the requirement for biotin in the cytotoxic T-cell response. DBA/2 or $B_6D_2F_1$ peritoneal cells served as stimulator cells, while C57BL/6 spleen cells were used as responding cells. [56]Cr-labeled P-815 mastocytoma cells were used as target cells, and the release of [56]Cr was used to assay cell-mediated cytotoxicity. They found that in vitro generation of cytotoxic T lymphocytes required a suitable synthetic medium supplemented with serum. Dialyzed calf serum was deficient in an essential factor, which was recognized to be biotin. It was proposed that biotin was essential in view of its role as the prosthetic group of ACC, the key enzyme of lipogenesis. Fatty acid synthesis is an essential component of the process of membrane genesis. A closer examination of their results indicates that the generation of cytotoxic T cells is partially inhibited by avidin when it was added to a fatty acid-supplemented fetal calf serum containing Eagle's minimum essential medium. Mammalian cells cultured in a serum containing medium are capable of using albumin-bound fatty acids for the *de novo* synthesis of structural lipids (Mackenzie *et al.*, 1978). In view of this, the authors suggested that the primary function of biotin is in the "modulation of the fatty acid pool destined for structural lipid synthesis." Thus, biotin seems to be required during proliferation and emergence of cytotoxicity in the clone of responding T cells.

Further understanding of the role of biotin in immune function comes from studies on the biotin-dependent single and multiple carboxylase deficiency syndromes. Immunodeficiency has been described in one patient with propionic acidemia (Mueller *et al.*, 1980). Cowan *et al.* (1979) and Saunders *et al.* (1980) studied patients with central nervous system dysfunction, immunodeficiencies, conjunctivitis, and alopecia. These deficiences were attributed to a biotin-responsive MCD. The immune system defects included a decrease in serum immunoglobulin A (IgA) concentration, lack of antibody production after pneumococcal polysaccharide vaccine, absence of delayed dermal hypersensitivity reaction, and a diminished T-cell response to stimulation with *Candida* antigens. Chronic mucocutaneous candidiasis is a consistent clinical feature of infants with biotin-responsive carboxylase deficiency. Bacteremia and candidiasis are also seen in children with protein calorie malnutrition. Multiple vitamin deficiencies are always associated with this condition. Dietary biotin deficiency in children resulted in similar clinical symptoms (Sweetman *et al.*, 1979). The association of immune dysfunction with carboxylase deficiency is of great clinical importance. It is not clear whether this is due to a direct effect of biotin on the functioning of the immune system or to an indirect effect of the accumulated organic acids. If the latter were the reason, patients with organic acidemia unrelated to biotin deficiency or dependency would also be defective in immunocompetence. Patients with methylmalonic acidemia, however, do not consistently show abnormalities in immunofunction (Church *et al.*, 1984), thus indicating a more direct function of biotin.

Petrelli *et al.* (1981) reported that in biotin-deficient guinea pigs there was an increase in the number of leukocytes, specifically in the number of circulating neutrophils. Lymphocytes carrying B- and T-cell markers were decreased. Incubation of lymphocytes from deficient animals with biotin increased the number of lymphocytes carrying Band T-cell markers. Rabin (1983) studied the inhibition of experimentally induced autoimmunity in biotin-deficient rats. Biotin deficiency produced a marked reduction in thymus size and cellularity. It also prevented the development of experimental allergic encephalomyelitis following immunization with guinea pig myelin basic protein. Lymphocytes from rats fed a biotin-supplemented diet and immunized to myelin basic protein were capable of producing this disease in animals fed a biotin-deficient or biotin-supplemented diet. However, lymphocytes from biotin-deficient rats could not produce this disease in recipient animals, indicating that the afferent limb of immune response is impaired in biotin deficiency. Biotin is necessary for the generation of cytotoxic T lymphocytes. A lack of this function has been suggested as an explanation for the lack of development of experimental allergic encephalomyelitis in biotin-deficient animals.

Although the role of biotin in immune function has generally been ascribed to its effects on lipid synthesis, it is clear that fatty acid synthesis is not the only function of biotin. It is possible that the immune deficiencies could result from impairment of DNA synthesis in T cells. Addition of dibutyryl-cGMP to *in vitro* cultures restored both Peyer's patch lymphocyte IgM and IgA anti-sheep erythrocyte responses of mice fed a low-protein diet, whereas it had no effect on mice fed a high-protein diet (Weiss and Petro, 1986). A role for cGMP in cell activation in general and lymphocyte activation in particular has been suggested (Christman *et al.*, 1978). In view of our findings on the effect of biotin on guanylate cyclase activity and cGMP concentrations (Singh and Dakshinamurti, 1988), it is possible that the effect of biotin deficiency or dependency on immune dysfunction might be related to its effect on cGMP. This remains to be investigated further.

C. NEUROLOGICAL ABNORMALITIES

Isolated deficiencies of each of the biotin-dependent carboxylases have been reported. Intolerance to higher levels of protein intake or intercurrent infections leads to episodes of organic acidemia in these conditions. Failure to adequately treat these conditions leads to mental retardation, seizure, coma, and death. Some patients with isolated PCC deficiency have been successfully treated with biotin (Barnes *et al.*, 1970). The clinical features of PC deficiency include metabolic acidosis, hypotonia, delayed physical and mental development, and seizures. Administration of large doses of biotin has not been successful in the treatment of this condition (Hommes *et al.*, 1980). Leonard *et al.* (1981) described a 1-month-old with spasms that progressed to generalized seizures; urinary β-hydroxyisovaleric and lactic acids were elevated. There was improvement upon treatment with biotin by mouth. A case of isolated ACC deficiency in a newborn female with hypotonic myopathy and neurological damage has been reported (Blom et al., 1981).

Since the recognition of both neonatal (early-onset) and infantile (late-onset) forms of MCD syndromes, most reports of MCD include dermatological, immunological, and neurological disorders in the afflicted patients (Wolf and Feldman, 1982). Zak and D'Ambrosio (1985) described a 12-month-old male who underwent surgical correction of a short bowel syndrome at 6 months of age and had been maintained by total parenteral nutrition. The child had severe seizures and showed developmental delay. Ophthalmologic diagnosis of a Wernicke's type nystagmus was made. Daily biotin supplementation (100 mg) led to marked improvement. Suchy et al. (1985) and DiRocco et al. (1984) have described the neurological symptoms of biotinidase deficiency and suggest that these symptoms may be due to the accumulation of toxic metabolites in the brain. Low et al. (1986) have reported a patient with a progressive neurological disorder and metabolic acidosis, with an elevated urinary excretion of p-hydroxyisovaleric acid. Within 36 hours of the first biotin dose, there was a dramatic clinical improvement. Yatsidis et al. (1984) studied patients on chronic hemodialysis for 2–10 years who suffered from dialysis dementia and peripheral neuropathy. Treatment with biotin (10 mg/day) caused marked improvement in all patients within 3 months of the start of biotin therapy. The mechanism of the neurological defect in biotin-responsive carboxylase deficiencies is not known.

Suchy and Wolf (1986) suggest that since lipids are important structural components of both the brain and skin, the cutaneous and neurological disorders may be the result of defective lipid metabolism in biotin deficiency. In this study, total, free, and esterified cholesterol contents of the liver and the brain in biotin-deficient rats were not altered, confirming our earlier report in which we found no change in the rate of cholesterol synthesis (Dakshinamurti and Desjardins, 1968). Thus, it is unlikely that the neurological symptoms might be caused by disturbances in cholesterol or lipoprotein metabolism. It is possible that in the biotin-deficient condition the decrease in fatty acid synthesis might affect the formation of long-chain fatty acids, including nervonic acid. Lipids are essential in central nervous system function but the central role of pyruvate in cerebral oxidative metabolism must also be considered. Both pyruvate dehydrogenase, which forms acetyl-CoA from pyruvate, and pyruvate carboxylase, which forms oxaloacetate from pyruvate, are crucial enzymes for the smooth functioning of the tricarboxylic acid cycle (Fig. 2). Decreased activity of PC would cause decreased availability of oxaloacetate for the Kreb's cycle. Further, when oxidative metabolism is decreased, pyruvate would be reduced to lactate. The neurological symptoms of biotin deficiency are similar to those seen in other conditions of lactic acidosis, including Leigh's subacute necrotizing encephalomyelopathy (Murphy *et al.*, 1981). The quick response of the neurological condition in MCD syndrome to biotin therapy would also indicate that the defect is a reversible metabolic condition. Facci *et al.* (1985) have reported that central nervous system neurons, cultured as monolayers at low density, need exogeneous pyruvate for their survival and that the pyruvate requirement is reduced by low-molecular-weight components of DMEM. Among these are the vitamins pyridoxine, riboflavin, and biotin. The α-keto acid residues of the transamination process catalyzed by pyridoxal phosphate-containing enzymes are oxidatively degraded by dehydrogenases that utilize riboflavin-derived coenzymes, and biotin may be required in providing oxaloacetate through the PC reaction.

D. TERATOGENIC EFFECTS

Congenital malformations have been reported in chick embryos of domestic fowl maintained on a biotin-deficient diet (Cravens *et al.*, 1944). Kennedy and Palmer (1945) found that female rats given a biotin-deficient diet maintained a normal estrus cycle and progressed through gestation normally until the 11th–13th days of intrauterine life. From then on, and particularly around the 20th and 21st days of gestation, there was a high rate of fetal resorption, which coincided with the period of most rapid fetal growth. During this period the transfer of biotin from the mother to the fetus was very high. Rose *et al.* (1956) found that in the postnatal period lactation was arrested by the 15th day postpartum. However, Giroud *et al.* (1956) have reported that in the female rat 90% of the implanted eggs gave normal fetuses, although the maternal deficiency was acute. These contradictory observations cannot be explained.

In a more recent study, using mice, Watanabe (1983; Watanabe and Endo, 1984) found that more than 90% of the fetuses from biotin-deficient females showed external or skeletal congenital abnormalities. The predominant malformations included micrognathia, cleft palate, and micromelia. In spite of the fetal malformations and intrauterine growth retardation their dams did not exhibit any overt signs of biotin deficiency. Supplementation of biotin in the diet prevented the malformations. The specific cause of intrauterine growth retardation or teratogenesis is not known. In view of the suggested role of the biotin carboxylases in major metabolic pathways, it is not surprising that a deficiency of this vitamin would lead to reproductive failure or congenital malformations. A drastic deficiency of biotin obviously would be incompatible with life and would explain the high rate of fetal resorption in the deficient state.

VIII. Conclusion

Biotin is the prosthetic group of the carboxylases involved in CO_2 fixation. Of these carboxylases, only four are found in animal tissues. Nevertheless, the effect of biotin deficiency in animals, including humans, is quite severe. Apart from the scaly dermatitis characteristic of this deficiency, other functions including the neuromuscular and immune systems, are adversely affected. The biochemical implications of biotin deficiency are discussed in this context. In addition to a prosthetic group function, it appears that biotin might be involved in the synthesis of growth/transformation factors. Studies on the isolation, distribution, and characterization of biotinidase indicate that this might be the sought-after putative biotin-carrier protein.

REFERENCES

Alberts, A. W., and Vagelos, P. R. (1972). Acyl-CoA carboxylase. *Enzymes* **6,** 37–82.
Allen, R. W., and Moskowitz, M. (1973). Regulation of the rate of protein synthesis in BHK21 cells by exogenous serine, *Exp. Cell Res.* **116,** 139–152.
Anderson, K. M., Mendelson, I. S., and Gusik, G. (1975). Solubilized DNA-dependent nuclear RNA polymerases from the mammary glands of late-pregnant rats. *Biochim. Biophys. Acta* **343,** 56–66.
Argarana, C. E., Kuntz, I. D., Birken, S., Axel, R., and Cantor, C. R. (1986). Molecular cloning and nucleotide sequence of the streptavidin gene. *Nucleic Acids Res.* **14,** 1871–1882.
Axelrod, A. E. (1978). The role of nutritional factors in the antibody response of anamestic response. *Am. J. Clin. Nutr.* **6,** 119–125.
Bai, D. H., Pape, E., Lopex-Casilas, F., Luo, X. C., Dixon, J. E., and Kim, K. (1986). Molecular cloning of cDNA for acetyl-coenzyme A carboxylase. *J. Biol. Chem.* **261,** 12395–99.
Baker, H. (1985). Assessment of biotin status. *Ann. N.Y. Acad. Sci.* **447,** 129–132.
Ballard, F. J., and Hanson, R. W. (1967). The citrate cleavage pathway and lipogenesis in rat adipose tissue: Replenishment of oxaloacetate. *J. Lipid Res.* **8,** 73–79.
Balnave, D. (1971). The influence of biotin upon the utilization of acetate and palmitate by chick liver *in vitro. Int. J. Biochem.* **2,** 99–110.
Barnes, N. D., Hull, D., Balgobin, L., and Gompertz, D. (1970). Biotin-responsive propionic acidemia. *Lancet* **2,** 244–245.
Baumgartner, E. R., Suormala, T., Wick, H., Bausch, J., and Bonjour, J. P. (1985).

Biotinidase deficiency associated with renal loss of biocytin and biotin. *Ann. N.Y. Acad. Sci.* **447**, 272–287.

Baxter, R. M. and Quastel, J. H. (1953). The enzymatic breakdown of d-biotin *in vitro. J. Biol. Chem.* **201**, 751–764.

Beisel, W. R. (1982). Single nutrients and immunity. *Am. J. Clin. Nutr.* **35**, Suppl., 417–418.

Berger, E., Long, E., and Semenza, G. (1972). The sodium activation of biotin absorption in hamster small intestine. *Biochim. Biophys. Acta* **255**, 873–87.

Bernlohr, D. A., Bolanowski, M. A., Kelly, T. J., Jr., and Lane, M. D. (1985). Evidence for an increase in transcription of specific mRNA during differentiation of 3T3-L1 preadipocytes. *J. Biol. Chem.* **260**, 5563–5567.

Bhullar, R. P. (1985). Regulation of acetyl-CoA carboxylase and role of biotin in cellular functions. Ph.D. Thesis, University of Manitoba, Winnipeg, Canada.

Bhullar, R. P., and Dakshinamurti, K. (1985). The effects of biotin on cellular functions in HeLa cells. *J. Cell. Physiol.* **122**, 425–430.

Blom, W., DeMuinck Keizer, S. M. P. F., and Stolti, H. R. (1981). Acetyl CoA carboxylase deficiency: An inborn error of *de novo* fatty acid synthesis. *N. Engl. J. Med.* **305**, 465–466.

Boeckx, R. L. O., and Dakshinamurti, K. (1974). Biotin-mediated protein biosynthesis. *Biochem. J.* **140**, 549–556.

Boeckx, R. L. O., and Dakshinamurti, K. (1975). Effect of biotin on ribonucleic acid synthesis. *Biochim. Biophys. Acta* **383**, 282–289.

Bowers-Komro, D. M., and McCormick, D. B. (1985). Biotin uptake by isolated rat liver hepatocytes. *Ann. N.Y. Acad. Sci.* **447**, 350–358.

Bowman, B. B., Selhub, J., and Rosenberg, D. E. (1986). Intestinal absorption of biotin in the rat. *J. Nutr.* **116**, 1266–1271.

Brady, R. N., Ruis, H., McCormick, D. B., and Wright, L. D. (1966). Bacterial degradation of biotin. Catabolism of ^{14}C-biotin and its sulfoxides. *J. Biol. Chem.* **241**, 4717–4721.

Braughler, J. M., Mittal, C. K., and Murad, F. (1979). Purification of soluble guanylate cyclase from rat liver. *Proc. Natl. Acad. Sci. U.S.A.* **76**, 219–222.

Brewer, L. E., and Edwards, H. M. J. (1972). Studies on the biotin requirement of broiler breeders. *Poult. Sci.* **51**, 619–624.

Brownsey, R. W., and Denton, R. M. (1987). Acetyl-coenzyme A carboxylase. *Enzymes* **18**, 123–46.

Burri, J., Sweetman, L., and Nyhan, W. L. (1981). Mutant holocarboxylase synthetase. Evidence for the enzyme defect in early infantile biotin-responsive multiple carboxylase deficiency. *J. Clin. Invest.* **68**, 1491–1495.

Canas, P. E., and Congote, L. F. (1984). Effect of cGMP on RNA polymerase II activities in fetal calf liver nuclei and in purified enzyme preparations. *Exp. Biol.* **43**, 5–11.

Chalifour, L. E. (1982). The biotin requirement of cells in culture and the uptake of the avidin–biotin complex. Ph.D. Thesis, University of Manitoba, Winnipeg, Canada.

Chalifour, L. E., and Dakshinamurti, K. (1982a). The requirement of human fibroblasts in culture. *Biochem. Biophys. Res. Commun.* **104**, 1047–1053.

Chalifour, L. E., and Dakshinamurti, K. (1982b). The characterization of the uptake of avidin–biotin complex by HeLa cells. *Biochim. Biophys. Acta* **721**, 64–69.

Chalifour, L. E., and Dakshinamurti, K. (1983). The partial characterization of the binding of avidin–biotin complex to rat liver plasma membrane. *Biochem. J.* **210**, 121–128.

Chauhan, J., and Dakshinamurti, K. (1986). Purification and characterization of human serum biotinidase. *J. Biol. Chem.* **261**, 4268–4275.

Chauhan, J., and Dakshinamurti, K. (1988). Role of human serum biotinidase as biotin-binding protein. *Biochem. J.* **256**, 265–270.

Chauhan, J., Dakshinamurti, K., Dodd, J. G., and Matusik, R. J. (1988). Cloning and sequence of cDNA of human liver biotinidase. *Can. Fed. Biol. Soc.* **31**, 184 (abstr).

Cheng, D. K. S., and Moskowitz, M. (1982). Growth stimulation of Rous sarcoma virus-transformed BHK cells by biotin and serum lipids. *J. Cell. Physiol.* **113**, 487–493.

Christman, T. D., Garbers, D. L., Parks, M. A., and Hardman, J. G. (1978). Characterization of particulate and soluble guanylate cyclase from rat lung. *J. Biol. Chem.* **250**, 2329–2334.

Christner, J. E., Schlesinger, M. J., and Coon, M. J. (1964). Enzymatic activation of biotin. Biotinyl adenylate formation. *J. Biol. Chem.* **239**, 3997–4002.

Church, J. A., Koch, R., Shaw, K. N. F., Nye, C. A., and Donnell, G. N. (1984). Immunofunction in methyl malonic aciduria. *J. Inherited Metab. Dis.* **7**, 12–14.

Cohen, D. C., and Gospodarowicz, D. (1985). Biotin and choline replace the growth requirement of Madin–Darby canine kidney cells for high density lipoprotein. *J. Cell. Physiol.* **124**, 96–106.

Cohen, N. D., and Thomas, M. (1982). Biotin transport into fully differentiated 3T3-L1 cells. *Biochem. Biophys. Res. Commun.* **108**, 1508–1516.

Collins, J. C., Morell, A. G., and Stockert, R. J. (1987). Biotin is required for expression of the asiloglycoprotein receptor (ASGP-R) in HepG2. *J. Cell Biol.* **105**, 330 (abstr).

Couch, J. R., Craven, W. W., Elvehjem, C. A., and Halpin, J. G. (1949). Studies on the function of biotin in the domestic fowl. *Arch. Biochem.* **21**, 77–86.

Cowan, M. S., Packman, S., Wara, D. W., Ammann, A. J., Yashino, M., Sweetman, L., and Nyhan, W. (1979). Multiple biotin-dependent carboxylase deficiencies associated with defect in T cells and B-cell immunity. *Lancet* **2**, 115–118.

Craft, D. V., Goss, N. H., Chandramouli, N., and Wood, H. G. (1985). Purification of biotinidase from human plasma and its activity on biotinyl peptides. *Biochemistry* **24**, 2471–2476.

Cravens, W. W., McGibbon, W. H., and Sebesta, E. E. (1944). Effect of biotin deficiency on embryonic development in the domestic fowl. *Anat. Rec.* **90**, 55–64.

Dakshinamurti, K., and Bhagavan, H. N. E., eds. (1985). Biotin. *Ann. N.Y. Acad. Sci.* **447**.

Dakshinamurti, K., and Chalifour, L. E. (1981). The biotin requirement of HeLa cells. *J. Cell. Physiol.* **107**, 427–438.

Dakshinamurti, K. and Chauhan, J. (1986). Role of biotinidase as carrier protein in human plasma. *Fed. Proc., Fed. Am. Soc. Exp. Biol.* **45**, 584 (abstr.).

Dakshinamurti, K., and Chauhan, J. (1988). Regulation of biotin enzymes. *Annu. Rev. Nutr.* **8**, 211–233.

Dakshinamurti, K., and Chauhan, J. (1989). Non-avidin biotin-binding proteins. *In* "Methods in Enzymology" (M. Wilchek and A. Bayer, eds.). Academic Press, San Diego, California (in press).

Dakshinamurti, K., and Cheah-Tan, C. (1968a). Liver glucokinase of the biotin deficient rat. *Can. J. Biochem.* **46**, 75–80.

Dakshinamurti, K., and Cheah-Tan, C. (1968b). Biotin-mediated synthesis of hepatic glucokinase in the rat. *Arch. Biochem. Biophys.* **127**, 17–21.

Dakshinamurti, K. and Desjardins, P. R. (1968). Lipogenesis in biotin deficiency. *Can. J. Biochem.* **46**, 1261–1267.

Dakshinamurti, K. and Hong, H. C. (1969). Regulation of key hepatic glycolytic enzymes. *Enzymol. Biol. Clin.* **11**, 423–428.

Dakshinamurti, K. and Mistry, S. P. (1963a). Tissue and intracellular distribution of biotin-C¹⁴OOH in rats and chick. *J. Biol. Chem.* **238**, 294–296.

Dakshinamurti, K. and Mistry, S. P. (1963b). Amino acid incorporation and biotin deficiency. *J. Biol. Chem.* **238**, 297–301.

Dakshinamurti, K., and Rector, E. S. (1989). Monoclonal antibodies to biotin. *In* "Methods in Enzymology" (M. Wilchek and E. A. Bayer, eds.). Academic Press, San Diego, California (in press).

Dakshinamurti, K., Chalifour, L., and Bhullar, R. P. (1985). Requirement for biotin and the function of biotin in cells in culture. *Ann. N.Y. Acad. Sci.* **447**, 38–55.

Dakshinamurti, K., Bhullar, R. P., Scoot, A., Rector, E. S., Delespesse, G., and Sehon, A. H. (1986). Production and characterization of a monoclonal antibody to biotin. *Biochem. J.* **237**, 477–482.

Dakshinamurti, K., Chauhan, J., and Ebrahim, H. (1987). Intestinal absorption of biotin and biocytin in the rat. *Biosci. Rep.* **7**, 667–673.

Delange, R. J. (1970). Egg white avidin. I. Amino acid composition; sequence of the amino- and carboxyl-terminal cyanogen bromide peptides. *J. Biol. Chem.* **245**, 907–916.

Delost, P., and Terroine, T. (1956). Les troubles endocriniens dans la carence en biotin. *Arch. Sci. Physiol.* **10**, 17–51.

DiRocco, M. A., Superti-Furga, A., and Durand, P. (1984). Different organic acid patterns in urine and in cerebrospinal fluid in a patient with biotinidase deficiency. *J. Inherited Metab. Dis.* **7**, 119–120.

Dowling, D. T., Stewart, M. E., Wertz, P. W., Collon, S. W., VI, and Strauss, J. S. (1983). Skin lipids. *Comp. Biochem. Physiol. B* **76B**, 673–678.

Dupree, L. T., Sanford, K. K., Westfall, B. B., and Covalensky, A. B. (1962). Influence of serum protein on determination of nutritional requirement of cells in culture. *Exp. Cell Res.* **28**, 381–405.

Du Vigneaud, W., Dittmer, K., Hague, B., and Long, B. (1942a). Growth stimulating effect of biotin for diphtheria bacillus in absence of pimelic acid. *Science* **96**, 186–187.

Du Vigneaud, W., Melville, D. B., Folkers, K., Wolf, D. E., and Mozingo, R. (1942b). The structure of biotin: A study of desthiobiotin. *J. Biol. Chem.* **146**, 475–85.

Eagle, H. (1955). The minimum requirement of the L and HeLa cells in tissue culture, the production of specific vitamin deficiencies and their cure. *J. Exp. Med.* **102**, 595–600.

Eakin, R. E., and Eakin, E. A. (1942). Biosynthesis of biotin. *Science* **96**, 187–188.

Eakin, R. E., Snell, E. E., and Williams, R. J. (1940). A constituent of raw egg white capable of inactivating biotin *in vitro*. *J. Biol. Chem.* **136**, 801–802.

Earp, H. S. (1980). The role of insulin, glucagon, and cAMP in the regulation of hepatocyte guanylate cyclase activity. *J. Biol. Chem.* **255**, 8979–8982.

Eisenberg, M. A. (1962). The incorporation of 1,7 C¹⁴ pimelic acid into biotin vitamers. *Biochem. Biophys. Res. Commun.* **8**, 437–441.

Eisenberg, M. A. (1973). Biotin: Biogenesis, transport, and their regulation. *Adv. Enzymol.* **38**, 317–72.

Eisenberg, M. A. (1985). Regulation of biotin operon in *E. coli*. *Ann. N.Y. Acad. Sci.* **447**, 335–49.

Eisenberg, M. A., and Star, C. (1968). Synthesis of 7-oxo-8-aminopelargonic acid, a biotin vitamer, in cell free extracts of *Escherichia coli* biotin auxotrophs. *J. Bacteriol.* **96**, 1291–1297.

Eisenberg, M. A., Prakash, O., and Hsiung, S. C. (1982). Purification and properties of the biotin repressor. A bifunctional protein. *J. Biol. Chem.* **257**, 15167–73.

Elias, P. M. (1981). Epidermal lipids, membranes and keratinization. *Int. J. Dermatol.* **20**, 1–19.

Facci, L., Skaper, S. D., and Varon, S. (1985). Selected nutrients reduce the pyruvate requirement for survival *in vitro* of chick central nervous system neurons. *J. Neurosci. Res.* **14**, 293–302.

Frank, O., Luisada-Opper, A. V., Feingold, S., and Baker, H. (1970). Vitamin binding by humans and some animal plasma proteins. *Nutr. Rep. Int.* **1**, 161–168.

Freytag, S. O., and Collier, K. J. (1984). Molecular cloning of a cDNA for human pyruvate carboxylase. Structural relationship to other biotin-containing carboxylases and regulation of mRNA content in differentiating preadipocytes. *J. Biol. Chem.* **259**, 12831–37.

Gauthier, P., Gauthier, A., and Thelin, F. (1957). Dermatite seborrhoide et biotine. *Int. Z. Vitaminforsch.* **28**, 61–67.

Gehrig, D. and Leuthardt, F. (1976). A biotin-binding glycoprotein from human plasma: Isolation and characterization. *Proc. Int. Cong. Biochem., 10th, 1976* Abstr., p. 208.

Giroud, A., Lefebvres, J., and Dupuis, R. (1956). Carence en biotine et reproduction chezlaratte. *C.R. Seances Soc. Biol. Ses Fil.* **150**, 2066–2067.

Goldberg, N. D., Graft, G., Haddox, M. K., Stephenson, J. H., Glass, D. E., and Moser, M. E. (1978). Redox modulation of splenic cell soluble guanylate cyclase activity: Activation by hydrophilic and hydrophobic oxidants represented by ascorbic acid and dehydrophobic acids, fatty acid hydroperoxides, and prostagladin endoperoxides. *Adv. Cyclic Nucleotide Res.* **9**, 101–130.

Gore, J., Hoinard, C., and Mainganlt, P. (1986). Biotin uptake by isolated rat intestinal cells. *Biochim. Biophys. Acta* **856**, 357–361.

Gospodarowicz, D. and Cohen, D. C. (1988). MDCK cell growth in defind medium: Roles of high density lipoproteins, biotin, pyruvate and an autocrine growth factor. *FASEB J.* **2**, A726 (abstr).

Goss, N. H., and Wood, H. G. (1984). Formation of N^ε-(biotinyl) lysine in biotin enzymes. *In* "Methods in Enzymology" (G. Di Sabato, J. J. Langone, and H. Van Vunakis, eds.), Vol. 107, 261–278. Academic Press, Orlando, Florida.

Gravel, R. A., and Robinson, B. H. (1985). Biotin-dependent carboxylase deficineces (propionyl-CoA and pyruvate carboxylase). *Ann. N.Y. Acad. Sci.* **447**, 225–34.

Gravel, R. A., Lam, K.-F., Scully, K. J., and Hsia, Y. E. (1977). Genetic complementation of proionyl-CoA carboxylase deficiency in cultured human fibroblasts. *Am. J. Hum. Genet.* **29**, 378–88.

Green, H., and Kehinde, O. (1974). Subline of mouse 3T3 cells that accumulate lipid. *Cell (Cambridge, Mass.)* **1**, 113–16.

Green, N. M. (1962). Spectroscopic evidence for the participation of tryptophan residues in the binding of biotin by avidin. *Biochim. Biophys. Acta* **59**, 244–246.

Green, N. M. (1963a). The use of [^{14}C] biotin for kinetic studies and for assay. *Biochem. J.* **89**, 585–591.

Green, N. M. (1963b). Stability at extremes of pH and dissociation into subunits by guanidine hydrochloride. *Biochem. J.* **89**, 609–620.

Green, N. M. (1964a). The nature of the biotin-binding site. *Biochem. J.* **89**, 599–609.

Green, N. M. (1964b). The molecular weight of avidin. *Biochem. J.* **92**, 16c–17c.

Green, N. M. (1975). Avidin. *Adv. Protein Chem.* **29**, 85–133.

Green, N. M. and Toms, E. J. (1970). Purification and crystallization of avidin. *Biochem. J.* **118**, 67–70.

Guillerm, G., Frappier, F., Gaudry, M., and Marquet, A. (1977). On the mechanism of conversion of dethiobiotin to biotin in *Escherichia coli*. *Biochimie* **59**, 119–121.

György, P. (1939). The curative factor (vitamin H) for egg white injury, with particular reference to its presence in different foodstuffs and in yeast. *J. Biol. Chem.* **131**, 733–44.

György, P., and Rose, C. S. (1949). Distribution of biotin and avidin in hen's egg. *Proc. Soc. Exp. Biol. Med.* **49**, 294–298.

György, P., Rose, C. S., Eakin, R. E., Snell, E. E., and Williams, R. J. (1941). Egg-white injury as result of nonabsorption or inactivation of biotin. *Science* **93**, 477–478.

György, P., Harris, R. S., and Langer, B. W. J. (1968). Biotin. *In* "The Vitamins" (W. H. Sebrell, Jr. and R. S. Harris, eds.). Vol. 2, pp. 336–350. Academic Press, New York.

Hansen, A. E., Wiese, H. F., and Boelsche, A. N., Haggard, M. E., Adam, D. J. D., and Davis, H. (1963). Role of linoleic acid in infant nutrition. Clinical and chemical study of 428 infants fed on mixtures varying in kind and amount of fat. *Pediatrics* **31**, 171–192.

Harris, S. A., Wolf, D. E., Mozingo, R., and Folkes, K. (1943). Synthetic biotin. *Science* **97**, 447–48.

Hertz, R., and Sebrell, W. H. (1942). Occurrence of avidin in oviduct and secretion of genital tract of several species. *Science* **96**, 257.

Holmes, R. (1959). Long-term cultivation of human cells (Chang) in chemically defined medium and effect of added peptone fraction. *J. Biophys. Biochem. Cytol.* **6**, 535–536.

Hommes, F. A., Kuipers, J. R., Elema, J. D., Janse, J. F., and Janxis, J. P. (1968). Propionic acidemia, a new inborn error of metabolism. *Pediatr. Res.* **2**, 519–524.

Hommes, F. A., Scheyver, J., and Dias, T. (1980). Pyruvate carboxylase deficiency. Studies on patients and animal models system. *In* "Inherited Disorders of Carbohydrate Metabolism" (D. Burman, J. B. Holton and C. A. Pennock, eds.), pp. 269–289. University Park Press, Baltimore.

Howard, P. K., Shaw, J., and Otsuka, A. J. (1985). Nucleotide sequence of the *bir A* gene encoding the biotin operon repressor and biotin holoenzyme synthetase function of *Escherichia coli*. *Gene* **35**, 321–331.

Innis, S. M., and Sllardya, D. B. (1983). Possible biotin deficiency in adults receiving long term total parenteral nutrition. *Am. J. Clin. Nutr.* **37**, 185–187.

Izumi, Y., Morita, Y., Sato, K., Tani, Y., and Ogata, K. (1972a). Synthesis of biotin-vitamers from pimelic acid and coenzyme A by cell-free extraction of various bacteria. *Biochim. Biophys. Acta* **264**, 210–213.

Izumi, Y., Morita, Y., Tani, Y., and Ogata, K. (1972b). Partial purification and some properties of 7-keto-8-aminopelargonic acid synthetase, an enzyme involved in biotin biosynthesis. *Agric. Biol. Chem.* **36**, 510–521.

Izumi, Y., Sato, K., Tani, Y., and Ogata, K. (1973). Distribution of 7-keto-8-amino-pelargonic acid synthetase in bacterial and the control mechanism of the enzyme activity. *Agric. Biol. Chem.* **37**, 1335–1337.

Izumi, Y., Sato, K., Tani, Y., and Ogata, K. (1975). Diaminopelargonic acid aminotransferase, an enzyme involved in biotin biosynthesis by microorganisms. *Agric. Biol. Chem.* **39**, 175–181.

Johnson, L. D., and Haddon, J. M. (1975). cGMP and lymphocyte proliferation: Effects on DNA-dependent RNA polymerase I and II activities. *Biochem. Biophys. Res. Commun.* **65**, 1498–1505.

Kaplan, P. L., Anderson, M., and Ozanne, B. (1982). Transforming growth factor(s) production enables cells to grow in the absence of serum: An autocrine system. *Proc. Natl. Acad. Sci. U.S.A.* **79**, 485.

Kasturi, R., and Wakil, S. J. (1983). Increased synthesis and accumulation of phospholipids during differentiation of 3T3-L1 cells into adipocytes. *J. Biol. Chem.* **258**, 3559–4832.

Kennedy, C., and Palmer, L. S. (1945). Biotin deficiency in relation to reproduction and lactation. *Arch. Biochem.* **7**, 9–13.

Keranen, A. J. A. (1972). The biotin synthesis of HeLa cells *in vitro. Cancer Res.* **32**, 119–124.

Knappe, J., Brummer, W., and Biederbick, K. (1963). Reinigung und eigenschaften der biotinidase aus schweinenieren und *Lactobacillus casei. Biochem. Z.* **338**, 599–613.

Kogl, F., and Tonnis, B. (1936). Uber das Bios-Problem. Darstellung von krystallisiertem Biotin aus Eigelb. *Hoppe-Seyler's Z. Physiol. Chem.* **242**, 43–73.

Korpela, J. (1984). Avidin, a high affinity biotin-binding protein, as a tool and subject of biological research. *Med. Biol.* **62**, 5–26.

Kosow, D. B., Huang, S. C., and Lane, M. D. (1962). Propionyl holocarboxylase syntheis. I. preparation and properties of the enzyme system. *J. Biol. Chem.* **237**, 3633–3639.

Kramer, T. R., Briske-Anderson, M., Johnson, S. B., and Holman, R. T. (1984). Effects of biotin deficiency on polyunsaturated fatty acid metabolism in rats. *J. Nutr.* **114**, 2047–2052.

Kraus, J. P., Williamson, C. L., Firgaira, F. A., Yang-Feng, T. L., Munke, M., Francke, U., and Rosenberg, L. E. (1986a). Cloning and screening with nanogram amounts of immunopurified mRNAs: cDNA cloning and chromosomal mapping of cystathionine synthetase and the subunit of propionyl-CoA carboxylase. *Proc. Natl. Acad. Sci. U.S.A.* **83**, 2047–2051.

Kraus, J. P., Firgaira, F., Novotny, J., Kalousek, F., Williams, K. R., Williamson, C., Ohura, T., and Rosenberg, L. E. (1986b). Coding sequence of the precursor of the subunit of rat propionyl-CoA carboxylase. *Proc. Natl. Acad. Sci. U.S.A.* **83**, 8049–8053.

Krause, K. H., Bonjour, J. P., Berlit, P., and Kochen, W. (1985). Biotin status of epileptics. *Ann. N.Y. Acad. Sci.* **447**, 297–313.

Kumar, M., and Axelrod, A. E. (1978). Cellular antibody synthesis in thiamine, riboflavine, biotin and folic acid deficient rats. *Proc. Soc. Exp. Biol. Med.* **157**, 421–423.

Kung, J. T., Cosmo, G., Mackenzie, G., and Talmage, D. W. (1979). The requirement for biotin and fatty acids in the cytotoxic T-cell response. *Cell. Immunol.* **48**, 100–110.

Kuri-Harcuch, W., and Green, H. (1978). Adipose conversion of 3T3 cells depends on a serum factor. *Proc. Natl. Acad. Sci. U.S.A.* **75**, 6107–6109.

Kuri-Harcuch, W., and Marsch-Moreno, M. (1983). DNA synthesis and cell division related to adipose differentiation of 3T3 cells. *J. Cell. Physiol.* **114**, 39–44.

Kuri-Harcuch, W., Wise, L. S., and Green, H. (1978). Interruption of the adipose conversion of 3T3 cells by biotin deficiency: Differentiation without triglyceride accumulation. *Cell (Cambridge, Mass.)* **14**, 53–59.

Lamhonwah, T. A. M., Barankiewicz, T., Willard, H. F., Mahuran, D., and Quan, F. (1985). Propionic acidemia: Absence of alpha chain mRNA in pccA complementation group. *Am. J. Hum. Genet.* **37**, A164 (abstr.).

Lamhonwah, A., Barankiewicz, T. J., Willard, H. F., Mahuran, D. J., and Quan, F. (1986). Isolation of cDNA clones coding for the α and β chains of human propionylcoA carboxylase: Chromosomal assignments and DNA polymorphisms associated with PCCA and PCCB genes. *Proc. Natl. Acad. Sci. U.S.A.* **83**, 4864–68.

Lane, M. D., Moss, J., and Polakis, S. E. (1974). Acetyl coenzyme A carboxylase. *Curr. Top. Cell. Regul.* **8,** 139–95.

Leonard, J. V., Seakins, J. W. T., Bartlett, K., Hyde, J., Wilson, J., and Clayton, B. (1981). Inherited disorders of 3-methylcrotonyl CoA carboxylation. *Arch. Dis. Child.* **56,** 53–59.

Low, L. C. K., Stephenson, J. B. P., Bartlet, K., Seakins, J. W. T., and Shaikh, S. A. (1986). Biotin-reversible neurodegenerative disease in infancy. *Aust. Paediatr. J.* **22,** 65–68.

Lynen, F. (1967). The role of biotin-dependent carboxylation in biosynthetic reactions. *Biochem. J.* **102,** 381–400.

Mackall, J. C., and Lane, M. D. (1977). Role of pyruvate carboxylase in fatty acid synthesis: Alterations during preadipocyte differentiation. *Biochem. Biophys. Res. Commun.* **79,** 720–725.

Mackall, J. C., Student, A. K., Polakis, S. E., and Lane, M. D. (1976). Induction of lipogenesis during differentiation in a "preadipocyte" cell line. *J. Biol. Chem.* **251,** 6462–6464.

Mackenzie, C. G., Moritz, E., Wisneski, J. A., Reiss, O. K., and Mackenzie, J. B. (1978). Fatty acid ester turnover: A control factor in triacylglycerol and lipid-rich particle accumulation in cultured mammalian cells. *Mol. Cell. Biochem.* **19,** 7–15.

Maloy, W. L., Bowien, B. U., Zwolinski, G. K., Kumar, G. K., Wood, H. G., Ericsson, L. H., and Walsh, K. A. (1979). Amino acid sequence of the biotinyl subunit from transcarboxylase. *J. Biol. Chem.* **254,** 11615–22.

Mandella, R. D., Meslar, H. W., and White, H. B., III. (1978). Relationship between biotin-binding proteins from chicken plasma and egg yolk. *Biochem. J.* **175,** 629–633.

McAllister, H. C. and Coon, M. J. (1966). Further studies on the properties of liver propionyl coenzyme A holocarboxylase synthetase and the specificity of holocarboxylase formation. *J. Biol. Chem.* **241,** 2855–2861.

McCormick, D. B., and Wright, L. D. (1971). The metabolism of biotin and analogues. *In* "Comprehensive Biochemistry" (M. Florkin and E. H. Stotz, eds.), p. 81–110. Am. Elsevier, New York.

McDonnell, D. P., Mangelsdorf, D. J., Pike, J. W., Haussler, M. R., and O'Malley, B. W. (1987). Molecular cloning of complementary DNA encoding the avian receptor for vitamin D. *Science* **238,** 1214–1217.

McElroy, L. W., and Jukes, T. H. (1940). Formation of the anti egg-white-injury factor (biotin) in the rumen of the cow. *Proc. Soc. Exp. Biol. Med.* **45,** 296–297.

Meglasson, M. D., and Matschnisky, F. M. (1984). New perspective on pancreatic islet glucokinase. *Am. J. Physiol.* **246,** E1–E13.

Menton, D. N. (1970). The effect of essential fatty acid deficiency on fine structure of mouse skin. *J. Morphol.* **132,** 181–206.

Meslar, H. W., Camper, S. A., and White, H. B., III. (1978). Biotin-binding protein from egg yolk. A protein distinct from egg white avidin. *J. Biol. Chem.* **253,** 6979–6982.

Messmer, T. O., and Young, D. V. (1977). The effects of biotin and fatty acids on SV 3T3 cells growth in the presence of normal calf serum. *J. Cell. Physiol.* **90,** 265–270.

Mistry, S. P., and Dakshinamurti, K. (1964). Biochemistry of biotin. *Vitam. Horm. (N.Y.)* **22,** 1–55.

Mock, D. M., deLorrioner, A., Leibman, N. M., Sweetman, L., and Baker, H. (1981). Biotin deficiency: An unusual complication of parenteral alimentation. *N. Engl. J. Med.* **304,** 820–823.

Moskowitz, M., and Cheng, D. K. S. (1985). Stimulation of growth factor production in cultured cells by biotin. *Ann. N.Y. Acad. Sci.* **447,** 212–221.

Moss, J., and Lane, M. D. (1971). The biotin-dependent enzymes. *Adv. Enzymol.* **35,** 321–342.

Mueller, S., Falkenbers, N., Morch, E., and Jakobs, C. (1980). Propionacidaemia and immunodeficiency. *Lancet* **1,** 551–552.

Munnich, A., Saudnbray, J. M., Conde, F. X., Charpentier, C., Saurat, J. H., and Frezal, J. (1980). Fatty acid responsive alopecia in multiple carboxylase deficiency. *Lancet* **2,** 1080–1081.

Murphy, J. V., Isolioshi, F., Weinberg, M. B., and Utter, M. F. (1981). Pyruvate carboxylase deficiency: An alleged biochemical-caused Leigh's disease. *Pediatrics* **68,** 401–404.

Murty, C. V. R., and Adiga, P. R. (1985). Estrogen induction of biotin-binding protein in immature chicks: Kinetics, hormonal specificity and modulation. *Mol. Cell. Endocrinol.* **40,** 79–86.

Nakano, E. T., Ciampi, N. A., and Young, D. V. (1982). The identification of a serum viability factor for SV3T3 cells as biotin and its possible relationship to the maintenance of krebs cycle activity. *Arch. Biochem. Biophys.* **215,** 556–563.

Nisenson, A. (1969). Seborrheic dermatitis of infants: Treatment with biotin injection for the nursing mother. *Pediatrics* **44,** 1014–1016.

Nishimura, H., Yoshoka, K., and Iwashima, A. (1984). A method for determining binding kinetics applied to thiamine-binding protein. *Anal. Biochem.* **139,** 373–376.

Parry, R. J., and Kunitani, M. G. (1976). Biotin biosynthesis. I. The incorporation of specifically tritiated dethiobiotin into biotin. *J. Am. Chem. Soc.* **98,** 4024–4026.

Paulose, C. S., Thliveris, J., and Dakshinamurti, K. (1989). Testicular function in biotin deficiency. *Horm. Metab. Res.,* (in press).

Petkovich, M., Brand, N. J., Krust, A., and Chambon, P. (1987). A human retinoic acid receptor which belongs to the family of nuclear receptors. *Nature (London)* **330,** 444–450.

Petrelli, F., Moretti, P., and Champarate, G. (1981). Studies on the relationship between biotin and the behavior of B and T lymphocytes in the guinea pig. *Experientia* **37,** 1204–1206.

Pispa, J. (1965). Animal biotinidase. *Ann. Med. Exp. Biol. Fenn.* **43,** Suppl. 5, 5–39.

Prazansky, J., and Axelrod, A. E. (1955). Antibody production to diphthesia toxoid in vitamin deficient states. *Proc. Soc. Exp. Biol. Med.* **89,** 323–325.

Rabin, B. S. (1983). Inhibition of experimentally induced autoimmunity in rats by biotin deficiency. *J. Nutr.* **113,** 2316–2322.

Rolfe, B., and Eisenberg, M. A. (1968). Genetic and biochemical analysis of the biotin loci of *Escherichia coli* K-12. *J. Bacteriol.* **96,** 515–524.

Rose, M. R., Commural, R., and Mazella, O. (1956). Heriditary deficiencies. *Arch. Sci. Physiol.* **10,** 381–421.

Rosen, O. M., Smith, C. J., Hirsch, A., Lai, E., and Rubin, C. S. (1979). Recent studies of the 3T3-L1 adipocyte-like cell line. *Recent Prog. Horm. Res.* **35,** 477–499.

Rosenberg, L. E. (1983). Disorders of propionate and methylmalonate metabolism. *In* "The Metabolic Basis of Inherited Disease" (J. B. Stanbury, J. B. Wyngaarden, D. S. Fredrickson, J. I. Goldstein, and M. S. Brown, eds.), 5th ed., pp. 474–497. McGraw-Hill, New York.

Roth, K. S. (1985). Prenatal treatment of multiple carboxylase deficiency. *Ann. N.Y. Acad. Sci.* **447,** 263–271.

Roth, K. S., Yang, W., Allan, L., Saunders, M., Gravel, R. A., and Dakshinamurti, K.

(1982). Prenatal administration of biotin in biotin responsive multiple carboxylase deficiency. *Pediatr. Res.* **16**, 126–129.

Rudland, P. S., Gospodarowicz, D., and Seifert, W. (1974). Activation of guanylate cyclase and intracellular cyclic GMP by fibroblast growth factor. *Nature (London)* **250**, 771–773.

Rylatt, D. B., Keech, D. B., and Wallace, J. C. (1977). Pyruvate carboxylase: Isolation of the biotin-containing tryptic peptide and the determination of its primary sequence. *Arch. Biochem. Biophys.* **183**, 113–122.

Said, S. M., and Redha, R. (1987). A carrier-mediated system for transport of biotin in rat intestine *in vitro*. *Am. J. Physiol.* **252**, G52–G55.

Saunders, J. E., Malamud, N., Cowan, M. J., Packman, S., Amman, A. J., and Wara, D. W. (1980). Intermittent ataxia and immunodeficiency with multiple carboxylase deficiencies: A biotin responsive disorder. *Ann. Neurol.* **8**, 544–547.

Scatchard, G. (1949). The attractions of proteins for small molecules and ions. *Ann. N.Y. Acad. Sci.* **51**, 660–672.

Scheiner, J., and DeRitter, E. (1975). Biotin contents of feedstuffs. *J. Agric. Food Chem.* **23**, 1157–1162.

Sharma, C., Manjeshwar, R., and Weinhouse, S. (1963). Effects of diet and insulin on glucose-adenosine triphosphate phosphotransferase of rat liver. *J. Biol. Chem.* **238**, 3840–3845.

Shaw, J. H., and Phillips, P. H. (1942). Pathological studies of acute biotin deficiency in the rat. *Proc. Soc. Exp. Biol. Med.* **51**, 406–407.

Singh, I., and Dakshinamurti, K. (1988). Stimulation of guanylate cyclase and RNA polymerase II activities in HeLa cells and fibroblasts by biotin. *Mol. Cell. Biochem.* **79**, 47–55.

Sorrell, M. F., Frank, O., Thomas, A. D., Aquino, A., and Baker, H. (1971). Absorption of vitamins from large intestine *in vivo*. *Nutr. Rep. Int.* **3**, 143–48.

Spence, J. T., and Koudelka, A. P. (1984). Effects of biotin upon the intracellular level of cGMP and the activity of glucokinase in cultured rat hepatocytes. *J. Biol. Chem.* **259**, 6393–6396.

Spence, J. T., Merrill, M. J., and Pitot, H. C. (1981). Role of insulin, glucose, and cyclic GMP in the regulation of glukokinase in cultured hepatocytes. *J. Biol. Chem.* **256**, 1598–1603.

Spencer, R. P., and Brody, K. R. (1964). Biotin transport by small intestine of rat, hamster, and other species. *Am. J. Physiol.* **206**, 653–57.

Spiegelman, B. M., and Farmer, S. R. (1982). Decrease in tubulin and actin gene expression prior to morphological differentiation of 3T3 adipocytes. *Cell (Cambridge, Mass.)* **29**, 53–60.

Suchy, S. F., McVoy, J. S., and Wolf, B. (1985). Neurological symptoms of biotinidase deficiency: Possible explanation. *Neurology* **35**, 1510–1511.

Suchy, S. F., and Wolf, B. (1986). Effect of biotin deficiency and supplementation on lipid metabolism in rats: Cholesterol and lipoproteins. *Am. J. Clin. Nutr.* **43**, 831–838.

Sutton, M. R., Fall, R. R., Nervi, A. M., Alberts, A. W., Vagelos, P. R., and Bradshaw, R. A. (1977). Amino acid sequence of *Escherichia coli* carboxyl carrier protein (9100).*J. Biol. Chem.* **252**, 3934–3940.

Sweetman, L. (1981). Two forms of biotin-responsive multiple carboxylase deficiency. *J. Inherited Metab. Dis.* **4**, 53–54.

Sweetman, L., and Nyhan, W. L. (1986). Inheritable biotin-treatable disorders and associated phenomena. *Annu. Rev. Nutr.* **6**, 317–343.

Sweetman, L., Suhr, L., and Nyhan, W. L. (1979). Deficiencies of propionyl CoA and 3-methylcrotonyl-CoA carboxylase in a patient with dietary deficiency of biotin. *Clin. Res.* **27,** 118A (abstr.).

Sweetman, L., Burri, B. J., and Nyhan, W. L. (1985). Biotin holocarboxylase synthetase deficiency. *Ann. N.Y. Acad. Sci.* **447,** 288–296.

Swim, H. E., and Parke, R. F. (1958). Vitamin requirements of uterine fibroblasts, strain U12-79; their replacement by related compounds. *Arch. Biochem. Biophys.* **78,** 46–53.

Tanaka, K. (1981). New light on biotin deficiency. *N. Engl. J. Med.* **304,** 839–840.

Tatum, E. L. (1945). Desthiobiotin in the biosynthesis of biotin. *J. Biol. Chem.* **160,** 455–459.

Terroine, T. (1960). Physiology and biochemistry of biotin. *Vitam. Horm. (N.Y.)* **18,** 1–42.

Thoene, J. G., Lemons, R., and Baker, H. (1983). Impaired intestinal absorption of biotin in juvenile multiple carboxylase deficiency. *N. Engl. J. Med.* **308,** 639–642.

Thoma, R. W., and Peterson, W. H. (1954). The enzymatic degradation of soluble bound biotin. *J. Biol. Chem.* **210,** 569–579.

Thomson, R. C., Eakin, R. E., and Williams, R. J. (1941). The extraction of biotin from tissues. *Science* **94,** 589–590.

Tranter, H. S., and Board, R. G. (1982). The antimicrobial defence of avian eggs: biological perspective and chemical basis. *J. Appl. Biochem.* **4,** 295–338.

Turner, J. B., and Hughes, D. E. (1962). The absorption of some B-group vitamers by surviving rat intestine preparations. *Q. J. Exp. Physiol. Cogn. Med. Sci.* **47,** 107–123.

Ureta, T., Radojkovic, J., and Niemeyer, H. (1970). Inhibition by catecholamines of the induction of rat liver glucokinase. *J. Biol. Chem.* **245,** 4819–4824.

Utter, M. F., Barden, R. E., and Taylor, B. L. (1975). Pyruvate carboxylase: An evaluation of the relationship between structures and mechanisms and between structure and catalytic activity. *Adv. Enzymol.* **42,** 1–72.

Vallotton, M., Hess-Sander, U., and Leuthardt, F. (1965). Fixation spontanée de la biotine a une protéine dans le serum humain. *Helv. Chim. Acta* **48,** 126–133.

Vesely, D. L. (1981). Human and growth hormones enhance guanylate cyclase activity. *Am. J. Physiol.* **240,** E79–E82.

Vesely, D. L. (1982). Biotin enhances guanylate cyclase activity. *Science* **216,** 1329–1330.

Vesely, D. L., Wormser, H. C., and Abramson, H. N. (1984). Biotin analogs activate guanylate cyclase. *Mol. Cell. Biochem.* **60,** 109–114.

Watanabe, T. (1983). Teratogenic effect of biotin deficiency in mice. *J. Nutr.* **113,** 574–581.

Watanabe, T., and Endo, A. (1984). Teratogenic effects of avidin-induced biotin deficiency in mice. *Teratology* **30,** 91–94.

Watkins, B. A. (1988). Conversion of ^{14}C linoleate to dihomo-τ-linoleate is depressed in biotin-deficient chick. *FASEB J.* **2,** A1531.

Wegner, M. I., Booth, A. N., Elvejhem, C. A., and Hart, E. B. (1940). Formation of the anti egg-white-injury factor (biotin) in the rumen of the cow. *Proc. Soc. Exp. Biol. Med.* **45,** 769–771.

Weinhowe, S. (1976). Regulation of glucokinase in liver. *Curr. Top. Cell. Regul.* **11,** 1–50.

Wess, J. A., and Petro, T. M. (1987). Modulation of murine Peyer's patch immunoglobulin A response by Enterotoxic *Escherichia coli. Infect. Immun.* **55,** 1085–1099.

White, H. B., III, and Whitehead, C. C. (1987). Role of avidin and other biotin-binding proteins in the deposition and distribution of biotin in chicken eggs: Discovery of a new biotin-binding protein. *Biochem. J.* **241**, 677–684.

White, L. D., and George, W. J. (1981). Increased concentrations of cGMP in fetal liver cells stimulated by erythroprotein. *Proc. Soc. Exp. Biol. Med.* **166**, 186–193.

Wilchek, M., and Bayer, A., eds. (1989). "Methods in Enzymology." Academic Press, San Diego, California.

Williams, M. L., and Elias, P. M. (1987). The extracellular matrix of stratum corrium: Role of lipids in hormonal and pathological function. *CRC Crit. Rev. Ther. Drug Carrier Syst.* **3**, 95–122.

Williams, M. L., Packman, S., and Cowman, M. J. (1983). Alopecia and periorificial dermatitis in biotin-responsive multiple carboxylase deficiency. *J. Am. Acad. Dermatol.* **9**, 97–103.

Wise, L. S., Sul, H. S., and Rubin, C. S. (1984). Coordinate regulation of the biosynthesis of ATP-citrate lyase and malic enzyme during adipocyte differentiation. Studies on 3T3-L1 cells. *J. Biol. Chem.* **259**, 4827–4832.

Wisniesky, B. J., Williams, R. E., and Fox, C. F. (1973). Manipulations of fatty acid composition in animal cells grown in culture. *Proc. Natl. Acad. Sci. U.S.A.* **70**, 3669–3673.

Wolf, B. (1978). Biochemical characterization of mutant propionyl-CoA carboxylases from two minor genetic complementation groups. *Biochem. Genet.* **17**, 703–07.

Wolf, B., and Feldman, G. L. (1982). The biotin-dependent carboxylase deficiencies. *Am. J. Hum. Genet* **34**, 699–716.

Wolf, B., Hsia, Y. E., and Rosenberg, L. E. (1978). Biochemical differences between mutant propionyl-CoA carboxylases from two complementation groups. *Am. J. Hum. Genet.* **30**, 455–64.

Wolf, B., Willard, H. F., and Rosenberg, L. E. (1980). Kinetic analysis of genetic complementation in heterokaryons of propionyl CoA carboxylase-deficient human fibroblasts. *Am. J. Hum. Genet.* **32**, 16–25.

Wolf, B., Hsia, Y. E., Sweetman, L., Gravel, R., Harris, D. J., and Nyhan, W. L. (1981). Propionic acidemia: A clinical update. *J. Pediatr.* **99**, 835–46.

Wolf, B., Grier, R. E., Allen, R. J., Goodman, S. I., and Kien, C. L. (1983a). Biotinidase deficiency: The enzymatic defect in late-onset multiple carboxylase deficiency. *Clin. Chim. Acta* **131**, 273–281.

Wolf, B., Grier, R. E., Allen, R. J., Goodman, S. I., Kien, C. L., Parker, W. D., Howell, D. M., and Hurst, D. L. (1983b). Phenotype variation in biotinidase deficiency. *J. Pediatr.* **103**, 233–237.

Wolf, B., Heard, G. S., McVoy, J. R. S., and Grier, R. E. (1985). Biotinidase deficiency. *Ann. N.Y. Acad. Sci.* **447**, 252–261.

Wood, H. G., and Barden, R. E. (1977). Biotin enzymes. *Annu. Rev. Biochem.* **46**, 385–413.

Wood, H. G., and Harmon, F. R. (1980). Comparison of the biotination of apotranscarboxylase and its aposubunit. Is assembly essential for biotination. *J. Biol. Chem.* **255**, 7397–7409.

Wood, H. G., and Kumar, G. K. (1985). Transcarboxylase: Its quaternary structure and the role of the biotinyl subunit in the assembly of the enzyme and in catalysis. *Ann. N.Y. Acad. Sci.* **447**, 1–21.

Woolley, D. W., and Longsworth, L. G. (1942). Isolation of an antibiotin factor from egg white. *J. Biol. Chem.* **142**, 285–290.

Wray, W. (1978). Parallel isolation procedures for metaphase chromosomes, mitotic apparatus, and nuclei. *Methods Enzymol.* **50**, 75–89.

Wright, L. D., Driscoll, C. A., and Boger, W. P. (1954). Biocytinase, an enzyme concerned with hydrolytic cleavage of biocytin. *Proc. Soc. Exp. Biol. Med.* **86,** 335–337.

Yanofsky, C. (1981). Attenuation in control of expression of bacterial operons. *Nature (London)* **289,** 751–758.

Yatsidis, H., Koutsinas, D., Agrayannis, B., Papastephanidis, C., Francos-Phemanis, M., and Delatala, Z. (1984). Biotin in the management of uremic neurologic disorders. *Nephron* **36,** 183–85.

Zak, T. A., and D'Ambrosio, J. F. A. (1985). Nutritional nystagmus in infants. *J. Pediatr. Ophthalmol. Strabismus* **22,** 140–142.

Zeilberg, C. E., and Goldberg, N. D. (1977). Cell-cycle-related changes of 3′,5′-cyclic GMP levels in Novikoff hepatoma cells. *Proc. Natl. Acad. Sci. U.S.A.* **74,** 1052–1056.

Index

A

Acetyl-CoA carboxylase, biotin and, 340–342
  deficiency symptoms, 365, 367, 370
  nonprosthetic group functions, 344, 347
Acetylcholine, experimental obesity and, 28
Adenosine triphosphate (ATP)
  biotin and, 340
  calcium homeostasis in birds and, 200
  experimental obesity and, 62
  folypolyglutamate synthesis and, 302
  pyrroloquinoline quinone and, 255
Adenylate cyclase, calcium homeostasis in birds and, 183–185
Adipsin, experimental obesity and, 33, 34, 88
Adrenal corticosteroids, experimental obesity and, 82–85, 89, 90
Adrenal steroids, experimental obesity and, 27, 63, 64, 81, 83
Adrenalectomy
  dietary obesity and, 63, 64, 68
  experimental obesity and, 2, 90
    efferent signals, 79, 81
    mechanism, 83–85
  genetic obesity and
    afferent signals, 36, 37
    central integration, 40, 43, 46
    controlled system, 53
  hypothalamic obesity and, 11, 27
Adrenocortical cells, calcium homeostasis in birds and, 183
Adrenocorticotropin (ACTH), experimental obesity and, 83, 84, 89
  genetic obesity, 36, 37, 41, 46
Afferent signals, experimental obesity and, 32–37, 76–78, 82

Afferent systems, experimental obesity and
  dietary obesity, 57–65
  hypothalamic obesity, 6, 16–20
Aldosterone, calcium homeostasis in birds and, 183
Alkaline phosphatase, calcium homeostasis in birds and, 190, 196
Amine oxidases, pyrroloquinoline quinone and
  cofactor research, 229, 230, 241
  distribution, 245, 246
Amino acids
  biotin and
    biotin-binding proteins, 354–356
    enzymes, 340
    nonprosthetic group functions, 343, 344
  breast cancer and, 133, 137, 140, 149, 154
  calcium homeostasis in birds and, 180, 190
  experimental obesity and, 3, 78, 89
    dietary obesity, 67
    hypothalamic obesity, 13, 14, 17
  folypolyglutamate synthesis and, 263
    folate, 265–269
    γ-glutamylhydrolases, 310
    role, 277, 280–283
  pyrroloquinoline quinone and
    biosynthesis, 248, 250, 251
    cofactor research, 229
    properties, 231, 232, 236–238
γ-Aminobutyric acid, experimental obesity and, 79
  dietary obesity, 67
  genetic obesity, 47
  hypothalamic obesity, 13, 14
Amphetamine, experimental obesity and, 11, 15, 16, 47, 69
Amygdala, experimental obesity and, 2, 10